Pharmaceutical Calculations

TENTH EDITION

Pharmaceutical Calculations

Mitchell J. Stoklosa, A. M., Sc.D.

Professor of Pharmacy Emeritus
Massachusetts College of Pharmacy
and Allied Health Sciences,
Boston, Massachusetts

Howard C. Ansel, Ph. D.

Professor of Pharmacy
College of Pharmacy
The University of Georgia
Athens, Georgia

A Lea & Febiger Book

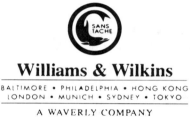

Williams & Wilkins

BALTIMORE • PHILADELPHIA • HONG KONG
LONDON • MUNICH • SYDNEY • TOKYO

A WAVERLY COMPANY
1996

**WILLIAMS
&WILKINS**

Executive Editor: Donna Balado
Managing Editor: Vicki Vaughn
Production Coordinator: Danielle Santucci
Book Project Editor: Susan Rockwell
Typesetting: Maryland Composition
Printing: Hamilton Printing Company
Binding: Hamilton Printing Company
Text Designer: Karen Klinedinst
Cover Designer: Karen Klinedinst

Copyright © 1996
Williams & Wilkins
Rose Tree Corporate Center
1400 North Providence Road
Building II, Suite 5025
Media, PA 19063-2043 USA

The use of portions of the text of The United States Pharmacopeia 23 / The National Formulary 18, is by permission of the United States Pharmacopeial Convention, Inc. The Convention is not responsible for any inaccuracy of quotation or for any false or misleading implications that may arise by reason of the separation of excerpts from the original texts.

Accurate indications, adverse reactions, and dosage schedules for drugs are provided in this book, but it is possible they may change. The reader is urged to review the package information data of the manufacturers of the medications mentioned.

Printed in the United States of America

First Edition 1945

Library of Congress Cataloging-in-Publication Data

Stoklosa, Mitchell J.
     Pharmaceutical calculations. — 10th ed. / Mitchell J. Stoklosa
and Howard C. Ansel.
        p.   cm.
     Includes bibliographical references and index.
     ISBN 0-683-08001-6
     1. Pharmaceutical arithmetic.   I. Ansel, Howard C., 1933– .
II. Title.
     [DNLM: 1. Weights and Measures.   2. Pharmacy.   3. Mathematics.
4. Drug Compounding.   5. Dosage Forms.   QV 16 S874p 1995]
RS57.S86   1996
615'.14'01513—dc20
DNLM/DLC
for Library of Congress   95-36483
                                                              CIP

The Publishers have made every effort to trace the copyright holders for borrowed material. If they have inadvertently overlooked any, they will be pleased to make the necessary arrangements at the first opportunity.

96 97 98 99
1 2 3 4 5 6 7 8 9 10

Reprints of chapters may be purchased from Williams & Wilkins in quantities of 100 or more. Call Isabella Wise, Special Sales Department, (800) 358-3583.

Preface

This Tenth Edition of *Pharmaceutical Calculations* represents the most complete revision of this widely used textbook in its fifty-year history. Each chapter has been revised completely to reflect the dramatic changes in the practice of pharmacy and the requirements of today's and tomorrow's students and practitioners.

Among the changes, and the most significant, is the elimination of the apothecaries' system from the body of the text and the use throughout of the metric system. This is in recognition of contemporary practice in the United States and throughout the world and is in conformance with the new edition of the *United States Pharmacopeia*. For reference, the apothecaries' and avoirdupois systems and factors for intersystem conversion appear in an Appendix chapter along with the recommendation to convert to metric quantities in problem-solving.

Another new and useful reference Appendix chapter includes definitions and brief descriptions of the various pharmaceutical dosage forms and drug delivery systems. This is intended to assist the beginning pharmacy student in understanding the terminology and the purpose of calculations in the preparation of extemporaneously compounded and prefabricated dosing forms. A new section on the techniques of pharmaceutical measurement also has been included to assist beginning students, and may be of special benefit to those programs in which instruction in calculations is integrated with an initial pharmacy laboratory experience.

The introduction of *dimensional analysis* as a problem-solving technique has been added to the traditional approach of using ratio and proportion. A retitled chapter "Constituted Solutions, Intravenous Admixtures, and Rate of Flow Calculations," offers a new array of calculations for the constitution of dry powders for oral solution or suspension, for pediatric drops, and for parenteral use. A completely revised section on total parenteral nutrition includes standard formulas, parameters for use, and new and expanded treatment of problems involving electrolyte and caloric requirements. Another retitled chapter, "Some Calculations Involving Use of Prefabricated Dosage Forms in Compounding Procedures," presents a variety of problems involving the use of tablets, capsules, and injections as the drug-source in the extemporaneous compounding of prescriptions and medication orders.

Other changes include: an expanded discussion and related dosage problems for the pediatric and elderly patient; new material on the use of creatinine clearance dosage tables and the adjustment of dosage based on body surface area; a new section covering calculations based on parts-per-million; additional treatment of millimoles; the introduction of freezing-point data in solving isotonicity problems; and, the introduction of problems involving *tissue culture infectious dose ($TCID_{50}$), flocculating units (Lf)* and other measures of potency used in the dosing of biologic products. Where applicable, the International System (SI) of units of measure is integrated in the text and in problem sets.

As is the case with each of the primary chapters of the text, the Appendix chapters have been thoroughly evaluated and retained when considered useful, excluded when not, revised as needed, and new chapters added as noted. Throughout the text, new example and practice problems have replaced older ones and the comprehensive section of review problems has been completely revised to reflect modern therapies.

On this, the golden anniversary of this textbook, the authors acknowledge the wonderful heritage to this work provided by Professors Willis T. Bradley and Carroll B. Gustafson, and express with gratitude the many helpful comments and suggestions of colleagues and students so thoughtfully and generously provided during the preparation of this revision.

Special appreciation is extended to Keith N. Herist for his contributions in the area of dimensional analysis.

Boston, Massachusetts   Mitchell J. Stoklosa
Athens, Georgia   Howard C. Ansel

Contents

Introduction

SCOPE OF PHARMACEUTICAL CALCULATIONS

The use of calculations in pharmacy is varied and broad-based. It encompasses calculations performed by pharmacists in traditional as well as in specialized practice settings and within operational and research areas in industry, academia, and government.

In the broad context, the scope of pharmaceutical calculations includes computation of:

- Chemical purity, physical characteristics, and biological parameters of drug substances, pharmaceutical ingredients, dosage forms and drug delivery systems;
- Drug stability, rates of drug degradation, and shelf-life of pharmaceutical preparations;
- Rates of drug absorption, bodily distribution, metabolism, and elimination;
- Dosage, based on individual patient characteristics;
- Pharmaceutical formulations of various production batches;
- Individual prescriptions and medication orders requiring extemporaneous compounding;
- Various parameters of drug dynamics, clinical effectiveness, and safety in patient populations; and,
- Epidemiologic, sociologic, and economic impact of drugs and drug therapy, with statistical presentation and analysis.

For each of these, there is a body of knowledge upon which the premise and understanding of the calculation is based. Certain of these areas are more specialized or advanced than others and constitute separate and distinct areas of study. Others are more foundational, providing the basic underpinnings of pharmacy practice. It is upon the latter that this textbook is based.

The chapters and appendices in this text present an array of pharmaceutical calculations which have direct application to pharmacy practice in a variety of practice settings, including community, institutional, and industrial pharmacy.

In each of these settings, pharmacists provide for the medication needs of patients. In the community pharmacy, this is accomplished through the filling of a *prescription,* written by a physician or other authorized health care professional, and through the provision of appropriate clinical information to assure the safe and effective use of the medication. The prescription may call for a *prefabricated* pharmaceutical product manufactured in industry, or, the prescription may be written for individual components to be weighed or measured by the pharmacist and *compounded* extemporaneously into a finished product. In the hospital and other institutional settings, a *medication order* entered on the patient's chart constitutes the prescription.

Whether the pharmaceutical product provided to a patient is produced in the industrial setting or prepared in a community or institutional pharmacy, pharmacists engage in calculations to determine quantities of the various ingredients used to achieve standards of quality and proper dosage upon administration. The difference between industrially prepared pharmaceuticals and those extemporaneously compounded by the pharmacist is the *quantity* of product prepared. In the community and institutional pharmacy, prescriptions and medication orders call for relatively small quantities of medications for individual patients. In the hospital setting, the pharmacy may additionally engage in the *small-scale* manufacture of frequently prescribed medications for institutional use. However, in industry, there is the routine *large-scale* production to meet the requirements of pharmacists and their patients on a national and even international basis. This involves the production of hundreds of thousands or even millions of dosage units (e.g. tablets) of a given drug product during a production cycle. The calculations involved in the compounding of a single prescription to the large-scale production of pharmaceuticals is an important component of pharmacy calculations and of this textbook.

In the preparation of prescriptions or product formulations various medicinal and non-medicinal *(pharmaceutic)* materials are used. Some are solid materials, as powders, which are accurately weighed on a pharmaceutical balance prior to use. Other materials are liquids, which are usually measured volumetrically prior to use, although they may also be weighed. The primary components of any prescription or pharmaceutical product are the *active ingredients* or the *medicinal substances,* which provide the basis for the product in preventing, treating, or curing the target illness or disease. Other components are *inactive ingredients* which are included in a formulation to produce the desired physical form, for convenience and safety of dosage administration, and the desired pharmaceutical qualities, including chemical and physical stability, rates of drug release, product appearance, taste, and smell. Active and inactive ingredients are obtained in *bulk* quantities for use in the pharmaceutical manufacture of *finished pharmaceuticals,* that is, *dosage forms* (e.g. tablets) and *drug delivery systems* (e.g. transdermal skin patches). In the extemporaneous filling of compounded prescriptions in the community pharmacy, in instances in which the active ingredient is unavailable in bulk, pharmacists may utilize prefabricated dosage forms as tablets, capsules, or injections of the drug as the source of active ingredient.

With very few exceptions, drugs are prepared and administered to patients in various dosage forms and drug delivery systems to assure accurate dosing. It is important for the pharmacy student to have an appreciation for the various dosage forms and drug delivery systems utilized in patient care. Calculations common to each involve the determination of the quantities of active and inactive ingredients required to achieve the desired strength, concentration, or quantity of drug per dosage unit. Additionally, there are calculations which are specific to particular dosage forms, pharmaceutical techniques, and patient requirements. The various types of pharmaceutical dosage forms and drug delivery systems are briefly defined and described in Appendix M, "Glossary of Pharmaceutical Dosage Forms and Drug Delivery Systems."

1 Some Fundamentals of Measurement and Calculation

NUMBERS AND NUMERALS

A *number* is a total quantity, or amount, of units. A *numeral* is a word or sign, or a group of words or signs, expressing a number. For example, *3, 6,* and *48* are Arabic numerals expressing numbers that are, respectively, *3 times, 6 times,* and 48 times the unit *1.*

KINDS OF NUMBERS

In *arithmetic,* the science of calculating with positive, real numbers, a number is usually (a) a natural or *whole* number, or *integer,* such as *549;* (b) a *fraction,* or subdivision of a whole number, such as $4/7$; or (c) a *mixed* number, consisting of a whole number plus a fraction, such as $3\frac{7}{8}$.

A number such as *4, 8,* or *12,* taken by itself, without application to anything concrete, is called an *abstract* or *pure* number. It merely designates how many times the unit *1* is contained in it, without implying that anything else is being counted or measured. An abstract number may be added to, subtracted from, multiplied by, or divided by any other abstract number. The result of any of these operations is always an abstract number designating a new total of units.

A number that designates a quantity of objects or units of measure, such as *4 grams, 8 ounces,* or *12 grains,* is called a *concrete* or *denominate* number. It designates the total quantity of whatever has been measured. A denominate number may be added to or subtracted from any other number of the same denomination, but a denominate number may be multiplied or divided only by a pure number. The result of any of these operations is always a number of the same denomination.

Examples:

$$10 \; grams \; + \; 5 \; grams \; = \; 15 \; grams$$
$$10 \; grams \; - \; 5 \; grams \; = \; 5 \; grams$$
$$300 \; grains \; \times \; 2 \; = \; 600 \; grains$$
$$12 \; ounces \; \div \; 3 \; = \; 4 \; ounces$$

If any one rule of arithmetic may take first place in importance, this is it: *Numbers of different denominations have no numeric connection with each other and cannot be used together in any direct arithmetical operation.* We will see again and again that if quantities are to be added, or if one quantity is to be subtracted from another, they must be expressed in the same denomination. When we apparently multiply or divide a denominate number by a number of different denomination, we are in fact using the multiplier or divisor as an abstract number. If, for example, *1 ounce* costs *5¢* and we want to find the cost of *12 ounces,* we do not multiply *5¢* by *12 ounces,* but by the abstract number *12.*

ARABIC NUMERALS

The so-called "Arabic" system of notation is properly called a *decimal system.* With only *10 figures*—*a zero* and *nine digits* (1,2,3,4,5,6,7,8,9)—any number can be expressed by an ingenious system in which different values are assigned to the digits according to the *place* they occupy in a row. The central place in the row is usually identified by a sign placed to its right called the *decimal point.* Any digit occupying this place expresses its own value—in other words, a certain number of *ones.* The former value of a digit is increased 10-fold each time it moves one place to the left, and, conversely, its value is one-tenth of its preceding value each time it moves one place to the right. *Zero* marks a place not occupied by one of the digits.

The simplicity of the system is further demonstrated by the fact that these *10 figures* serve all our needs in dealing with positive integers, and with the aid of a few signs, are adequate for expressing fractions, negative numbers, and irrational and imaginary numbers.

The practical range of the system is represented by the following scheme (which can be extended to the left or right into even higher or lower reaches):

Scheme of the decimal system:

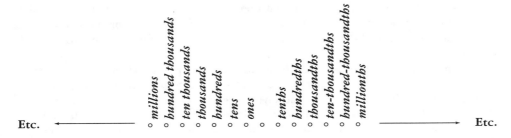

The total value of any number expressed in the Arabic (decimal) system, then, is the sum of the values of its digits as determined by their position.

Example:

> 5,083.623 *means:*
> 5,000.000 or 5 thousands
> + 000.000 plus 0 hundreds
> + 080.000 plus 8 tens
> + 003.000 plus 3 ones
> + 000.600 plus 6 tenths
> + 000.020 plus 2 hundredths
> + 000.003 plus 3 thousandths

The universal use of this system has resulted from the ease with which it can be adapted to the various purposes of arithmetical calculations.

ROMAN NUMERALS

The Roman system of notation expresses a fairly large range of numbers by the use of a few letters of the alphabet in a simple "positional" notation indicating adding to or subtracting from a succession of bases extending from 1 through *5, 10, 50, 100,* and *500* to *1000.* Roman numerals merely record quantities: they are of no use in computation.

To express quantities in the Roman system, eight letters of fixed values are used:

ss   = ½
I or i   = 1
V or v   = 5
X or x   = 10
L or l   = 50
C or c   = 100
D or d   = 500
M or m   = 1000

Other quantities are expressed by combining these letters by the general rule that when the second of two letters has a value equal to or smaller than that of the first, their values are to be added; when the second has a value greater than that of the first, the smaller is to be subtracted from the larger. This rule may be illustrated as follows:

1. Two or more letters express a quantity that is the *sum* of their values *if they are successively equal or smaller in value:*

ii	= 2	xv	= 15	lxxvii	= 77	dv	= 505	mc	= 1100
iii	= 3	xx	= 20	lxxxviii	= 88	dx	= 510	md	= 1500
vi	= 6	xxii	= 22	ci	= 101	dl	= 550	mdclxvi	= 1666
vii	= 7	xxxiii	= 33	cv	= 105	dc	= 600	mm	= 2000
viii	= 8	li	= 51	cx	= 110	mi	= 1001		
xi	= 11	lv	= 55	cl	= 150	mv	= 1005		
xii	= 12	lx	= 60	cc	= 200	mx	= 1010		
xiii	= 13	lxvi	= 66	di	= 501	ml	= 1050		

2. Two or more letters express a quantity that is the *sum* of the values remaining *after the value of each smaller letter has been subtracted from that of a following greater letter:*

iv	= 4	xxiv	= 24	xliv	= 44	cdi	= 401	cm	= 900
ix	= 9	xxxix	= 39	xc	= 90	cdxl	= 440	cmxcix	= 999
xiv	= 14	xl	= 40	xcix	= 99	cdxliv	= 444	MCDXCII	= 1492
xix	= 19	xli	= 41	cd	= 400	cdxc	= 490	MCMXCV	= 1995

Roman numerals are used in pharmacy only occasionally on prescriptions: (1) to designate the number of dosage units prescribed (e.g., *capsules no. C*), (2) to indicate the quantity of medication to be administered (e.g., *teaspoonfuls ii*), and (3) in rare instances in which the common or apothecaries' systems of measurement are used (e.g., *grains iv*).[1]

Practice Problems

1. Write the following in Roman numerals:
   (*a*) 18   (*f*) 37
   (*b*) 64   (*g*) 84
   (*c*) 72   (*h*) 48
   (*d*) 126   (*i*) 1989
   (*e*) 99

---

[1] On prescriptions, physicians tend to use capitals except for the letter *i*, which they dot for the sake of clarity; they may use *j* for a final *i*. Following the Latin custom, they put the symbol for the denomination first and the Roman numeral second (e.g., gr iv). Dates are customarily expressed in capitals.

2. Write the following in Arabic numerals:
    (*a*) Part IV
    (*b*) Chapter XIX
    (*c*) MCMLIX
    (*d*) MDCCCXIV

3. Interpret the *quantity* in each of these phrases taken from prescriptions:
    (*a*) Caps. no. xlv
    (*b*) Gtts. ij
    (*c*) Tabs. no. xlviii
    (*d*) Pil. no. lxiv
    (*e*) Pulv. no. xvi
    (*f*) Caps. no. lxxxiv

4. Interpret the *quantities* in each of these prescriptions:
    (*a*) ℞   Zinc Oxide   parts v
              Wool Fat   parts xv
              Petrolatum   parts lxxx
              Disp. ℥iv
              Sig. Apply.
    (*b*) ℞   Dilaudid   gr iss
              Ammonium Chloride   gr xl
              Syrup ad   ℥vi
              Sig. ℨss pro tuss.

COMMON AND DECIMAL FRACTIONS

The arithmetic of pharmacy requires facility in the handling of common fractions and decimal fractions. Even if the student already has a good working knowledge of their use, the following brief review of certain principles and rules should be helpful, and the practice problems should provide a means of gaining accuracy and speed in their manipulation.

Common Fractions

A number in the form $\frac{1}{8}$, $\frac{3}{16}$, and so on, is called a *common fraction,* or often simply a *fraction*. Its *denominator,* or second or lower figure, always indicates the number of aliquot parts into which *1* is divided; its *numerator,* or first or upper figure, specifies the number of those parts with which we are concerned.

The *value* of a fraction is the *quotient* (i.e., the result of dividing one number by another) when its numerator is divided by its denominator. If the numerator is smaller than the denominator, the fraction is called *proper,* and its value is less than *1*. If the numerator and denominator are alike, its value is *1*. If the numerator is larger than the denominator, the fraction is called *improper,* and its value is greater than *1*.

Two principles must be understood by anyone attempting to calculate with common fractions. In the **first principle,** multiplying the numerator increases the value of a fraction, and multiplying the denominator decreases the value, but *when both numerator and denominator are multiplied by the same number, the value does not change.*

$$\frac{2}{7} = \frac{3 \times 2}{3 \times 7} = \frac{6}{21}$$

This principle allows us to reduce two or more fractions to a common denomination when necessary. We usually want the *lowest common denominator,* which is the smallest number divisible by all the other given denominators. It is found most easily by testing successive multiples of the largest given denominator until we reach a number divisible by all the other given denominators. Then we multiply both numerator and denominator of each fraction by the number of times its denominator is contained in the common denominator.

Example:

Reduce the fractions ³⁄₄, ⁴⁄₅, and ¹⁄₃ to a common denomination.

By testing successive multiples of 5, we discover that 60 is the smallest number divisible by 4, 5, and 3; 4 is contained 15 times in 60; 5, 12 times; and 3, 20 times.

$$\left.\begin{array}{l}\dfrac{3}{4} = \dfrac{15 \times 3}{15 \times 4} = \dfrac{45}{60}, \\[2ex] \dfrac{4}{5} = \dfrac{12 \times 4}{12 \times 5} = \dfrac{48}{60}, \\[2ex] \dfrac{1}{3} = \dfrac{20 \times 1}{20 \times 3} = \dfrac{20}{60},\end{array}\right\} answers$$

In the **second principle,** dividing the numerator decreases the value of a fraction, and dividing the denominator increases the value, but *when both numerator and denominator are divided by the same number, the value does not change.*

$$\frac{6}{21} = \frac{6 \div 3}{21 \div 3} = \frac{2}{7}$$

This principle allows us to reduce an unwieldy fraction to more convenient lower terms, either at any time during a series of calculations or when recording a final result. To reduce a fraction to its *lowest terms,* divide both the numerator and the denominator by the largest common divisor.

Example:

Reduce ³⁶⁄₂₈₈₀ to its lowest terms.

The largest common divisor is 36.

$$\frac{36}{2880} = \frac{36 \div 36}{2880 \div 36} = \frac{1}{80}, answer.$$

In addition to developing a firm grasp of these two principles, the student should follow two rules before indulging in any short cuts.

Rule 1. Before performing any arithmetical operation involving fractions, *reduce every mixed number to an improper fraction.* To do so, multiply the integer, or whole number, by the denominator of the fractional remainder, add the numerator, and write the result over the denominator. For example, before attempting to multiply ³⁄₄ by 1¹⁄₅, first reduce the 1¹⁄₅ to an improper fraction:

$$1\tfrac{1}{5} = \frac{(1 \times 5) + 1}{5} = \tfrac{6}{5}$$

If the final result of a calculation is an improper fraction, you may, if you like, reduce it to a mixed number. To do so, simply divide the numerator by the denominator and express the remainder as a common, not a decimal fraction:

$$\tfrac{6}{5} = 6 \div 5 = 1\tfrac{1}{5}$$

Rule 2. When performing an operation involving a fraction and a whole number, *express (or at least visualize) the whole number as a fraction having 1 for its denominator.*

Think of 3, as $^3/_1$, 42 as $^{42}/_1$, and so on. This visualization is desirable when a fraction is subtracted from a whole number, and it is necessary when a fraction is divided by a whole number.

Adding Fractions. To add common fractions, reduce them to a common denomination, add the numerators, and write the sum over the common denominator. If whole and mixed numbers are involved, the safest (although not the quickest) procedure is to apply *Rules 1 and 2.* If the sum is an improper fraction, you may want to reduce it to a mixed number.

Example:

In preparing batches of a formula, a pharmacist used $^1/_4$ ounce, $^1/_{12}$ ounce, $^1/_8$ ounce, and $^1/_6$ ounce of a chemical. Calculate the total quantity of chemical used.

The lowest common denominator of the fractions is 24.

$$^1/_4 = ^6/_{24}, \ ^1/_{12} = ^2/_{24}, \ ^1/_8 = ^3/_{24}, \text{ and } ^1/_6 = ^4/_{24}$$

$$\frac{6 + 2 + 3 + 4}{24} \text{ ounce } = \frac{15}{24} \text{ ounce}$$

$$^{15}/_{24} \text{ ounce } = ^5/_8 \text{ ounce, } answer.$$

Subtracting Fractions. To subtract one fraction from another, reduce them to a common denomination, subtract, and write the difference over the common denominator. If a whole or mixed number is involved, first apply *Rule 1 or 2.* If the difference is an improper fraction, you may want to reduce it to a mixed number.

Examples:

A hospitalized patient received $^7/_{12}$ liter of a prescribed intravenous infusion. If he had not received the final $^1/_8$ liter, what fraction of a liter would he have received?

The lowest common denominator is 24.

$$^7/_{12} = ^{14}/_{24} \text{ and } ^1/_8 = ^3/_{24}$$

$$\frac{14 - 3}{24} \text{ liter } = \frac{11}{24} \text{ liter, } answer.$$

If 3 fl. oz. of a liquid mixture are to contain $^1/_{24}$ fl. oz. of ingredient A, $^1/_4$ fl. oz. of ingredient B, and $^1/_3$ fl. oz. of ingredient C, how many fluidounces of ingredient D are required?

The lowest common denominator is 24.

$$^1/_{24} = ^1/_{24}, \ ^1/_4 = ^6/_{24}, \text{ and } ^1/_3 = ^8/_{24}$$

$$\frac{1 + 6 + 8}{24} \text{ fl. oz. } = \frac{15}{24} \text{ fl. oz. } = \frac{5}{8} \text{ fl. oz.}$$

Interpret the given 3 fl. oz. as $^3/_1$ fl. oz., and reduce it to a fraction with 8 for a denominator:

$$^3/_1 \text{ fl. oz. } = ^{24}/_8 \text{ fl. oz.}$$

Subtracting:

$$\frac{24 - 5}{8} \text{ fl. oz. } = \frac{19}{8} \text{ fl. oz.}$$

Change the difference to a mixed number:

$$^{19}\!/_8 \text{ fl. oz. } = (19 \div 8) \text{ fl. oz. } = 2\tfrac{3}{8} \text{ fl. oz., } \textit{answer.}$$

Multiplying Fractions. To multiply fractions, multiply the numerators and write the product over the product of the denominators. If either is a mixed number, first apply *Rule 1*. If the multiplier is a whole number, simply multiply the numerator of the fraction and write the product over the denominator.

Examples:

What fraction of a grain of nitroglycerin is present in 24 Nitrostat® tablets labeled to contain
0.4 milligram ($^1\!/_{150}$ grain) of nitroglycerin per tablet?

$$24 \times \frac{1}{150} \text{ gr } = \frac{24 \times 1}{150} \text{ gr } = \frac{24}{150} \text{ gr } = \frac{4}{25} \text{ gr, } \textit{answer.}$$

If the adult dose of a medication is $^1\!/_2$ fluidounce, calculate the dose for a child if it is $^1\!/_8$ of the adult dose.

$$\frac{1}{8} \times \frac{1}{2} \text{ fl. oz. } = \frac{1 \times 1}{8 \times 2} \text{ fl. oz. } = \frac{1}{16} \text{ fl. oz., } \textit{answer.}$$

Dividing Fractions. In the division of fractions, it is important for the student to grasp the meaning of *reciprocal*. By definition, the *reciprocal* of a number is *1* divided by the number. For example, the reciprocal of 3 is $^1\!/_3$. If you apply *Rule 2* and regard 3 as the same as the fraction $^3\!/_1$, its reciprocal equals the inversion of this fraction. In general, therefore, when *a* is a fraction, its reciprocal is $^1\!/_a$ and proves to have the same value as the fraction inverted. So, the reciprocal of $^1\!/_4$ is $^4\!/_1$ or 4, and the reciprocal of $2\tfrac{1}{2}$ or $^5\!/_2$ is $^2\!/_5$.

Now, if the fraction $^3\!/_4$ is interpreted as meaning 3 divided by 4, then it should be emphasized that dividing by 4 is exactly the same as multiplying by the reciprocal of 4, or $^1\!/_4$. This method of handling division when fractions are involved is called the *reciprocal method*, and it points out the reciprocal relation, or inverse relation, between multiplication and division.

To divide by a fraction, then, simply invert its terms and multiply. When a fraction is to be divided by a whole number, first interpret the whole number as a fraction, having 1 for its denominator, invert to get its reciprocal, and multiply.

Examples:

If $^1\!/_2$ ounce is divided into 4 equal parts, how much will each part contain?
Interpreting 4 as $^4\!/_1$:

$$\frac{1}{2} \text{ oz } \div \frac{4}{1} = \frac{1}{2} \text{ oz } \times \frac{1}{4} = \frac{1 \times 1}{2 \times 4} \text{ oz } = \frac{1}{8} \text{ oz, } \textit{answer.}$$

A manufacturer wishes to prepare samples of an ointment in sealed foil envelopes, each containing $^1\!/_{32}$ ounce of ointment. How many samples may be prepared from 1 pound (16 ounces) of ointment?

$$\frac{16}{1} \div \frac{1}{32} = \frac{16}{1} \times \frac{32}{1} = \frac{16 \times 32}{1 \times 1} = 512 \text{ samples, } \textit{answer.}$$

If a child's dose of a cough syrup is $^3\!/_4$ teaspoonful and represents $^1\!/_4$ of the adult dose, what is the adult dose?

$$\frac{3}{4} \text{ tsp. } \div \frac{1}{4} = \frac{3}{4} \text{ tsp. } \times \frac{4}{1} = \frac{3 \times 4}{4 \times 1} \text{ tsp. } = 3 \text{ tsp., } \textit{answer.}$$

Decimal Fractions

A fraction with a denominator of 10 or any power of 10 is called a *decimal fraction,* or simply a *decimal.* The denominator of a decimal fraction is never written, because the decimal point indicates the place value of the numerals. The numerator and the decimal point are sufficient to express the fraction. Therefore, $\frac{1}{10}$ is written 0.1, $\frac{45}{100}$ is written 0.45, and $\frac{65}{1000}$ is written 0.065.

All operations with decimal fractions are carried out in the same manner as with whole numbers, but care is needed when putting the decimal point in its proper place in the results.

Three familiar operations worth recalling are as follows:

1. As a direct consequence of the place value in the decimal notation, moving the decimal point one place to the right multiplies a number by 10, two places to the right multiplies it by 100, and so on. Likewise, moving the point one place to the left divides a number by 10, two places to the left it divides it by 100, and so on.

2. A decimal fraction may be changed to a common fraction by writing the numerator over the denominator and (if desired) reducing to lowest terms:

$$0.125 = \frac{125}{1000} = \frac{1}{8}$$

3. A common fraction may be changed to a decimal by dividing the numerator by the denominator (note that the result may be a repeating or endless decimal fraction):

$$\frac{3}{8} = 3 \div 8 = 0.375$$

$$\frac{1}{3} = 1 \div 3 = 0.3333 \ldots .$$

Practice Problems

1. Add each of the following:
    (a) $\frac{5}{8} + \frac{9}{32} + \frac{1}{4}$
    (b) $\frac{1}{150} + \frac{1}{200} + \frac{1}{100}$
    (c) $\frac{1}{60} + \frac{1}{20} + \frac{1}{16} + \frac{1}{32}$

2. Find the difference:
    (a) $3\frac{1}{2} - \frac{15}{64}$
    (b) $\frac{1}{30} - \frac{1}{40}$
    (c) $2\frac{1}{3} - 1\frac{1}{2}$

3. Find the product:
    (a) $\frac{30}{75} \times \frac{15}{32} \times 25$
    (b) $2\frac{1}{2} \times 12 \times \frac{7}{8}$
    (c) $\frac{1}{125} \times \frac{9}{20}$

4. What is the reciprocal of each of the following?
    (a) $\frac{1}{10}$
    (b) $3\frac{1}{3}$
    (c) $\frac{12}{1}$
    (d) $\frac{3}{2}$
    (e) $1\frac{7}{8}$
    (f) $\frac{1}{64}$

5. Find the quotient:
    (a) $\frac{2}{3} \div \frac{1}{24}$
    (b) $\frac{1}{5000} \div 12$
    (c) $6\frac{1}{4} \div \frac{1}{2}$

6. Solve each of the following:

    (a) $(\frac{1}{120} \div \frac{1}{150}) \times 50 = ?$

    (b) $\dfrac{1\frac{1}{2}}{100} \times 1000 = ?$

    (c) $\frac{3}{4} \times ? = 48.$

    (d) $\dfrac{\frac{1}{500}}{5} \times ? = 5.$

7. What fractional part:
    (a) of 64 is 2?
    (b) of $\frac{1}{16}$ is $\frac{1}{20}$?
    (c) of $\frac{1}{32}$ is 2?

8. What decimal fraction:
    (a) of 18 is $2\frac{1}{4}$?
    (b) of 25 is 0.005?
    (c) of 7000 is 437.5?

9. Write the following as decimals and add:

    $$\frac{3}{1000}, \; \frac{75}{100}, \; \frac{3}{20}, \; \frac{5}{8}, \; \frac{13}{25}$$

10. Write the following as decimals and add:

    $$\frac{3}{5}, \; \frac{1}{20}, \; \frac{65}{1000}, \; \frac{19}{40}, \; \frac{3}{8}$$

11. How many 0.000065-gram doses can be made from 0.130 gram of a drug?

12. Calculate the fractional difference between a $\frac{1}{400}$-grain and a $\frac{1}{150}$-grain tablet of nitroglycerin.

13. A pharmacist had 3 ounces of hydromorphone hydrochloride. He used the following:

    $\frac{1}{8}$ ounce
    $\frac{1}{4}$ ounce
    $1\frac{1}{2}$ ounce

    How many ounces of hydromorphone hydrochloride were left after he prepared the capsules?

14. A pharmacist had 5 grams of codeine sulfate. He used it in preparing the following:

    8 capsules each containing 0.0325 gram
    12 capsules each containing 0.015 gram
    18 capsules each containing 0.008 gram

    How many grams of codeine sulfate were left after he had prepared the capsules?

RATIO, PROPORTION, AND VARIATION

Ratio. The relative magnitude of two like quantities is called their *ratio*. Ratio is sometimes defined as *the quotient of two like numbers.* To avoid losing sight of the fact that *two* quantities are being *compared,* this quotient is always expressed as an *operation,* not as a *result:* in other words, it is expressed as a *fraction,* and the fraction is interpreted as indicating the operation of dividing the numerator by the denominator. Thus, a ratio presents us with the concept of a common fraction as expressing the relation of its two numbers.

The ratio of *20* and *10,* for example, is not expressed as *2* (that is, the quotient of *20* divided by *10*), but as the fraction $^{20}\!/_{10}$. Similarly, when the fraction $\frac{1}{2}$ is to be interpreted as a ratio, it is traditionally written *1 :2,* and it is read not as *one-half* but as *1 to 2.*

All the rules governing common fractions equally apply to a ratio. Of particular importance is the principle that *if the two terms of a ratio are multiplied or are divided by the same number, the value is unchanged,* the *value* being the quotient of the first term divided by the second. For example, the ratio *20 :4* or $^{20}\!/_4$ has a value of *5;* if both terms are divided by *2,* the ratio becomes *10 :2* or $^{10}\!/_2$, again the value of *5.*

The terms of a ratio must be of the same kind, for the *value* of a ratio is an abstract number expressing how many *times* greater or smaller the first term (or numerator) is than the second term (or denominator).[2] The terms may themselves be abstract numbers, or they may be concrete numbers of the same denomination. Thus, we can have a ratio of *20* to *4 ($^{20}\!/_4$)* or *20 grams* to *4 grams* (20 grams/4 grams). To recognize this relationship clearly, it is useful to interpret a ratio as expressing in its *denominator* a number of parts that a certain quantity (used for comparison) is conveniently taken to contain, and in its *numerator* the number of *those parts* that the quantity we are measuring is found to contain.[3]

When two ratios have the same value, they are *equivalent.* An interesting fact about equivalent ratios is that the *product of the numerator of the one and the denominator of the other always equals the product of the denominator of the one and the numerator of the other;* i.e., *the cross products are equal:*

$$\text{Because } \tfrac{2}{4} = \tfrac{4}{8},$$

$$2 \times 8 \text{ (or } 16) = 4 \times 4 \text{ (or } 16)$$

It is also true that *if two ratios are equal, their* reciprocals are equal:

$$\text{Because } \tfrac{2}{4} = \tfrac{4}{8}, \text{ then } \tfrac{4}{2} = \tfrac{8}{4}$$

We discover further that the *numerator of the one fraction equals the product of its denominator and the other fraction:*

$$\text{If } ^6\!/_{15} = \tfrac{2}{5},$$

$$\text{then } 6 = 15 \times \tfrac{2}{5} \left(\text{or } \frac{15 \times 2}{5} \right) = 6,$$

$$\text{and } 2 = 5 \times ^6\!/_{15} \left(\text{or } \frac{5 \times 6}{15} \right) = 2.$$

And the denominator of the one equals the quotient of its numerator divided by the other fraction:

---

[2] The ratio of *1* gallon to *3* pints is surely not *1 :3,* for the gallon contains *8* pints, and the ratio therefore is *8 :3.* To ignore this principle is to invite disaster in calculations.

[3] Ratios are expressed or implied everywhere in mathematics, "the science of measure." A common fraction may always be understood to designate in its denominator the number of equal parts into which *1* is divided, and in its numerator the number of those parts with which we are concerned. Decimal fractions are ratios with a fixed series of denominators: *10, 100, 1000,* and so on. We have observed that every whole number implies a ratio with *1,* our unit of counting. Percentage is a convenient ratio that expresses a number of parts in every hundred of the kind.

$$15 = 6 \div \tfrac{2}{5} \ (\text{or } 6 \times \tfrac{5}{2}) = 15,$$

$$\text{and } 5 = 2 \div \tfrac{6}{15} \ (\text{or } 2 \times \tfrac{15}{6}) = 5.$$

An extremely useful practical application of these facts is found in *proportion*.

Proportion. A *proportion* is the expression of the equality of two ratios. It may be written in any one of three standard forms:

(1) $a:b = c:d$

(2) $a:b :: c:d$

(3) $\dfrac{a}{b} = \dfrac{c}{d}$

Each of these expressions is read: *a is to b as c is to d*, and *a* and *d* are called the *extremes* (meaning "outer members") and *b* and *c* the *means* ("middle members").

In any proportion, *the product of the extremes is equal to the product of the means*. This principle allows us to find the missing term of any proportion when the other three terms are known. If the missing term is a *mean*, it will be *the product of the extremes divided by the given mean*, and if it is an *extreme*, it will be *the product of the means divided by the given extreme*. Using this information, we may derive the following fractional equations:

$$\text{If } \frac{a}{b} = \frac{c}{d}, \text{ then}$$

$$a = \frac{bc}{d}, \ b = \frac{ad}{c}, \ c = \frac{ad}{b}, \text{ and } d = \frac{bc}{a}.$$

Most experienced calculators are indifferent to the order of terms in the proportions they devise. For the sake of the greater mechanical accuracy gained by routine discipline, some teachers still prefer the old pattern of putting the unknown term in the fourth place; that is, in the denominator of the second fraction.

Few arithmetical problems, save for the simplest, cannot be solved most directly by proportion. Provided we correctly interpret the relationships implied by the data, *given any three terms of a proportion, by appeal to the facts set forth above, we may easily calculate the value of the fourth*. Because the missing fourth is usually the desired answer, proportion takes us to it without any intermediate steps.

Examples:

If 3 tablets contain 975 milligrams of aspirin, how many milligrams should be contained in 12 tablets?

$$\frac{3 \text{ (tablets)}}{12 \text{ (tablets)}} = \frac{975 \text{ (milligrams)}}{\text{x (milligrams)}}$$

$$x = \frac{12 \times 975}{3} \text{ milligrams} = 3900 \text{ milligrams}, \textit{ answer.}$$

If 3 tablets contain 975 milligrams of aspirin, how many tablets should contain 3900 milligrams?

$$\frac{3 \text{ (tablets)}}{\text{x (tablets)}} = \frac{975 \text{ (milligrams)}}{3900 \text{ (milligrams)}}$$

$$x = 3 \times \frac{3900}{975} \text{ tablets} = 12 \text{ tablets}, \textit{ answer.}$$

If 12 tablets contain 3900 milligrams of aspirin, how many milligrams should 3 tablets contain?

$$\frac{12 \ (\text{tablets})}{3 \ (\text{tablets})} = \frac{3900 \ (\text{milligrams})}{x \ (\text{milligrams})}$$

$$x = 3 \times \frac{3900}{12} \text{ milligrams} = 975 \text{ milligrams}, \textit{answer.}$$

If 12 tablets contain 3900 milligrams of aspirin, how many tablets should contain 975 milligrams?

$$\frac{12 \ (\text{tablets})}{x \ (\text{tablets})} = \frac{3900 \ (\text{milligrams})}{975 \ (\text{milligrams})}$$

$$x = \frac{12 \times 975}{3900} \text{ tablets} = 3 \text{ tablets}, \textit{answer.}$$

Some calculators set up "mixed" ratios in their proportions, invoking the principle that if the ratios are regarded as abstract numbers, *the means or the extremes may be interchanged without destroying the validity of the equation.*

So that if:

$$\frac{3 \ (\text{tablets})}{12 \ (\text{tablets})} = \frac{975 \ (\text{milligrams})}{3900 \ (\text{milligrams})}$$

then:

$$\frac{3 \ (\text{tablets})}{975 \ (\text{milligrams})} = \frac{12 \ (\text{tablets})}{3900 \ (\text{milligrams})}$$

and:

$$\frac{3900 \ (\text{milligrams})}{12 \ (\text{tablets})} = \frac{975 \ (\text{milligrams})}{3 \ (\text{tablets})}$$

and:

$$\frac{3900 \ (\text{milligrams})}{975 \ (\text{milligrams})} = \frac{12 \ (\text{tablets})}{3 \ (\text{tablets})}$$

However true this principle may be of abstract numbers, it is nevertheless illogical (and never necessary) to make a ratio between, say, a number of tablets and a number of milligrams. It is risky to ignore the rule that *ratios should express the relationship of denominate numbers of the same kind.* In many problems, the quantities given must be reduced or converted to a common denomination before we can proceed with the solution.

Proportions need not contain whole numbers. If common or decimal fractions are supplied in the data, they may be included in the proportion without changing the method.

Because calculating with common fractions is more complicated than with whole numbers or decimal fractions, however, it is useful to know—and wherever possible to apply—these two facts:

1. *Two fractions having a common denominator are directly proportional to their numerators.*

$$\frac{^{60}\!/_{100}}{^{50}\!/_{100}} = \frac{60}{50}$$

$$\text{Proof: } \frac{60}{100} \div \frac{50}{100} = \frac{60}{100} \times \frac{100}{50} = \frac{60}{50}$$

2. *Two fractions having a common numerator are inversely proportional to their denominators.*

$$\frac{\frac{2}{3}}{\frac{2}{7}} = \frac{7}{3}$$

$$\text{Proof: } \frac{2}{3} \div \frac{2}{7} = \frac{2}{3} \times \frac{7}{2} = \frac{7}{3}$$

Example:

If 30 milliliters represent $\frac{1}{6}$ of the volume of a prescription, how many milliliters will represent $\frac{1}{4}$ of the volume?

$$\frac{\frac{1}{6} \text{ (volume)}}{\frac{1}{4} \text{ (volume)}} = \frac{30 \text{ (mL)}}{\text{x (mL)}}$$

$$\text{Or: } \frac{4}{6} = \frac{30}{\text{x}} \text{ (mL)}$$

$$\text{x} = \frac{6 \times 30}{4} \text{ mL} = 45 \text{ mL, } answer.$$

Variation. In the preceding examples, the relationships were clearly *proportional.* Most pharmaceutical calculations deal with simple, *direct* relationships: twice the cause, double the effect, and so on. Occasionally, they deal with *inverse* relationships: twice the cause, half the effect, and so on, as when you *decrease* the strength of a solution by *increasing* the amount of diluent.[4]

Here is a typical problem involving inverse proportion:

If 10 *pints of a 5% solution are diluted to 40 pints, what is the percentage strength of the dilution?*

$$\frac{10 \text{ (pints)}}{40 \text{ (pints)}} = \frac{\text{x (\%)}}{5 \text{ (\%)}}$$

$$\text{x} = \frac{10 \times 5}{40}\% = 1.25\%, answer.$$

DIMENSIONAL ANALYSIS

When performing certain types of calculations, some students prefer to use a method termed *dimensional analysis*, which involves the logical sequencing and placement into an equation of all of the arithmetical terms (both quantities and units) involved in the problem such that all of the units cancel out except the unit(s) of the desired answer (e.g., milliliters, milligrams per milliliter, etc.). By this method, ratios of the data are used, conversion factors added as necessary, and individual terms inverted (to their reciprocals) to permit the cancellation of like units in the numerator(s) and denominators(s), leaving only the desired term(s) of the answer. An advantage to the use of dimensional analysis is the consolidation of multiple arithmetical steps to a single expression.

Example:

How many fluidounces are in 2.5 liters if there are 1000 milliliters in 1 liter and 29.57 milliliters in 1 fluidounce?

---

[4] In expressing an inverse proportion, we must not forget that *every* proportion asserts the equivalence of two fractions, and therefore the numerators must both be smaller or both larger than their respective denominators.

Solving by ratio and proportion:
Step 1:

$$\frac{2.5 \text{ L}}{1 \text{ L}} = \frac{x \text{ mL}}{1000 \text{ mL}}$$

$$x = 2500 \text{ mL}$$

Step 2:

$$\frac{1 \text{ fl. oz.}}{x \text{ fl. oz.}} = \frac{29.57 \text{ mL}}{2500 \text{ mL}}$$

$$x = 84.5 \text{ fl. oz.}, \textit{answer.}$$

Solving by dimensional analysis:

$$2.5 \text{ L} \times \frac{1000 \text{ mL}}{1 \text{ L}} \times \frac{1 \text{ fl. oz.}}{29.57 \text{ mL}} = 84.5 \text{ fl. oz.}, \textit{answer.}$$

A medication order calls for 1000 milliliters of a dextrose intravenous infusion to be administered over an 8-hour period. Using an intravenous administration set that delivers 10 drops/milliliter, how many drops per minute should be delivered to the patient?
Solving by ratio and proportion:
Step 1:

$$8 \text{ hours} = 480 \text{ minutes}$$

$$\frac{1000 \text{ mL}}{x \text{ mL}} = \frac{480 \text{ min.}}{1 \text{ min.}}$$

$$x = 2.1 \text{ mL (per minute)}$$

Step 2:

$$\frac{2.1 \text{ mL (per min.)}}{1 \text{ mL}} = \frac{x \text{ drops (per min.)}}{10 \text{ drops}}$$

$$x = 21 \text{ drops per minute}, \textit{answer.}$$

Solving by dimensional analysis:
(NOTE: arrange terms to have "drops" in the numerator and "minutes" in the denominator to result in the desired answer in drops per minute.)

$$1000 \text{ mL} \times \frac{1}{480 \text{ min.}} \times \frac{10 \text{ drops}}{1 \text{ mL}} = 21 \text{ drops per minute}, \textit{answer.}$$

The use of proportion in pharmaceutical problems is abundantly illustrated in the text. The following miscellany reveals a variety of application of the method.

Practice Problems

1. *Make valid ratios between these familiar quantities:*
    (*a*) 3 gallons and 2 quarts
    (*b*) 1 yard and 2 feet
    (*c*) ½ mile and 1760 feet

(*d*) 4 hours and 120 minutes

(*e*)   2 feet and 6 inches

Solve by proportion:

2. If 250 pounds of a chemical cost \$480, what will be the cost of 135 pounds?

3. In a clinical study, the drug triazolam produced drowsiness in 30 of the 1500 patients studied. How many patients of a certain pharmacy could expect similar effects, based on a patient count of 100 patients?

4. A formula for 1250 tablets contains 3.25 grams of diazepam. How many grams of diazepam should be used in preparing 350 tablets?

5. If 100 capsules contain ⅜ grain of an active ingredient, how many grains of the ingredient will 48 capsules contain?

6. If 450 pounds of Green Soap cost \$310.50, what will be the cost of 33 pounds?

7. A cough syrup contains 2 milligrams of brompheniramine maleate in each 5-milliliter dose. How many milligrams of brompheniramine maleate would be contained in a 120-milliliter container of syrup?

8. If 24 pounds of a chemical cost \$46.80, how many pounds can be bought for \$78.00?

9. If 15 gallons of a certain liquid cost \$36.25, how much will 4 gallons cost?

10. If 125 gallons of a mouth rinse contain 20 grams of a coloring agent, how many grams will 160 gallons contain?

11. If 50 tablets contain 1.5 grams of active ingredient, how many grams of the ingredient will 1375 tablets contain?

12. If a diarrhea remedy contains 3.7 milliliters of paregoric in each 30 milliliters of mixture, how many milliliters of paregoric would be contained in or 1 teaspoonful (5 milliliter) dose of the mixture?

13. A metered dose inhaler contains 225 milligrams of metaproterenol sulfate, which is sufficient for 300 inhalations. How many milligrams of metaproterenol sulfate would be administered in each inhalation?

14. How many grains of a substance are needed for 350 tablets if 75 tablets contain 3 grains of the substance?

15. Ipecac syrup contains the equivalent of 32 grains of ipecac in each fluidounce (480 minims) of the syrup. How many minims would provide the equivalent of 20 grains of ipecac?

16. A pediatric vitamin drug product contains the equivalent of 0.5 milligrams of fluoride ion in each milliliter. How many milligrams of fluoride ion would be provided by a dropper that delivers 0.6 milliliter?

17. If a pediatric vitamin contains 1500 units of vitamin A per milliliter of solution, how many units of vitamin A would be administered to a child given 2 drops of the solution from a dropper calibrated to deliver 20 drops per milliliter of solution?

18. An elixir of aprobarbital contains 40 milligrams of aprobarbital in each 5 milliliters. How many milligrams would be used in preparing 4000 milliliters of the elixir?

19. An elixir of ferrous sulfate contains 220 milligrams of ferrous sulfate in each 5

milliliters. If each milligram of ferrous sulfate contains the equivalent of 0.2 milligram of elemental iron, how many milligrams of elemental iron would be represented in each 5 milliliters of the elixir?

20. At a constant temperature, the volume of a gas varies inversely with the pressure. If a gas occupies a volume of 1000 milliliters at a pressure of 760 millimeters, what is its volume at a pressure of 570 millimeters?

21. If an ophthalmic solution contains 1 milligram of dexamethasone phosphate in each milliliter of solution, how many milliliters of solution would be needed to deliver 0.15 milligram of dexamethasone phosphate?

22. How many $\frac{1}{100}$-grain tablets will yield the same amount of nitroglycerin as 50 tablets each containing $\frac{1}{200}$-grain?

23. A 15-milliliter package of nasal spray delivers 20 sprays per milliliter of solution, with each spray containing 1.5 milligrams of drug. (a) How many total sprays will the package deliver? (b) How many milligrams of drug are contained in the 15-milliliter package of the spray?

24. A penicillin V potassium preparation provides 400,000 units of activity in each 250-milligram tablet. How many total units of activity would a patient receive from taking four tablets a day for 10 days?

25. A solution of digitoxin contains 0.2 milligrams per milliliter. How many milliliters will contain 0.03 milligram of digitoxin?

26. A pharmacist prepared a solution containing 5 million units of penicillin per 10 milliliters. How many units of penicillin will 0.25 milliliter contain?

27. If a 5.0-gram packet of a potassium supplement provides 20 milliequivalents of potassium ion and 3.34 milliequivalents of chloride ion, (a) how many grams of the powder would provide 6 milliequivalents of potassium ion, and (b) how many milliequivalents of chloride ion would be provided by this amount of powder?

28. If an intravenous fluid is adjusted to deliver 15 milligrams of medication to a patient per hour, how many milligrams are delivered per minute?

29. If a potassium chloride elixir contains 20 milliequivalents of potassium ion in each 15 milliliters of elixir, how many milliliters will provide 25 milliequivalents of potassium ion to the patient?

30. The blood serum concentration of the antibacterial drug ciprofloxacin increases proportionately with the dose of drug administered. If a 250-milligram dose of the drug results in a serum concentration of 1.2 micrograms of drug per milliliter of serum, how many micrograms of drug would be expected per milliliter of serum following a dose of 500 milligrams of drug?

31. If a syringe contains 5 milligrams of medication in each 10 milliliters of solution, how many milligrams would be administered when 4 milliliters of solution are injected?

32. The dosage of the drug Mintezol® is determined in direct proportion to a patient's weight. If the dose of the drug for a patient weighing 150 pounds is 1.5 grams, what would be the dose for a patient weighing 110 pounds?

33. If 0.5 milliliters of a mumps virus vaccine contains 5000 units of antigen, how

many units would be present in each milliliter if the 0.5 milliliter of vaccine was diluted to 2 milliliters with water for injection?

SIGNIFICANT FIGURES

When we *count* objects accurately, *every* figure in the numeral expressing the total number of objects must be taken at its face value. Such figures may be said to be *absolute*. When we record a *measurement*, the last figure to the right must be taken to be an *approximation*, an admission that the limit of possible precision or of necessary accuracy has been reached, and that any further figures to the right would be nonsignificant, i.e., either meaningless or, for a given purpose, needless.

We should learn to interpret a denominate number like 325 *grams* as follows: The 3 means *300 grams,* neither more nor less, and the 2 means *exactly 20 grams more;* but the final 5 means *approximately 5 grams more,* i.e., *5 grams plus or minus some fraction of a gram.* Whether this fraction is, for a given purpose, negligible depends on how precisely the quantity was (or is to be) weighed.

Significant figures, then, are consecutive figures that express the value of a denominate number accurately enough for a given purpose. The accuracy varies with the number of significant figures, which are all absolute in value except the last, and this is properly called *uncertain.*

Two-figure accuracy is liable to a deviation as high as 5% from the theoretic absolute measurement. For example, if a substance is reported to weigh *10 grams* to the nearest *gram,* its actual weight may be anything between *9.5* and *10.5 grams.* Three-figure accuracy is liable to a deviation as high as 0.5%; four-figure accuracy may deviate 0.05%; and five-figure accuracy, 0.005%.

Any of the digits in a valid denominate number must be regarded as significant. Whether *zero* is significant, however, depends on its position or on known facts about a given number. The interpretation of *zero* may be summed up as follows:

1. Any zero between digits is significant.
2. Initial zeros to the left of the first digit are never significant; they are included merely to show the location of the decimal point and thus give place value to the digits that follow.
3. One or more final zeros to the right of the decimal point may be taken to be significant.
4. One or more final zeros in a whole number, i.e., immediately to the left of the decimal point, sometimes merely give place value to digits to the left, but the data may show them to be significant.

Examples:

Assuming that the following numbers are all denominate:

1. In *12.5,* there are *three* significant figures; in 1.256, *four* significant figures; and in *102.56, five* significant figures.
2. In *0.5,* there is *one* significant figure. The digit 5 tells us how many *tenths* we have. The nonsignificant *0* simply calls attention to the decimal point.
3. In *0.05,* there is still only *one* significant figure, and again in *0.005.*
4. In *0.65,* there are *two* significant figures, and likewise *two* in *0.065* and *0.0065.*
5. In *0.0605,* there are *three* significant figures. The first *0* calls attention to the decimal

point; the second *0* shows the number of places to the right of the decimal point occupied by the remaining figures; and the third *0* significantly contributes to the value of the number. In *0.06050*, there are *four* significant figures, because the final *0* also contributes to the value of the number.

6. In *20000*, there are *five* significant figures; but *20000* ± *50* or, to express the same quantity another way, *20000 to the nearest 100*, contains only *three* significant figures.

As noted previously, one of the factors determining the degree of approximation to perfect measurement is the precision of the instrument used. It would be absurd to claim that *7.76 milliliters* had been measured in a graduate calibrated in units of *1 milliliter*, or that *25.562 grains* had been weighed on a balance sensitive to $\frac{1}{10}$ *grain*.

Other Examples:

1. If a substance weighs *0.06 gram*, according to a balance sensitive to *0.001 gram*, we may record the weight as *0.060 gram*. But if the balance is sensitive only to *0.01 gram*, the value should be recorded as *0.06 gram*, and a record of *0.060 gram* would be invalid.
2. When recording a length of *10 millimeters* found by use of an instrument accurate to *0.1 millimeter*, the value may be recorded as *10.0 millimeters*.
3. If a volume of *5 milliliters* is measured with an instrument calibrated in *tenths of a milliliter*, the volume may be recorded as *5.0 milliliters*.

We must clearly distinguish *significant figures* from *decimal places*. When recording a measurement, the number of decimal places we include indicates *the degree of precision with which the measurement has been made*, whereas the number of significant figures retained indicates *the degree of accuracy* that is sufficient for a given purpose.

Sometimes we are asked to record a value "correct to (so-many) decimal places". We should never confuse this familiar expression with the expression "correct to (so-many) significant figures."

Examples:

1. If the value of *27.625918* is rounded off to *five decimal places*, it is written *27.62592;* but when this value is rounded off to *five significant figures*, it is written *27.626*.
2. The value *54.3265*, when rounded off to *54.3*, is precise to *one decimal place* but it is accurate to *three significant figures*.

The principle that *the result of any calculation involving an approximate number should be rounded off so as to contain only one uncertain figure* holds for quotients and products as well as for sums and differences.

With this principle in mind, we can get valid results, and save a good deal of time, by obeying the following rules for recording measurements, calculating with approximate numbers, and recording the results of such calculations.

First, *when recording a measurement, retain as many figures as will give only one uncertain figure.* The uncertain figure will sometimes represent an estimate between graduations on a scale. Thus, if you use a ruler calibrated in centimeters, you might record a measurement as approximately *11.3 centimeters,* but not as approximately *11.32 centimeters.* Because the 3 is uncertain, no other figure should follow it.

Second, *when rejecting superfluous figures in the result of a calculation, add 1 to the last figure retained if the following figure is 5 or more.* Thus, 2.43 may be rounded off to 2.4, but 2.46 should be rounded off to 2.5. Note that if a number like 2.597 is rounded off to three significant figures, the 1 added to the 9 makes 10, and 0 should be recorded, for it is significant: 2.60.

Third, *when adding or subtracting approximate numbers, include only as many decimal places as are in the number with the least decimal places.*

Example:

Add these approximate weights: 162.4 grams, 0.489 gram, 0.1875 gram, and 120.78 grams.

Incorrect	Correct
162.4	162.4
0.489	0.5
0.1875	0.2
120.78	120.8
283.8565, answer.	283.9, answer.

It is important to note that in filling a prescription, the pharmacist *must* assume that the physician means each quantity to be measured with *the same degree of precision.* Hence, if we add these quantities taken from a prescription:

5.5   *grams*
0.01   *grams*
0.005 *gram*

we must *not* round off the total to one decimal place. Rather we must retain at least *three* decimal places in the total by interpreting the given quantities to mean 5.500 *grams,* 0.010 *gram,* and 0.005 *gram.* When greater precision is required, we may interpret the given quantities to mean 5.5000, 0.0100, and 0.0050, etc.

Fourth, *when multiplying or dividing one approximate number by another approximate number, round off the component with the greater number of significant figures to the number contained in the component having fewer significant figures. Retain no more significant figures in the product or quotient than in the number with the least significant figures.*

Example:

Multiply 1.65370 grams by 0.26.
1.65370 grams is rounded off to 1.65 grams
1.65 grams × 0.26 = 0.4290 or
0.43 grams, *answer.*

When multiplying or dividing with denominate numbers taken from a prescription or official formula, assuming that each quantity is meant to be measured with the same degree of accuracy, we must interpret each quantity as having at least as many significant figures as appear in the quantity containing the greatest number of significant figures. So, if the quantities 0.25 *gram,* 0.5 *gram,* and 5 *grams* are included in a prescription, they should be interpreted as 0.25 *gram,* 0.50 *gram,* and 5.0 *grams* for purposes of multiplication or division (as when we enlarge or reduce a formula), and results should be rounded off to contain two significant figures. Where greater accuracy is required, we may interpret the given quantities to mean 0.2500, 0.5000, and 5.000, etc.

It should be noted that in multiplication and division, we are concerned with the number of significant figures, whereas in addition and subtraction, the number of decimal places is important.

Fifth, *after multiplying or dividing an approximate number by an absolute number, round off the result to the same number of significant figures as are contained in the approximate number.* This rule is consistent with the fourth rule, for the denominate number contains fewer significant figures if the absolute number is interpreted as being followed by significant zeros to an infinite number of decimal places.

Example:

If a patient has taken 96 doses, each containing 2.54 mg of active ingredient, how many milligrams of the active ingredient has he taken in all?

$$\begin{array}{r} 2.54 \text{ milligrams} \\ \times\ 96 \\ \hline 1524 \\ 2286\ \ \ \ \\ \hline \end{array}$$

243.84 or 244 milligrams, *answer.*

Practice Problems

1. State the number of significant figures in each of the *italicized* quantities:
   (*a*) One gram equals *15.4324* grains.
   (*b*) One liter equals *1000* milliliters.
   (*c*) One inch equals *2.54* centimeters.
   (*d*) The chemical costs *$1.05* per pound.
   (*e*) One gram equals *1,000,000* micrograms.
   (*f*) One microgram equals *0.001* milligram.

2. Assuming these numbers to be denominate, how many significant figures are in each?
   (*a*) 35
   (*b*) 609
   (*c*) 2.7
   (*d*) 9004
   (*e*) 506.03
   (*f*) 0.0047
   (*g*) 40.07
   (*h*) 350 (to nearest 1)
   (*i*) 350 (to nearest 10)
   (*j*) 5000 (to nearest 100)

3. Round off each of the following to three significant figures:
   (*a*) 32.75
   (*b*) 200.39
   (*c*) 0.03629
   (*d*) 21.635
   (*e*) 0.00944
   (*f*) 1.0751
   (*g*) 27.052
   (*h*) 0.86249
   (*i*) 3.14159
   (*j*) 1.00595632

4. Round off each of the following to three decimal places:
   (*a*) 0.00083
   (*b*) 34.79502
   (*c*) 0.00494
   (*d*) 6.12963
   (*e*) 14.8997
   (*f*) 1.00595632

5. If a mixture of seven ingredients contains the following approximate weights, what can you validly record as the approximate total combined weight of the ingredients?

   26.83 grams, 275.3 grams, 2.752 grams, 4.04 grams, 5.197 grams, 16.64 grams, and 0.085 gram.

6. If each of a batch of tablets contains 0.050 grain of active ingredient, what approximate weight of active ingredient will be contained in 750 tablets?

7. If each tablet contains 0.05 grain of active ingredient, what will be the approximate weight of active ingredient in 750 tablets?

8. Perform the following computations and retain only significant figures in the results:
   (a) 6.39 − 0.008
   (b) 7.01 − 6.0
   (c) 97.1 − 6.9368
   (d) 5.0 × 48.3 grains
   (e) 24 × 0.25 gram
   (f) 350 × 0.60156 gram
   (g) 0.720 × 0.095 grain
   (h) 0.056 × 0.9626 gram
   (i) 56.824 ÷ 0.0905
   (j) 250 ÷ 1.109
   (k) 5.0001 ÷ 1.9
   (l) 0.00729 ÷ 0.2735
   (m) 71.455 ÷ 0.512
   (n) 71.955 ÷ 3.0

9. What is the difference in meaning between a volume recorded as 473 milliliters and one recorded as 473.0 milliliters?

10. What is the difference in meaning between a weight recorded as 0.65 gram and one recorded as 0.6500 gram?

11. The answers in the following computations are arithmetically correct. In each case, if the answer does not contain the proper number of significant figures, rewrite it so that all the figures retained are significant.
    (a) 15.432 grains × 0.26 = 4.01232 grains
    (b) 0.2350 grain ÷ 0.55 = 0.42727 grain
    (c) 1.25500 grams + 0.650 gram + 0.125 gram + 12.78900 grams = 14.81900 grams
    (d) 16.23 minims × 0.75 = 12.1725 minims
    (e) 437.5 grains ÷ 1.25 = 350.000 grains

ESTIMATION

One of the best checks of the reasonableness of a numeric computation is an estimation of the answer. If we arrive at a wrong answer by using a wrong method, a thoughtless, mechanical final verification of our figuring may not reveal the error. But an absurd result, such as occurs when the decimal point is put in the wrong place, will not likely slip past if we check it against a preliminary estimation of what the result should be.

Because it is imperative that pharmacists ensure the accuracy of their calculations by every possible means, pharmacy students are urged to adopt *estimation* as one of those means. Proficiency in estimating comes only from constant practice. Therefore, pharmacy students are urged to acquire the habit of estimating the answer to every problem encountered before attempting to solve it. Estimation serves not only as a means for judging the reasonableness of the final result, but also as a guide in the solution of the problem.

Checking the accuracy of every calculation, of course, such as by adding a column first upward and then downward, is important. Hence the student should follow this invariable procedure: (1) *estimate*, (2) *compute*, (3) *check*.

The estimating process is basically simple. First, the numbers given in a problem are mentally rounded off to slightly larger or smaller numbers containing fewer significant figures; e.g., 59 would be rounded off to 60, and 732 to 700. Then, the required computations are performed, as far as possible mentally, and the result, although known to be somewhat greater or smaller than the exact answer, is close enough to serve as an estimate.

No set rules for estimating can be given to cover all the computations in arithmetic. But examples can illustrate some of the methods that can be used.

In *addition,* one way to obtain a reasonable estimate of the total is first to add the figures in the leftmost column. The neglected remaining figures of each number are equally likely to express more or less than one-half the value of a unit of the order we have just added, and hence to the sum of the leftmost column is added $\frac{1}{2}$ for every number—or *1* for every two numbers—in the column.

Examples:

Add the following numbers: 7428, 3652, 1327, 4605, 2791, and 4490.
Estimation:
The figures in the thousands column add up to 21000, and with each number on the average contributing 500 more, or every pair 1000 more, we get 21000 + 3000 = 24000, *estimated answer.*
Calculation:
```
   7428
   3652
   1327
   4605
   2791
   4490
```
24293, *answer.*
Add the following numbers: 2556, 449, 337, 1572.
Estimation:
The figures of the thousands column add up to 3000, and with each pair of numbers contributing approximately another 1000, we get 3000 + 2000 = 5000, *estimated answer.*
Calculation:
```
2556
 449
 337
1572
```
4914, *answer.*

In *multiplication,* the product of the two leftmost digits plus a sufficient number of *zeros* to give the right place value serves as a fair estimate. The number of *zeros* supplied must equal the total number of all discarded figures to the left of the decimal point. Approximation to the correct answer is closer if the discarded figures are used to round off the value of those retained.

Examples:

Multiply 612 by 413.
Estimation:
$4 \times 6 = 24$, and because we discarded four figures, four zeros must be supplied, giving 240,000, *estimated answer.*
Calculation:
```
   612
 × 413
  1836
   612
  2448
```
252756, *answer.*

Multiply 2889 by 209.

Estimation:

The given numbers round off to 3000 and 200. $3 \times 2 = 6$, and supplying five zeros we get 600,000, *estimated answer.*

Calculation:

```
   2889
 × 209
  26001
  5778
```
603801, *answer.*

The correct place value is easier to keep track of if relatively insignificant decimal fractions are ignored. When the multiplier is a decimal fraction, the possibility of error is reduced if we first convert it to a common fraction of approximately the same place.

Examples:

Multiply 41.76 by 20.3.
Estimate: $42 \times 20 = 840$.

Multiply 730.5 by 321.
Estimate: $700 \times 300 = 210,000$.

Multiply 314.2 by 0.18.
Estimate: Because 0.18 or $^{18}/_{100}$ lies between $\frac{1}{6}$ and $\frac{1}{5}$, the answer will lie between 50 and 60.

Multiply 48.16 by 0.072.
Estimate: $^{7}/_{100}$ equals about $\frac{1}{15}$, and $\frac{1}{15}$ of 48 is about 3.

In *division,* the given numbers may be rounded off to convenient approximations, but again care is needed to preserve the correct place values.

Example:

Divide 2456 by 5.91.
Estimate: The numbers may be rounded off to 2400 and 6. We may divide 24 by 6 mentally, but we must remember the two zeros substituted for the given 56 in 2456. The estimated answer is 400.

The use of short cuts and variations in arithmetical computations contributes to both speed and accuracy in mental calculation. Facility in the use of short cuts can be developed only if we select or devise variations that appeal to us and practice them constantly. The following are some short cuts that may suggest other possibilities:

1. To multiply by 10, 100, 1000, etc., move the decimal place one, two, three places to the right, etc. To divide by 10, 100, 1000, etc., move the decimal place one, two, three places to the left, etc.
2. To multiply by 200, 300, 500, etc., multiply by 2, 3, 5, etc., and then multiply by 100. To divide by the same numbers, divide by 2, 3, 5, etc., and divide by 100.
3. To multiply by 2000, 4000, 6000, etc., multiply by 2, 4, 6, etc., and then multiply

by 1000. To divide by these numbers, divide by 2, 4, 6, etc., and divide by 1000.

4. To multiply by 75, which is ¾ of a hundred, multiply by 300 and divide by 4. To divide by 75, multiply by 4 and divide by 300.

5. To multiply by 66⅔, which is ⅔ of 100, multiply by 200 and divide by 3. To divide by 66⅔, multiply by 3 and divide by 200.

6. To multiply by 50, which is ½ of 100, multiply by 100 and divide by 2. To divide by 50, multiply by 2 and divide by 100.

7. To multiply by 33⅓, which is ⅓ of 100, multiply by 100 and divide by 3. To divide by 33⅓, multiply by 3 and divide by 100.

8. To multiply by 25, which is ¼ of 100, multiply by 100 and divide by 4. To divide by 25, multiply by 4 and divide by 100.

9. To multiply by 12½, which is ⅛ of a hundred, multiply by 100 and divide by 8. To divide by 12½, multiply by 8 and divide by 100.

10. To multiply any *two-digit* number by 11, first add the two digits. If the sum is less than 10, place it between the digits; if the sum is 10 or more, place the unit figure between the digits and add 1 to the left digit.

$$11 \times 43: 4 + 3 = 7, \text{ hence } 473$$
$$11 \times 83: 8 + 3 = 11, \text{ hence } 913$$

To multiply *any* number by 11, multiply by 10 and add the multiplicand.

Practice Problems

1. In estimating the result of multiplying 8,329 by 7,242, how many zeros will follow 56?

2. In estimating the result of dividing 811,500 by 16.23, how many zeros will follow 5?

3. How many terminal zeros are there in the product obtained by multiplying 5.100 by 90,000?

4. How many terminal zeros are there in the quotient obtained by multiplying 8.100 by 0.009?

Estimate the sums:

5.	5641	7.	3298	9.	$ 75.82
	2177		368		37.92
	294		5192		14.69
	8266		627		45.98
	3503		4835		28.91
					49.87
6.	9874	8.	7466	10.	$ 49.55
	6018		5288		9.75
	459		9013		12.98
	1297		8462		53.36
	3361		716		29.79
	396		4369		14.56

Estimate the products:

11. $17 \times 22 =$

12. $28 \times 31 =$

13. $8 \times 48 =$

14. $19 \times 38 =$

15. $28 \times 62 =$

16. $39 \times 77 =$

17. $42 \times 39 =$

18. $125 \times 92 =$

19. $365 \times 98 =$

20. $473 \times 102 =$

21. $596 \times 204 =$

22. $604 \times 122 =$

23. $675 \times 19 =$

24. $998 \times 13 =$

25. $6549 \times 830 =$

26. $1073 \times 972 =$

27. $8431 \times 9760 =$

28. $7183 \times 19 =$

29. $5106 \times 963 =$

30. $2349 \times 5907 =$

31. $2\frac{1}{2} \times 14\frac{1}{2} =$

32. $\frac{2}{3} \times 400 =$

33. $21\frac{1}{3} \times 6\frac{2}{3} =$

34. $\frac{3}{4} \times 816 =$

35. $\frac{2}{3} \times 425.65 =$

36. $5.8 \times 7165 =$

37. $2.04 \times 705.3 =$

38. $0.016 \times 589.4 =$

39. $0.0726 \times 6951 =$

40. $98 \times 0.0031 =$

41. $6.1 \times 67.39 =$

42. $7569 \times 0.0963 =$

Estimate the quotients:

43. $171 \div 19 =$

44. $165 \div 15 =$

45. $184 \div 2300 =$

46. $3080 \div 144 =$

47. $160 \div 3200 =$

48. $36900 \div 41 =$

49. $86450 \div 72 =$

50. $1078 \div 98 =$

51. $98000 \div 49 =$

52. $17015 \div 57 =$

53. $1.0745 \div 500 =$

54. $18.954 \div 0.39 =$

55. $1.9214 \div 0.026 =$

56. $19.223 \div 47 =$

57. $458.4 \div 8 =$

58. $448.32 \div 0.048 =$

Estimate the final results:

59. $\dfrac{272103 \times 300}{901} =$

60. $\dfrac{750 \times 300 \times 380.5}{760 \times 375} =$

61. $\dfrac{270 \,(15 - 10)}{91 \times 5} =$

62. $\frac{1}{120} \times \frac{1}{10} \times 11.95 =$

63. $\dfrac{437.5}{8.05} \times \frac{1}{16} =$

64. $\dfrac{809 \times (35 - 25)}{4.01 \times 20} =$

65. $\dfrac{\frac{1}{100}}{\frac{1}{2}} \times 5123 =$

66. $\dfrac{627 \times (25 - 10)}{30 \times 15} =$

67. $\dfrac{750 \times 380 \times 319.53}{760 \times 750} =$

68. What should be the approximate total cost of 625,250 tablets at $\frac{3}{5}$¢ each?

69. Estimate the approximate cost of 32,560 capsules at $12.50 per thousand.

70. Estimate the approximate cost of 30,125 capsules at $1.50 per hundred.

71. What should be the approximate cost of 120,050 tablets at 66$\frac{2}{3}$¢ per hundred?

72. A formula for 1,250 capsules contains 3.635 grams of a medicament. Estimate the amount of medicament that should be used in preparing 325 capsules.

73. Approximately how many teaspoonful- (5-milliliter) doses can be obtained from 1 gallon (3,785 milliliters) of a liquid?

74. The cost of 1000 capsules is $30.50. If they are sold at the rate of $3.25 for 48 capsules, estimate the profit that can be realized from the sale of 1000 capsules.

75. The cost of 5000 capsules is $256.00. If they are sold at the rate of $3.95 for 24 capsules, estimate the profit that can be realized from the sale of 500 capsules.

PERCENTAGE OF ERROR

Because measurements are never absolutely accurate, it is important for the pharmacist to recognize the limitations of the instruments used and the magnitude of the errors that may be incurred. When a pharmacist measures a volume of liquid or weighs a material, two quantities become important: (1) the *apparent* weight or volume measured, and (2) the possible excess or deficiency in the actual quantity obtained.

Percentage of error may be defined as *the maximum potential error multiplied by 100 and divided by the quantity desired.* The calculation may be formulated as follows:

$$\frac{\text{Error} \times 100\%}{\text{Quantity desired}} = \text{Percentage of error}$$

Calculating Percentage Error in Volumetric Measurement. As described in the following section concerning measurement of volume, the precision obtained in a given measurement depends on the selection of the measuring device used (e.g., pipet, graduated cylinder), the volume of liquid being measured, and the skill and care of the pharmacist.

The percentage error in a measurement of volume may be calculated from the preceding formula, relating the volume in error (determined through devices of greater precision) to the volume desired (or apparently measured).

Example:

Using a graduated cylinder, a pharmacist measured 30 milliliters of a liquid. On subsequent examination, using a narrow-gauge burette, it was determined that the pharmacist had actually measured 32 milliliters. What was the percentage of error in the original measurement?

32 milliliters − 30 milliliters = 2 milliliters, the volume of error

$$\frac{2 \text{ mL} \times 100\%}{30 \text{ mL}} = 6.7\%, \text{ answer.}$$

Calculating Percentage Error in Weighing. The various scales and balances used in pharmaceutical weighing have ascribed to them different degrees of precision. The *sensitivity* of a balance may be defined in several ways. Balance manufacturers use the term to designate the smallest weight that will cause a perceptible movement of the balance, shown by the balance's indicator scale.

As described in the following section concerning measurement of weight, prescription balances have established standards of precision based on a *Sensitivity Requirement (SR)*, defined by the *United States Pharmacopeia* as "the maximum change in load that will cause a specified change, one subdivision on the index plate, in the position of rest of the indicating element or elements of the balance." Prescription balances should have a SR (or maximum potential error) of 6 milligrams or less. Obviously, the smaller the weight required to move the indicating element, the more sensitive the balance.

Examples:

When the maximum potential error is ± 4 milligrams in a total of 100 milligrams, what is the percentage of error?

$$\frac{4 \times 100\%}{100} = 4\%, \textit{answer.}$$

A prescription calls for 800 milligrams of a substance. After weighing this amount on a balance, the pharmacist decides to check by weighing it again on a more sensitive balance, which registers only 750 milligrams. Because the first weighing was 50 milligrams short of the desired amount, what was the percentage or error?

$$\frac{50 \times 100\%}{800} = 6.25\%, \textit{answer.}$$

If a certain percentage of error is not to be exceeded, and the maximum potential error of an instrument is known, it is possible to calculate the smallest quantity that can be measured within the desired accuracy. A convenient formula follows:

$$\frac{100 \times \text{Maximum potential error}}{\text{Permissible percentage of error}} = \text{Smallest quantity}$$

Example:

What is the smallest quantity that can be weighed with a potential error of not more than 5% on a balance sensitive to 6 milligrams?

$$\frac{100 \times 6 \text{ milligrams}}{5} = 120 \text{ milligrams}, \textit{answer.}$$

Practice Problems

1. A pharmacist attempts to weigh 120 milligrams of codeine sulfate on a balance with a sensitivity requirement of 6 milligrams. Calculate the maximum potential error in terms of percentage.

2. In compounding a prescription, a pharmacist weighed 0.050 gram of a substance on a balance insensitive to quantities smaller than 0.004 gram. What was the maximum potential error in terms of percentage?

3. A pharmacist wants to weigh 5 grains of a substance on a balance with a sensitivity requirement of ¼ grain. Calculate the maximum potential error in terms of percentage.

4. A pharmacist weighed 825 milligrams of a substance. When checked on another balance, the weight was found to be 805 milligrams. Calculate the deviation from the original weighing in terms of percentage.

5. A pharmacist weighed 475 milligrams of a substance on a balance of dubious accuracy. When checked on a balance of high accuracy, the weight was found to be 445 milligrams. Calculate the percentage of error in the first weighing.

6. A 10-milliliter graduate weighs 42.745 grams. When 5 milliliters of distilled water are measured in it, the combined weight of graduate and water is 47.675 grams. By definition, 5 milliliters of water should weigh 5 grams. Calculate the weight of the measured water and express any deviation from 5 grams as percentage of error.

7. A graduate weighs 35.825 grams. When 10 milliliters of water are measured in it, the weight of the graduate and water is 45.835 grams. Calculate the weight of the water and express any deviation from 10 grams as percentage of error.

8. In preparing a certain ointment, a pharmacist used 28.35 grams of zinc oxide instead of the 31.1 grams called for. Calculate the percentage of error on the basis of the desired quantity.

9. A pharmacist attempts to weigh 0.375 gram of morphine sulfate on a balance of dubious accuracy. When checked on a highly accurate balance, the weight is found to be 0.400 gram. Calculate the percentage of error in the first weighing.

10. On a prescription balance with a sensitivity requirement of 0.012 gram, what is the smallest amount that can be weighed with a maximum potential error of not more than 5%?

11. On a torsion prescription balance with a sensitivity requirement of $\frac{1}{16}$ grain, what is the smallest amount that can be weighed with a potential error of not more than 2%?

12. If an accuracy of 2% is desired, what is the minimum amount that should be weighed on a torsion prescription balance with a sensitivity requirement of 0.004 gram?

13. A pharmacist measured 60 milliliters of glycerin by difference, starting with 100 milliliters. After completing the measurement, he noted that the graduate that he used contained 45 milliliters of glycerin. Calculate the percentage of error incurred in the measurement.

14. A pharmacist failed to place the balance in equilibrium before weighing 200 milligrams of codeine sulfate. Later, he discovered that the balance was out of equilibrium and that a 20% error was incurred. If the balance pan on which he placed the codeine sulfate was heavy, how many milligrams of codeine sulfate did he actually weigh?

15. In compounding a prescription for a nasal spray, a pharmacist weighed 30 milligrams of menthol on a balance with a sensitivity requirement of 3 milligrams. Calculate the percentage of error that may have been incurred.

16. Using a torsion balance with a sensitivity requirement of 4 milligrams (or $\frac{1}{16}$ grain), state which of the following weights could be made with a dispensing error not greater than plus or minus 5%:
    (a) $\frac{5}{8}$ grain
    (b) 0.085 gram

(c) $1\frac{1}{2}$ grains

(d) 50,000 micrograms (1 microgram = 0.001 milligrams)

(e) 65 milligrams

(f) $1\frac{1}{4}$ grains

17. A certain prescription balance is not to be used in weighing loads of less than 648 milligrams. If its sensitivity requirement is 30 milligrams, calculate the percentage of error that might be incurred in weighing the minimum specified load.

18. The sensitivity requirement of a class A prescription balance is 0.006 gram. Calculate the percentage of error that might be incurred in weighing 0.1 gram on this balance.

19. A pharmacist measures 900 milliliters in a 1000-milliliter cylindric graduate calibrated in 10-milliliter units. Calculate the percentage of error that might be incurred in the measurement.

20. When substances are to be "accurately weighed" in an assay or a test, the *United States Pharmacopeia* directs that a quantity of 50 milligrams is to be weighed to the nearest 0.05 milligram. Calculate the percentage of error in the weighing.

21. You are directed to weigh 10 grams of a substance so as to limit the error to 0.2%. Calculate the maximum potential error, in terms of grams, that you would not be permitted to exceed.

22. In a certain assay, 100 milligrams of a substance are to be weighed so as to limit the error to 0.1%. Calculate the maximum potential error, in terms of milligrams, that the analyst must not exceed.

MEASUREMENT OF VOLUME

Common instruments for the pharmaceutical measurement of volume range from micropipets and burettes used in analytic procedures to large, industrial-size calibrated vessels. The selection of measuring instrument should be based on the level of precision required. In pharmacy practice, the most common instruments for measuring volume are cylindric and conical (cone-shaped) graduates (Fig. 1.1). For the measurement of small volumes, however, the pharmacist often uses a calibrated syringe or, when required, a pipette.

Whereas cylindric graduates are calibrated in metric units, conical graduates are usually dual-scale, i.e., calibrated in both metric and apothecary units of volume. Both glass and plastic graduates are commercially available in a number of capacities, ranging from 5 to 1000 milliliters and greater.

As a general rule, it is best to select the graduate with a capacity equal to or just exceeding the volume to be measured. Measurement of small volumes in large graduates tends to increase the size of the error. The design of a volumetric apparatus is an important factor in measurement accuracy; the narrower the bore or chamber, the lesser the error in reading the meniscus and the more accurate the measurement (Fig. 1.2). According to the *United States Pharmacopeia*, a deviation of $\pm$ 1 mm in the meniscus reading causes an error of approximately 0.5 milliliter when a 100-milliliter cylindric graduate is used and an error of 1.8 milliliter at the 100-milliliter mark in a comparable conical graduate. Conical graduates of less that 25-milliliter capacities are not recommended for use in pharmaceutical compounding. It is essential for the pharmacist to select the proper type and capacity of instrument for volumetric measure and to carefully observe the meniscus at eye level to achieve the desired measurement.

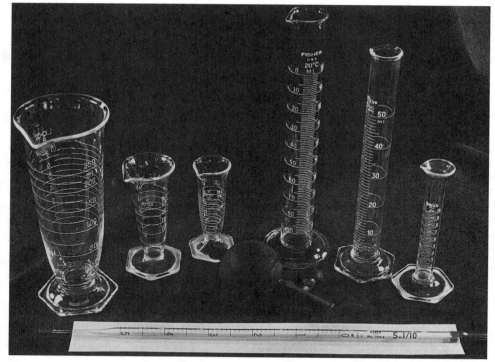

Fig. 1.1. Examples of conical and cylindric graduates, pipet, and a pipet-filling bulb for volumetric measurement.

MEASUREMENT OF WEIGHT

The selection of implements from the wide range of available weights, balances, and scales for pharmaceutical measurement depends on the task at hand, from highly sensitive electronic analytic balances in performing assay tests and prescription balances in extemporaneous compounding procedures to large capacity scales in the industrial manufacturing and production of pharmaceutical agents. Each instrument used must meet established standards for sensitivity, accuracy, and capacity.

Prescription balances (Fig. 1.3) are designed for the weighing of medicinal or other substances required in the filling of prescriptions or in small-scale compounding. Some prescription balances have a weighbeam and rider, and others a dial, to add up to 1 gram of weight. As required, additional external weights may be added to the right-hand balance pan. The material to be weighed is placed on the left-hand pan. Powder papers are added to each pan before any additions and the balance is leveled by leveling feet or balancing screws. Weighings are performed through the careful portion-wise (by spatula) addition and removal of the material being weighed, with the balance being *arrested* (pans locked in place by the control knob) during each addition and removal of material, and *un*arrested with the lid closed for determinations of balance rest points. When the unarrested pans neither ascend nor descend and the index plate shows the needle is in the center, the material and balance weights are considered equivalent. The student may wish to refer to other sources, such as the *United States Pharmacopeia*, for more detailed information on the proper use and testing of the prescription balance.

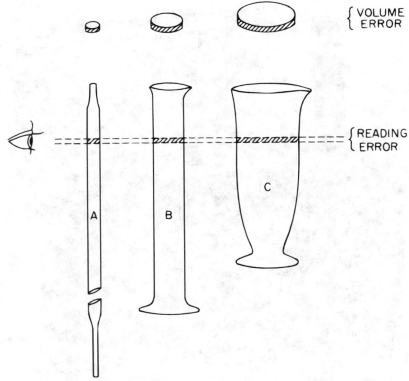

Fig. I.2. Volume error differentials due to instrument diameters.

Class III (previously called class A) prescription balances should be used in all prescription compounding procedures. Balances of this type have a sensitivity requirement (SR) of 6 milligrams or less with no load and with a load of 10 grams in each pan.[5] To avoid errors of greater than 5% when using this balance, the pharmacist should not weigh less than 120 milligrams of material (i.e., a 5% error in a weighing of 120 milligrams = 6 milligrams). Most commercially available class III balances have a capacity of 120 grams.

ALIQUOT METHOD OF WEIGHING AND MEASURING

When a degree of precision in measurement is required that is beyond the capacity of the instrument at hand, the pharmacist may achieve the desired precision by measuring and calculating in terms of aliquot parts.

---

[5] The term *sensitivity* as it applies to a prescription balance may be defined as the smallest weight that will disturb its equilibrium. This designation of the *sensitivity* of a prescription balance is not to be confused with the term *sensitivity requirement (SR)*, which is defined in the *United States Pharmacopeia* as "the maximum change in load that will cause a specified change, one subdivision on the index plate, in the position of rest of the indicating element or elements of the balance."

In view of the fact that the term *sensitivity* has various interpretations, the *United States Pharmacopeia* has adopted the term *sensitivity requirement* to designate the sensitiveness of a balance. In accordance with this adoption, the designation *sensitivity requirement* is used herein when reference is made to the sensitiveness of a prescription balance.

The *sensitivity requirement* may be determined by the following procedure:

1. Level the balance.

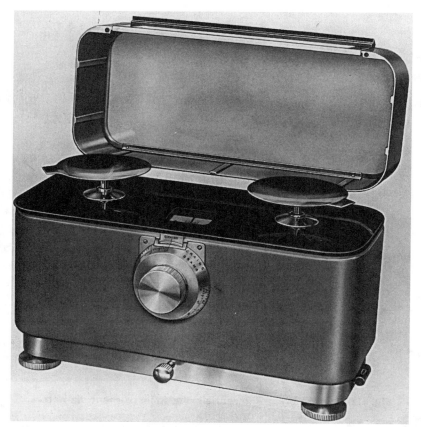

Fig. 1.3. Model DRX2 Torsion prescription balance. (Courtesy of Torsion Balance Company.)

An *aliquot part* is any part that is contained a whole number of times in a quantity. Thus, *2* is an aliquot part of *10*, and *because 10 ÷ 2 = 5*, *2* is called the *fifth aliquot* of *10*. Again, *4* is an aliquot part of *16*, and because *16 ÷ 4 = 4*, *4* is the *fourth aliquot of 16*.

Weighing by the Aliquot Method. *The aliquot method of weighing* is a method by which small quantities of a substance may be obtained within the degree of accuracy desired. A summary of the procedure follows:

Step 1. Select some multiple of the desired quantity that can be weighed with the required precision. Weigh this multiple.

Step 2. Using an inert substance that is compatible with the given preparation, dilute the multiple quantity.

Step 3. Weigh the aliquot part of the dilution that contains the desired quantity.

To select the multiple quantity in step 1, first calculate the smallest quantity of the substance that can be weighed with the required precision (see the preceding section concerning

---

2.   Determine the rest point of the balance.

3.   Determine the smallest weight that causes the rest point to shift one division on the index plate. (In accordance with the *United States Pharmacopeia*, 23rd revision.)

percentage of error). To ensure an error of no greater than 5%, for instance, a quantity at least 20 times the sensitivity requirement of the balance must be weighed; hence, if the sensitivity requirement of a balance is *4 milligrams, 20 × 4 milligrams,* or *80 milligrams,* is the smallest amount that can be weighed. If *50 milligrams* were weighed on such a balance, the maximum potential error would be 8% (see discussion of percentage of error). Convenience in multiplying, availability of weights, and the cost of the substance are other factors that help to determine the choice of the multiple quantity.

The amount of inert diluent used in Step 2 is determined by the fact that the aliquot part of the dilution to be weighed in *Step 3* must be a quantity large enough to be weighed within the desired degree of accuracy. In *Step 1,* we calculated the minimum quantity that satisfies this condition. The aliquot must weigh at least as much as the multiple quantity weighed in *Step 1;* to reduce the potential error, its weight should be somewhat greater. So, if the multiple quantity weighs *80 milligrams,* the aliquot must weigh at least *80 milligrams,* but preferably *100 milligrams* or more. When we multiply the chosen aliquot by the multiple selected in *Step 1,* we get the quantity of the dilution, and have only to add sufficient diluent to the multiple quantity to equal this weight of dilution.

The aliquot weighed in Step 3 will contain the quantity originally desired; e.g., if *20* times the original quantity is diluted, $\frac{1}{20}$ of the dilution will contain the original quantity. By arbitrarily selecting a sufficiently large multiple quantity and a sufficiently large dilution, we can be sure we have measured within the required degree of precision.

Example:

A torsion prescription balance has a sensitivity requirement of 4 milligrams. Explain how you would weigh 5 milligrams of atropine sulfate with an accuracy of ± 5%, using lactose as the diluent.

Because 4 milligrams is the potential balance error, 80 milligrams is the smallest amount that should be weighed to achieve the required precision.

If 100 milligrams, or 20 times the desired amount of atropine sulfate, is chosen as the multiple quantity to be weighed in Step 1, and if 150 milligrams is set as the aliquot to be weighed in Step 3, then:

1. Weigh 20 × 5 mg, or   100 mg of atropine sulfate
2. Dilute with   <u>2900</u> mg of lactose
   to make   3000 mg of dilution
3. Weigh $\frac{1}{20}$ of dilution, or 150 mg of dilution, which will contain 5 mg of atropine sulfate, *answer.*

In this example, the weight of the aliquot was arbitrarily set as *150 mg,* which exceeds the weight of the multiple quantity, as it preferably should. If *100 mg* had been set as the aliquot, the multiple quantity should have been diluted with *1900 mg* of lactose to get *2000 mg* of dilution, and its twentieth aliquot, or *100 mg,* would have contained *5 mg* of atropine sulfate. On the other hand, if *200 mg* had been set as the aliquot, the multiple quantity of atropine sulfate should have been diluted with *3900 mg* of lactose to get *4000 mg* of dilution.

Another Example:

A torsion prescription balance has a sensitivity requirement of $\frac{1}{10}$ grain. Explain how you would weigh $\frac{1}{4}$ grain of atropine sulfate with an accuracy of ± 5%, using lactose as the diluent.

Because $\frac{1}{10}$ grain is the potential balance error, 2 grains is the smallest amount that should be weighed to achieve the required precision.

If 12 is chosen as the multiple, and if 3 grains is set as the weight of the aliquot, then:

1. Weigh 12 × ¼ grains, or   3 grains of atropine sulfate.
2. Dilute with   33 grains of lactose
   to make   36 grains of dilution
3. Weigh ¹⁄₁₂ of dilution, or 3 grains of dilution, which will contain ¼ grain of atropine sulfate, *answer*.

Measuring Volume. *The aliquot method of measuring volume,* which is identical in principle to the aliquot method of weighing, may be used when relatively small volumes must be measured with great precision:

Step 1. Select a multiple of the desired quantity that can be measured with the required precision.

Step 2. Dilute the multiple quantity with a compatible diluent (usually a solvent for the liquid to be measured) to an amount evenly divisible by the multiple selected.

Step 3. Measure the aliquot of the dilution that contains the quantity originally desired.

In conformity with the legal requirements for pharmaceutical graduates, as stated in the *National Bureau of Standards Handbook 44*—Fourth Edition, a graduate shall have an initial interval that is not subdivided, equal to not less than one-fifth and not more than one-fourth of the capacity of the graduate.

Examples:

A prescription calls for 0.5 milliliter of hydrochloric acid. Using a 10-milliliter graduate calibrated from 2 to 10 milliliters in 1-milliliter divisions, explain how you would obtain the desired quantity of hydrochloric acid by the aliquot method.

If 4 is chosen as the multiple, and if 2 milliliters (mL) is set as the volume of the aliquot, then:

1. Measure 4 × 0.5 mL, or   2 mL of the acid
2. Dilute with   6 mL of water
   to make   8 mL of dilution
3. Measure ¼ of dilution, or 2 mL of dilution, which will contain 0.5 mL of hydrochloric acid, *answer*.

A prescription calls for 5 minims of clove oil. Using a 60-minim graduate calibrated from 15 to 60 minims in units of 5 minims, explain how you would obtain the clove oil by the aliquot method. Use alcohol as the diluent.

If 3 is chosen as the multiple, and if 20 minims is set as the volume of the aliquot, then:

1. Measure 3 × 5 minims, or   15 minims of clove oil
2. Dilute with   45 minims of alcohol
   to make   60 minims of dilution
3. Measure ⅓ of dilution, or 20 minims of dilution, which will contain 5 minims of clove oil, *answer*.

LEAST WEIGHABLE QUANTITY METHOD OF WEIGHING

This method may be used as an alternative to the aliquot method of weighing to obtain small quantities of a drug substance.

After determining the quantity of drug substance that is desired and the smallest quantity that can be weighed on the balance with the desired degree of accuracy, the procedure is as follows:

Step 1.   Weigh an amount of the drug substance that is *equal to or greater than* the least weighable quantity.

Step 2.   Dilute the drug substance with a calculated quantity of inert diluent such that a predetermined quantity of the drug-diluent mixture will contain the desired quantity of drug.

Example:

   If 20 *milligrams of a drug substance are needed to fill a prescription, explain how you would obtain this amount of drug with an accuracy of* ± 5% *using a balance with a sensitivity requirement of 6 milligrams. Use lactose as the diluent.*

   In the example, 20 milligrams is the amount of drug substance needed. The least weighable quantity would be 120 milligrams. The amount of drug substance to be weighed, therefore, must be equal to or greater than 120 milligrams. In solving the problem, 120 milligrams of drug substance is weighed. In calculating the amount of diluent to use, a predetermined quantity of drug-diluent mixture must be selected to contain the desired 20 milligrams of drug substance. The quantity selected must be greater than 120 milligrams because the drug-diluent mixture must be obtained accurately through weighing in the balance. An amount of 150 milligrams may be arbitrarily selected. The total amount of diluent to use may then be determined through the calculation of the following proportion:

$$\frac{20 \text{ mg (drug needed for } R\!\!\!/)}{150 \text{ mg (drug-diluent mixture to use in } R\!\!\!/)} = \frac{120 \text{ mg (total drug substance weighed)}}{x \text{ mg (total amount of drug-diluent mixture prepared)}}$$

   x = 900 milligrams (mg) of the drug-diluent mixture to prepare
   Hence, 900 mg − 120 mg = 780 mg of diluent (lactose) to use, *answer.*
   It should be noted that in this procedure, each weighing, including that of the drug substance, the diluent, and the drug-diluent mixture, must be determined to be equal to or greater than the least weighable quantity as determined for the balance used and accuracy desired.

Practice Problems

1.   If 1000 milliliters of a certain solution contain 30 milligrams of a dye, (a) what is the volume of the tenth aliquot, and (b) how many milligrams of the dye will the tenth aliquot contain?

2.   A prescription balance has a sensitivity requirement of 0.006 gram. Explain how you would weigh 0.012 gram of atropine sulfate with an error not greater than 5%, using lactose as the diluent.

3.   A torsion prescription balance has a sensitivity requirement of 4 milligrams. Explain how you would weigh 5 milligrams of hydromorphone hydrochloride with an error not greater than 5%. Use lactose as the diluent.

4.   The sensitivity requirement of a prescription balance is $\frac{1}{16}$ grain. Explain how you would weigh $\frac{1}{10}$ grain of atropine sulfate with an error not greater than 5%. Use milk sugar as the diluent.

5. A prescription balance has a sensitivity requirement of 6.5 milligrams. Explain how you would weigh 20 milligrams of a substance with an error not greater than 2%.

6. A prescription balance has a sensitivity requirement of $\frac{1}{6}$ grain. Explain how you would weigh 1 grain of a substance with an error not greater than 5%.

7. A torsion prescription balance has a sensitivity requirement of 0.004 g. Explain how you would weigh 0.008 g of a substance with an error not greater than 5%.

8. A prescription balance has a sensitivity requirement of $\frac{1}{8}$ grain. Explain how you would weigh $\frac{3}{4}$ grain of a substance with an error not greater than 5%.

9. A formula calls for 0.6 milliliter of a coloring solution. Using a 10-milliliter graduate calibrated from 2 to 10 milliliters in 1-milliliter units, how could you obtain the desired quantity of the coloring solution by the aliquot method? Use water as the diluent.

10. A pharmaceutical formula calls for 0.4 milliliter of the surfactant polysorbate 80. Using water as the diluent and a 10-milliliter graduate calibrated in 1-milliliter units, how could you obtain the desired quantity of polysorbate 80?

11. Using a 10-milliliter graduate calibrated in 1-milliliter units, explain how you would measure 1.25 milliliters of a dye solution by the aliquot method. Use water as the diluent.

12. The formula for 100 milliliters of pentobarbital sodium elixir calls for 0.75 milliliter of orange oil. Using alcohol as a diluent and a 10-milliliter graduate calibrated in 1-milliliter units, how could you obtain the desired quantity of orange oil?

13. A prescription calls for 50 milligrams of chlorpheniramine maleate. Using a prescription balance with a sensitivity requirement of 6 milligrams, explain how you would obtain the required amount of chlorpheniramine maleate with an error not greater than 5%.

2

Interpretation of the Prescription or Medication Order

By definition, a *prescription* is an order for medication issued by a physician, dentist, or other properly licensed medical practitioner. Prescriptions designate a specific medication and dosage to be prepared by a pharmacist and administered to a particular patient.

Prescriptions are usually written on preprinted forms containing the name, address, telephone number, and other pertinent information regarding the physician or other prescriber. In addition, blank spaces are used by the prescriber to provide information about the patient, the medication desired, and the directions for use. The information generally found on a completed prescription is shown in Figure 2.1.

In addition to the written form, prescription orders are frequently received by the pharmacist by telephone or by direct communication. In these instances, the pharmacist immediately reduces the order to a properly written form.

In hospitals and other institutions, the forms are somewhat different and are referred to as *medication orders.* A typical medication order sheet is shown in Figure 2.2. The orders shown in this example are typed; typically, these instructions are written by the physician in ink.

Prescriptions and medication orders written for infants, children, and sometimes the elderly may also include the age, weight, and/or body surface area (BSA) of the patient. This information is sometimes necessary in calculating the appropriate medication dosage.

It is not the purpose of this text to discuss all aspects of the prescription, but rather to address only those that are relevant to pharmaceutical calculations. It is important to recognize the following types of prescriptions: (1) those written for a single component or prefabricated product and *not requiring compounding* or admixture by the pharmacist, and (2) those written for more than a single component and *requiring compounding*.[1] Prescriptions may include the chemical or nonproprietary name of the substance or the manufacturer's brand or trademark name. Prescriptions requiring compounding contain the quantities of each ingredient required. Medications are prepared into various types of *dosage forms* (e.g., *tablets, syrups, injections*) and *drug delivery systems* (e.g., *transdermal patches*) to ensure that the medication is administered accurately and appropriately. Definitions and descriptions of dosage forms and drug delivery systems are presented in Appendix M.

Examples:

1. *Prescriptions not requiring compounding:*

    ℞   Phenobarbital Tablets, 30 mg
        Dispense 24 tablets.

---

[1] The extemporaneous compounding of prescriptions is an activity for which pharmacists are uniquely qualified by virtue of their education, training, and experience. By definition, *pharmacy compounding* involves the mixing, assembling, packaging, and labeling of a medication on receipt of a prescription order for a specific patient. In addition to the compounding of individual prescriptions as received, guidelines of the Food and Drug Administration permit the advance preparation of small quantities of compound products *in anticipation* of prescriptions for patients, based on regularly observed prescribing patterns. Unless licensed as a manufacturer, however, pharmacies may not engage in the large-scale production or *manufacturing* of drugs for other pharmacies or entities for resale.

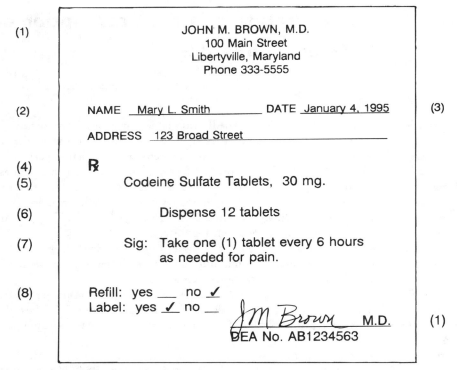

(1)

(2)

(3)

(4)
(5)

(6)

(7)

(8)

(1)

Fig. 2.1. Components of a typical prescription. Parts labeled are as follows:
(1) Prescriber information and signature
(2) Patient information
(3) Date prescription was written
(4) ℞ symbol (the Superscription) meaning "take thou,"
   "you take," or "recipe"
(5) Medication prescribed (the Inscription)
(6) Dispensing instructions to the pharmacist (the Subscription)
(7) Directions to the patient (the Signa)
(8) Special instructions

    ℞   Feosol Elixir
         Dispense 12 fluidounces.

2. *Prescriptions requiring compounding:*

    ℞   Aspirin   3.6 g
         Codeine Sulfate   0.4 g
         Mix and make 12 capsules.

    ℞   Paregoric   30 mL
         Kaopectate q.s. ad   120 mL
         Mix well.

The quantities of ingredients to be used may be expressed on the prescription in the metric or apothecaries' systems of weights and measures. These systems are covered in detail in Chapter 3 and Appendix A. In the use of the metric system, the decimal is often

CITY HOSPITAL
Athens, GA 30600

PATIENT NAME:	Thompson, Linda
ADDRESS:	2345 Oak Circle
CITY, STATE:	Athens, GA
AGE/SEX:	35 Female
PHYSICIAN:	J. Hardmer
HOSP. NO.:	900612345
SERVICE:	Medicine
ROOM:	220 East

PHYSICIAN'S ORDER

DATE	TIME	ORDERS
01/01/95	1200	1. Propranolol 40 mg po QID
		2. Furosemide 20 mg po q AM
		3. Flurazepam 30 mg at HS prn sleep
		4. D-5-W + 20 mEq KCL/L at 84 mL/hr
		Hardmer, MD

Unless "No substitution permitted" is clearly written after the order, a generic or therapeutic equivalent drug may be dispensed according to the Formulary policies of this hospital.

Fig. 2.2. Typical hospital medication order sheet.

replaced by a vertical line that may be imprinted on the prescription blank or drawn by the prescriber. In these instances, whole or subunits of grams of weight and milliliters of volume are separated by the vertical line. Sometimes the abbreviations g (for gram) and mL (for milliliter) are absent and must be presumed. Examples of prescriptions written in the apothecaries' and metric systems follow:

Apothecaries'

R̸   Codeine Sulfate   gr iv
      Ammonium Chloride   ℥i
      Ephedrine Sulfate Syrup   ad   f℥iii
      Sig. ℥i t.i.d. for cough.

R̸   Aminophylline   ℈i
      Ephedrine Hydrochloride   gr iv
      Amobarbital   gr iv
      Lactose as needed
      Mix and make capsules no. xii
      Sig. One capsule every 3 hours.

Table 2.1. Abbreviations Commonly Used in Prescriptions and Medication Orders

Abbreviation	Meaning	Abbreviation	Meaning
aa. or $\overline{aa}$	of each	IV	intravenous
a.c.	before meals	IVP	intravenous push
ad	up to	IVPB	intravenous piggy back
a.d.	right ear	M.	mix
ad lib.	at pleasure, freely	m^2 or M^2	square meter
a.m.	morning	mcg	microgram
amp.	ampul	mEq	milliequivalent
aq.	water	mg	milligram
a.s.	left ear	mg/kg	milligrams (of drug) per
ASA	aspirin		kilogram (of body
ATC	around the clock		weight)
a.u.	each ear	mg/m^2	milligrams (of drug) per
b.i.d.	twice a day		square meter (of body
BM	bowel movement		surface area)
BP	blood pressure	ml	milliliter
BS	blood sugar	ml/h	milliliters (of drug
BSA	body surface area		administered) per hour
c. or $\overline{c}$	with		(as through intravenous
cap.	capsule		administration)
cc. or cc	cubic centimeter	mOsm or	
CHF	congestive heart failure	mOsmol	milliosmoles
comp.	compound	MS	morphine sulfate
dil.	dilute	N&V	nausea and vomiting
disc. or D.C.	discontinue	NF	National Formulary
disp.	dispense	NMT	not more than
div.	divide	noct.	night
d.t.d.	give of such doses	non rep. or	
DW	distilled water	N.R.	do not repeat
D5LR	dextrose 5% in lactated	NPO	nothing by mouth
	Ringer's	N.S. or NS	normal saline
D5NS	dextrose 5% in normal	½NS	half-strength normal saline
	saline (0.9% sodium	NTG	nitroglycerin
	chloride)	O.	pint
D5W	dextrose 5% in water	o.d.	right eye
D10W	dextrose 10% in water	oint.	ointment
elix.	elixir	OJ	orange juice
et	and	o.l.	left eye
ex aq.	in water	o.s.	left eye
fl	fluid	o.u.	each eye
ft.	make	o_2	both eyes
g. or Gm. or	gram	p.c.	after meals
g		p.m.	afternoon; evening
GI	gastrointestinal	p.o.	by mouth
gr	grain	postop	postoperatively
gtt.	drop	p.r.n.	when required
GU	genitourinary	pulv.	powder
H	hypodermic	q.d.	every day
h. or hr.	hour	q.h.	every hour
HA	headache	q.i.d.	four times a day
HBP	high blood pressure	q.o.d.	every other day
HC	hydrocortisone	q.s.	a sufficient quantity
h.s.	at bedtime	q.s. ad	a sufficient quantity to
HT or HTN	hypertension		make
ID	intradermal	R	rectal
IM	intramuscular	R.L. or R/L	Ringer's Lactate
inj.	injection	s. or $\overline{s}$	without
IU	international units	Sig.	write on label

(continued)

Table 2.1. *Continued*

Abbreviation	Meaning	Abbreviation	Meaning
SL	sublingual	t.i.d.	three times a day
SOB	shortness of breath	t.i.w.	three times a week
sol.	solution	top	topically
s.o.s.	if there is need	TPN	total parenteral nutrition
ss. or s̄s̄	one-half	tr.	tincture
stat.	immediately	tsp.	teaspoonful
subc or subq	subcutaneously	U or u	unit
or s.c. or		u.d.	as directed
SQ		ung.	ointment
sup.	suppository	URI	upper respiratory infection
susp.	suspension	USP	United States
syr.	syrup		Pharmacopeia
tab.	tablet	UTI	urinary tract infection
tbsp.	tablespoonful	wk	week

Metric

R̸   Acetylsalicylic Acid   4.0 g

Phenacetin   0.8 g

Codeine Sulfate   0.5 g

Mix and make capsules no. 20

Sig. One capsule every 4 hours.

R̸   Phenobarbital   0 | 6

Belladonna Tincture   12 | 0

Aromatic Elixir ad   120 | 0

Sig. 5 mL in water a.c.

The portions of the prescription presenting directions to the pharmacist (the Subscription) and the directions to the patient (the Signa) commonly contain abbreviated forms of English or Latin terms as well as Roman numerals. The correct interpretation of these abbreviations and prescription notations plays an important part in pharmaceutical calculations and thus in the accurate filling and dispensing of medication.

Examples of Prescription Directions to the Pharmacist:
   (a) *M. ft. ung.*
       Mix and make an ointment.
   (b) *Ft. sup. no xii*
       Make 12 suppositories.
   (c) *M. ft. cap. d.t.d. no. xxiv*
       Mix and make capsules. Give 24 such doses.

Examples of Prescription Directions to the Patient:
   (a) *Caps. i. q.i.d. p.c. et h.s.*
       Take one (1) capsule four (4) times a day after each meal and at bedtime.
   (b) *gtt. ii o.d. q.d. a.m.*
       Instill two (2) drops in the right eye every day in the morning.
   (c) *tab. ii stat; tab. 1 q. 6 h. × 7 d.*
       Take two (2) tablets immediately, then take one (1) tablet every 6 hours for 7 days.

A list of abbreviations commonly used in prescriptions and medication orders is presented in Table 2.1.

MEDICATION SCHEDULING AND PATIENT COMPLIANCE

Medication scheduling may be defined as the frequency (i.e., times per day) and duration (i.e., length of treatment) of a drug's prescribed or recommended use. Some medications, because of their physical or chemical characteristics or their dosage formulation, may be taken just once daily for optimum benefit, whereas other drug products must be taken two, three, four, or more times daily for the desired effect. Frequency of medication scheduling is also influenced by the patient's physical condition and the nature and severity of the illness or condition being treated. Some conditions, such as indigestion, may require a single dose of medication for correction. Other conditions, such as a systemic infection, may require multiple daily, around-the-clock dosing for 10 days or more. Long-term maintenance therapy for such conditions as diabetes and high blood pressure may require daily dosing for life.

For optimum benefit from prescribed therapy or from the use of over-the-counter (nonprescription) medications, it is incumbent on the patient to adhere to the recommended medication schedule.

Patient compliance with prescribed and nonprescribed medications is defined as patient understanding and adherence to the directions for use. The compliant patient follows the label directions for taking the medication properly and adheres to any special instructions provided by the prescriber and/or pharmacist. Compliance includes taking medication at the desired strength, in the proper dosage form, at the appropriate time of day and night, at the proper interval for the duration of the treatment, and with proper regard to food and drink and consideration of other concomitant medications.

Patient noncompliance is the failure to comply with a practitioner's or labeled direction in the self-administration of any medication. Noncompliance may involve underdosage or overdosage, inconsistent or sporadic dosing, incorrect duration of treatment, and drug abuse or misadventuring with medications.

Patient noncompliance may result from a number of factors, including unclear or misunderstood directions, undesired side effects of the drug that discourage use, lack of patient confidence in the drug and/or prescriber, discontinued use because the patient feels better or worse, economic reasons based on the cost of the medication, absence of patient counseling and understanding of the need for and means of compliance, confusion over taking multiple medications, and other factors. Frequently, patients forget whether or not they have taken their medications. This situation is particularly common for patients who are easily confused, who have memory failure, or who are taking multiple medications scheduled to be taken at different times during the day or night. Special compliance aids are available to assist patients in their proper scheduling of medications. These devices include medication calendars, reminder charts, and special containers.

Patient noncompliance is not entirely the problem of ambulatory or noninstitutionalized patients. Patients in hospitals, nursing homes, and other inpatient settings are generally more compliant because of the efforts of health care personnel who are assigned the responsibility of issuing and administering medication on a prescribed schedule. Even in these settings, however, a scheduled dose of medication may be omitted or administered incorrectly or in an untimely fashion because of human error.

The consequences of patient noncompliance may include worsening of the condition, the requirement of additional and perhaps more expensive and extensive treatment methods or surgical procedures, otherwise unnecessary hospitalization, and increased total health care cost. Students interested in additional information on patient compliance are referred to other sources of information.[2]

Some of the different types of problems relating to patient compliance with medication are exemplified by the following examples.

Examples:

> ℞   Hydrochlorothiazide   50 mg
> No. XC
> Sig. i q AM for HBP

If the prescription was filled initially on April 15, on about what date should the patient return to have the prescription refilled?

Answer: 90 tablets, taken 1 per day, should last 90 days, approximately 3 months, and the patient should return to the pharmacy on or shortly before July 15 of the same year.

> ℞   Penicillin V Potassium Oral Solution   125 mg/5 mL
> Disp.————mL
> Sig. 5 mL q 6h ATC × 10 d

How many milliliters of medicine should be dispensed?

Answer: 5 mL times 4 (doses per day) equals 20 mL times 10 (days) equals 200 mL.

A pharmacist may calculate a patient's percent compliance rate as follows:

$$\% \text{ Compliance rate} = \frac{\text{Number of days supply of medication}}{\text{Number of days since last Rx refill}} \times 100$$

Example:

What is the percent compliance rate if a patient received a 30-day supply of medicine and returned in 45 days for a refill?

$$\% \text{ Compliance rate} = \frac{30 \text{ days}}{45 \text{ days}} \times 100 = 66.6\%, \textit{ answer.}$$

In determining the patient's actual (rather than apparent) compliance rate, it is important to determine if the patient had available and used extra days' dosage from some previous filling of the prescription.

Practice Exercises

1.   Interpret each of the following *Subscriptions* (directions to the pharmacist) taken from prescriptions:
     (*a*) Disp. sup. rect. no. xii
     (*b*) M. ft. isoton. sol. Disp. ℥i
     (*c*) M. et div. in pulv. no. xl
     (*d*) Disp. tal. dos. vi. Non rep.
     (*e*) M. et ft. ung. Disp. 10 g
     (*f*) M. et ft. Sol. DTD xlviii

---

[2] Bond, W.S. and Hussar, D.A.: Detection methods and strategies for improving medication compliance. Am. J. Hosp. Pharm., *48:*1978, 1991; Mackowiak, J. I.: *Enhancing Patient Compliance.* Ridgefield, CT, Boehringer Ingelheim Pharmaceuticals, Inc., 1990.

(g) M. et ft. sol. 1 g/tbsp.

(h) Ft. cap. #1. Disp. tal. no.xxxvi N.R.

(i) M. et ft. pulv. Div. in dos. #C

(j) M. et ft. inj. for I.V. use.

(k) Label: HC, 20 mg

2. Interpret each of the following *Signas* (directions to the patient) taken from prescriptions:

(a) Gtt. ii o.u. q. 4 h. p.r.n. pain.

(b) Tbsp. i in ⅓ gl. aq. q. 6 h.

(c) Appl. a.m. & p.m. for pain e.m.p.

(d) Gtt. iv a.d. m. & n.

(e) Tsp. i ex aq. q. 4 or 5 h. p.r.n. pain.

(f) Appl. ung. o.s. ad lib.

(g) Caps i c̄ aq. h.s. N.R.

(h) Gtt. v a.u. 3 × d. s.o.s.

(i) Tab. i sublingually, rep. p.r.n.

(j) Instill gtt. ii o.u. of neonate.

(k) Dil. c̄ = vol. aq. and use as gargle q. 5 h.

(l) Cap. ii 1 h. prior to departure, then cap. i after 12 h.

(m) Tab i p.r.n. SOB

(n) Tab i qAM HBP

(o) Tab ii q 6h ATC URI

3. Interpret each of the following taken from medication orders:

(a) Secobarbital sodium gr iss p.o. q.d. h.s. repeat s.o.s.

(b) 1000 mL D5W q. 8 h. IV c̄ 20 mEq KCI to every third bottle.

(c) Prochlorperazine 10 mg IM q. 3h. prn N&V

(d) Minocycline HCl susp. 1 tsp p.o. q.i.d. disc. after 5 d.

(e) Propranolol HCl 10 mg p.o. t.i.d. a.c. & h.s.

(f) NPH U-100 insulin 40 U subc q.d. A.M.

(g) Cefamandole nafate 250 mg IM q. 12 h.

(h) Potassium chloride 15 mEq p.o. b.i.d. p.c.

(i) Vincristine sulfate 1 mg/m^2 BSA.

(j) Flurazepam 30 mg at HS prn sleep.

(k) D5W + 20 mEq KCl/L at 84 mL/hour.

(l) 2.5 g/kg/d amino acids TPN.

4. (a) If a 10-mL vial of insulin contains 200 units of insulin per milliliter, and a patient is to administer 20 units twice daily, how many days will the product last the patient? (b) If the patient returned to the pharmacy in exactly 7 weeks for another vial of insulin, was the patient compliant as indicated by the percent compliance rate?

5. A prescription is to be taken as follows: 1 tablet q.i.d. the first day; 1 tablet t.i.d. the second day; 1 tablet b.i.d. × 5 d; and 1 tablet q.d. thereafter. How many tablets should be dispensed to equal a 30-day supply?

3 The Metric System

The *measure* of a quantity is the number of times that it contains a standard quantity taken as a *unit*. A 5-lb weight, for instance, contains five times the weight of a standard 1-lb unit. Some kinds of quantities measured are temperature, length, area, volume, and time, respectively measured in such familiar units as degrees, feet, square miles, gallons, and hours.

The standard subdivisions and multiples of the unit in any system of measurement are called *denominations*. As noted previously, figures specifying their number are called *denominate numbers*. So, in the expression "10 cents," the term "cents" designates a denomination in our monetary system, and 10 is a denominate number. We find it convenient, as a rule, to express large quantities in terms of large denominations and small quantities in small denominations—as great distances are measured by the common system in miles, short intervals in inches. Denominations are understood to stand in a fixed ratio with the unit on which the system is based; a cent has a fixed value of $\frac{1}{100}$ of a dollar, and therefore the cents and the dollar have a fixed ratio with each other. A statement of the mutual relationships of denominations of the same kind is called a *table of measure*.

The *metric system* of measure was formulated in France in the late eighteenth century. Its use in the United States was legalized in 1866. By act of Congress in 1893, it became our legal *standard* of measure, and all other systems are referred to it for official comparison.

Its acceptance by scientists the world over has resulted from these two merits: (1) its tables are simple, for they are based on the decimal system of notation, and the greater of two consecutive denominations of the same kind is always 10 times the less; (2) its tables of length, volume, and weight are conveniently correlated, for the meter is the fundamental unit of the system.

Each table of the metric system contains a definitive unit. The *meter* is the unit of length, the *liter* of volume, and the *gram* of weight. Subdivisions and multiples of these principal units are indicated respectively by the following prefixes:

atto-   denotes one quintillionth (10^{-18}) of the basic unit
femto-   denotes one quadrillionth (10^{-15}) of the basic unit
pico-   denotes one trillionth (10^{-12}) of the basic unit
nano-   denotes one billionth (10^{-9}) of the basic unit
micro-   denotes one millionth (10^{-6}) of the basic unit
milli-   denotes one-thousandth (10^{-3}) of the basic unit
centi-   denotes one-hundredth (10^{-2}) of the basic unit
deci-   denotes one-tenth (10^{-1}) of the basic unit
deka-   denotes 10 times the basic unit
hecto-   denotes 100 times (10^2) the basic unit
kilo-   denotes 1000 times (10^3) the basic unit
myria-   denotes 10,000 times (10^4) the basic unit
mega-   denotes 1 million times (10^6) the basic unit
giga-   denotes 1 billion times (10^9) the basic unit
tera-   denotes 1 trillion times (10^{12}) the basic unit
peta-   denotes 1 quadrillion times (10^{15}) the basic unit
exa-   denotes 1 quintillion times (10^{18}) the basic unit

Table 3.1. Prefixes for SI Units

Power of Ten	Prefix	Symbol
10^{18}	exa	E
10^{15}	peta	P
10^{12}	tera	T
10^{9}	giga	G
10^{6}	mega	M
10^{3}	kilo	k
10^{2}	hecto	h
10	deka	da
10^{-1}	deci	d
10^{-2}	centi	c
10^{-3}	milli	m
10^{-6}	micro	μ
10^{-9}	nano	n
10^{-12}	pico	p
10^{-15}	femto	f
10^{-18}	atto	a

It should be noted that the metric unit prefixes are taken from the International System of Units *(SI units)* as adopted by the 44 governments of the *Conference Generale des Poids et Mesures,* which was held in Paris in 1960. The objective of this adoption was to provide a single worldwide system of weights and measures. Table 3.1 lists the prefixes and symbols for decimal multiples and submultiples for SI units.

Anyone who wishes to become familiar with the system quickly should note that U.S. currency is "metrically" or decimally computed. The names of the chief fractions of the dollar unit are a clue to their value: a *mill* (for which we have no coin) is one-thousandth, a *cent is* one-hundredth, and a *dime* is one-tenth of the unit.

In the United States and Canada, the decimal marker (or decimal point) is placed as a dot (.) directly on the line adjacent to the figures. In many other countries, however, a comma or a raised dot is used.

Decimal fractions (e.g., 0.25 mg) are preferred with metric units rather than common fractions (e.g., ¼ mg). To avoid errors arising from the use of a faint or uncertain decimal point, a zero is placed before the decimal point of numbers less than 1 (e.g., 0.1 mg *and NOT .1 mg*), although neither a decimal point nor a zero should be placed following a whole number (e.g., 1 mg *and NOT 1.0 mg*). Pharmacists must be alert and check all prescriptions, medication orders, and calculations for the possibility of decimal placement errors. A misplaced decimal point leads *minimally to an error of one-tenth or ten times the desired quantity!*

The abbreviations in the tables of metric length, volume, and weight are those used commonly and include those adopted by the *United States Pharmacopeia.* In accordance with the SI system, metric symbols are the same in singular and plural; e.g., 1 mg, 2 mg, or 100 mg. In selecting among unit dimensions (e.g., mg, g, kg), the choice generally is based on selecting the unit that will result in a numeric value between 1 and 1000. For example: 500 *g,* rather than 0.5 *kg;* 1.96 *kg* rather than 1,960 *g;* 750 *mL* rather than 0.75 *L;* or 750 *mm* or 75 *cm* rather than 0.75 *meter.*

MEASURE OF LENGTH

The meter is the fundamental unit of this system. It has been determined as approximately one ten-millionth part of the distance from the earth's equator to the North Pole, and is, in fact, a little over 1 yard long.

The **table of metric length** follows:

1 kilometer (km)	= 1000.000 meters
1 hectometer (hm)	= 100.000 meters
1 dekameter (dam)	= 10.000 meters
1 meter (m)	= 1.000 meter
1 decimeter (dm)	= 0.100 meter
1 centimeter (cm)	= 0.010 meter
1 millimeter (mm)	= 0.001 meter
1 micrometer (μm)	= 0.000,001 meter
1 nanometer (nm)	= 0.000,000,001 meter

Formerly, the abbreviation μ (for *micron*) was used in expressing one millionth of a meter (micrometer); and the abbreviation mμ (for *millimicron*) was used to designate one thousandth of a micron (nanometer).

A small unit equal to one ten-thousandth of a micron is the *angstrom* (Å), which is used to express the length of light waves.

Square meter is abbreviated m^2, *square centimeter*, cm^2, *cubic meter*, m^3, and *cubic centimeter*, cm^3 or cc.

The table may also be written:

1 meter	= 0.001 kilometer
	= 0.01 hectometer
	= 0.1 dekameter
	= 10 decimeters
	= 100 centimeters
	= 1000 millimeters
	= 1,000,000 micrometers
	= 1,000,000,000 nanometers

The denominations used most commonly are the millimeter, centimeter, and meter, as if the table were:

1000 millimeters (mm)	= 100 centimeters (cm)
100 centimeters (cm)	= 1 meter (m)

MEASURE OF VOLUME

The *liter* is the metric unit of volume. It represents the volume of the cube of one-tenth of a meter, that is, of 1 dm^3.

The **table of metric volume** follows:

1 kiloliter (kL)	= 1000.000 liters
1 hectoliter (hL)	= 100.000 liters
1 dekaliter (daL)	= 10.000 liters
1 liter (L)	= 1.000 liter
1 deciliter (dL)	= 0.010
1 centiliter (cL)	= 0.010 liter
1 milliliter (mL)	= 0.001 liter
1 microliter (μL)	= 0.000,001 liter

This table may also be written:

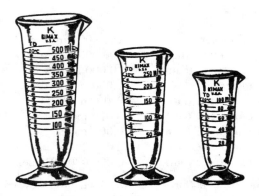

Fig. 3.1. Metric graduates. (Courtesy of Kimble Glassware Co.)

$$
\begin{aligned}
1 \text{ liter} \quad &= 0.001 \text{ kiloliter} \\
&= 0.010 \text{ hectoliter} \\
&= 0.100 \text{ dekaliter} \\
&= 10 \text{ deciliters} \\
&= 100 \text{ centiliters} \\
&= 1000 \text{ milliliters} \\
&= 1{,}000{,}000 \text{ microliters}
\end{aligned}
$$

Although in theory the liter was meant to have the volume of 1 dm^3 or 1000 cm^3, precise modern measurement has discovered that the standard liter contains slightly less than this volume. The discrepancy is insignificant for most practical purposes, however, and because the milliliter has so nearly the volume of 1 cm^3, the *United States Pharmacopeia* states: "One milliliter (mL) is used herein as the equivalent of 1 cubic centimeter (cc)."

The denominations used most commonly are the milliliter and liter, as if the table were simply:

$$1000 \text{ milliliters (mL)} = 1 \text{ liter (L)}$$

Examples of metric graduates for measuring volume are shown in Figure 3.1.

MEASURE OF WEIGHT

The unit of weight in the metric system is the *gram*, which is the weight of 1 cm^3 of water at 4° C, its temperature of greatest density.

The **table of metric weight** follows:

1 kilogram (kg)	= 1000.000 grams
1 hectogram (hg)	= 100.000 grams
1 dekagram (dag)	= 10.000 grams
1 gram (g)	= 1.000 gram
1 decigram (dg)	= 0.1000 gram
1 centigram (cg)	= 0.010 gram
1 milligram (mg)	= 0.001 gram
1 microgram (μg or mcg)	= 0.000,001 gram
1 nanogram (ng)	= 0.000,000,001 gram
1 picogram (pg)	= 0.000,000,000,001 gram

This table may also be written:

$$1 \text{ gram} \quad = 0.001 \text{ kilogram}$$
$$= 0.010 \text{ hectogram}$$
$$= 0.100 \text{ dekagram}$$
$$= 10 \text{ decigrams}$$
$$= 100 \text{ centigrams}$$
$$= 1000 \text{ milligrams}$$
$$= 1{,}000{,}000 \text{ micrograms}$$
$$= 1{,}000{,}000{,}000 \text{ nanograms}$$
$$= 1{,}000{,}000{,}000{,}000 \text{ picograms}$$

The denominations used most commonly are the microgram, milligram, gram, and kilogram, as if the table were:

1000 micrograms (μg or mcg)   = 1 milligram (mg)
1000 milligrams (mg)   = 1 gram (g)
1000 grams (g)   = 1 kilogram (kg)

An example of a metric set of weights is shown in Fig. 3.2.

The abbreviation *mcg* came into general use in pharmaceutical literature and labeling some years ago and was formerly used in pharmaceutical monographs. The symbol μg is now more widely accepted, however, and is presently used in the *United States Pharmacopeia*. The abbreviation *mcg* is still used to denote microgram(s) in labeling and prescription writing. The term *gamma*, symbolized by γ, is customarily used for microgram in biochemical literature.

When prescriptions are written in the metric system, Arabic numerals are always used and are written *before* the abbreviations for the denominations, if such abbreviations are used. Quantities of weight are usually written as grams and *decimals* of a gram, and volumes as milliliters and *decimals* of a milliliter.

Example:

℞   Codeine Sulfate   0.26 g
    Ammonium Chloride   6.0 g
    Cherry Syrup   ad   120.0 mL
    Sig. 5 mL as directed.

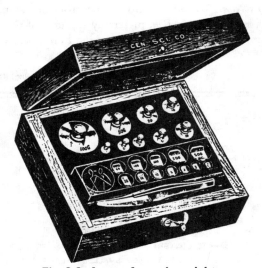

Fig. 3.2. A set of metric weights.

FUNDAMENTAL COMPUTATIONS

Reducing to Lower or Higher Denominations. The restatement of a given quantity in terms of a higher or lower denomination is called *reduction.* "Thirty minutes" may equally be expressed as a "half hour" or, if occasion requires, as "1800 seconds." The process of changing from higher to lower denominations is known as *reduction descending*; from lower to higher, *reduction ascending.*

A length, a volume, or a weight expressed in one denomination of the metric system may be expressed in another denomination by simply moving the decimal point. It is often best to reduce the given quantity first to the *unit* and then to the required denomination.

To change a metric denomination to the next smaller denomination, move the decimal point one place to the right. To change to the next larger denomination, move the decimal point one place to the left, as shown in Figure 3.3.

Examples:

> *Reduce 1.23 kilograms to grams.*
> 1.23 kg = 1230 g, *answer.*
>
> *Reduce 9876 milligrams to grams.*
> 9876 mg = 9.876 g, *answer.*

In the first example, 1.23 kg are to be converted to grams (g). On the scale, the gram position is three decimal positions from the kilogram position. Thus, the decimal point is moved three places toward the right. In the second example, the conversion from milligrams (mg) also requires the movement of the decimal point three places, but this time to the left.

Examples:

> *Reduce 85 micrometers to centimeters.*
> 85 μm = 0.085 mm = 0.0085 cm, *answer.*
>
> *Reduce 2.525 liters to microliters.*
> 2.525 L = 2525 mL = 2,525,000 μL, *answer.*

Addition and Subtraction. To add or subtract quantities in the metric system requires reducing them to a *common denomination*, preferably the unit of the table, and arranging their denominate numbers for addition or subtraction as ordinary decimals.

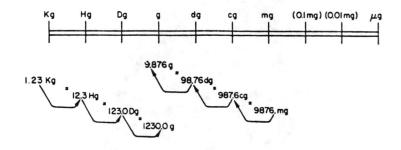

DECIMAL MOVEMENT

◉← TO CONVERT FROM LARGER TO SMALLER UNITS
→◉ TO CONVERT FROM SMALLER TO LARGER UNITS

Fig. 3.3. Metric weight scale.

Examples:

Add 1 kg, 250 mg, and 7.5 g. Express the total in grams.

$$
\begin{array}{llr}
1 \text{ kg} & = 1000. & \text{g} \\
250 \text{ mg} & = 0.250 & \text{g} \\
7.5 \text{ g} & = 7.5 & \text{g} \\
\hline
& 1007.750 \text{ g or } 1008 \text{ g, } \textit{answer.}
\end{array}
$$

Add 4 L, 375 mL, and 0.75 L. Express the total in milliliters.

$$
\begin{array}{lll}
4 \text{ L} & = 4000 \text{ mL} \\
375 \text{ mL} & = 375 \text{ mL} \\
0.75 \text{ L} & = \underline{750 \text{ mL}} \\
& 5125 \text{ mL, } \textit{answer.}
\end{array}
$$

A capsule contains the following amounts of medicinal substances: 0.075 g, 20 mg, 0.0005 g, 4 mg, and 500 μg. What is the total weight of the substances in the capsule?

$$
\begin{array}{lll}
0.075 \text{ g} & = 0.075 \text{ g} \\
20 \text{ mg} & = 0.020 \text{ g} \\
0.0005 \text{ g} & = 0.0005 \text{ g} \\
4 \text{ mg} & = 0.004 \text{ g} \\
500 \text{ μg} & = \underline{0.0005 \text{ g}} \\
& 0.1000 \text{ g or } 100 \text{ mg, } \textit{answer.}
\end{array}
$$

Subtract 2.5 mg from 4.850 g.

$$
\begin{array}{lll}
4.850 \text{ g} & = 4.850 \text{ g} \\
2.5 \text{ mg} & = \underline{0.0025 \text{ g}} \\
& 4.8475 \text{ g or } 4.848 \text{ g, } \textit{answer.}
\end{array}
$$

A prescription calls for 0.060 g of one ingredient, 2.5 mg of another, and enough of a third to make 0.5 g. How many milligrams of the third ingredient should be used?

Interpreting all quantities as accurate to the nearest tenth of a milligram:

$$
\begin{array}{lll}
\text{1st ingredient:} & 0.0600 \text{ g} & = 0.0600 \text{ g} \\
\text{2nd ingredient:} & 2.5 \text{ mg} & = \underline{0.0025 \text{ g}} \\
& & 0.0625 \text{ g}
\end{array}
$$

$$
\begin{array}{ll}
\text{Total weight:} & 0.5000 \text{ g} \\
\text{Weight of 1st and 2nd:} & \underline{0.0625 \text{ g}} \\
\text{Weight of 3rd:} & 0.4375 \text{ g or } 437.5 \text{ mg, } \textit{answer.}
\end{array}
$$

Multiplication and Division. Because every measurement in the metric system is expressed in a single given denomination, problems involving multiplication and division are solved by the methods used for any decimal numbers.

Examples:

Multiply 820 mL by 12.5 and express the result in liters.

$$820 \text{ mL} \times 12.5 = 10250 \text{ mL} = 10.25 \text{ L, } \textit{answer.}$$

Divide 0.465 g by 15 and express the result in milligrams.

$$0.465 \text{ g} \div 15 = 0.031 \text{ g} = 31 \text{ mg, } \textit{answer.}$$

RELATION OF METRIC TO OTHER SYSTEMS OF MEASUREMENT

In addition to the metric system, the pharmacy student should be aware of two other systems of measurement, the avoirdupois and apothecaries' systems. The avoirdupois system, widely used in United States in measuring body weight and in selling goods by the ounce or pound, is slowly giving way to the metric system. The apothecaries' system, once the predominant pharmacist's system of volumetric and weight measure, has largely been replaced in pharmacy by the metric system. The pharmacist must still appreciate the relationship between the various systems of measurement, however, and to deal effectively with them as the need arises.

The avoirdupois and apothecaries' systems of measurement, including all necessary equivalents and methods for intersystem conversion, are presented in Appendix A. The example equivalents presented in Table 3.2 are useful in gaining perspective and in solving certain problems in the text (e.g., dosing calculations based on body weight) by ratio and proportion or by dimensional analysis. These equivalents should be committed to memory.

> For prescriptions and all other problems stated in the apothecaries'
> or avoirdupois systems of measurement, it is suggested that stu-
> dents study Appendix A covering these systems and that all such
> quantities be converted to equivalent metric quantities before
> solving problems in the usual manner described in this text.

Table 3.2. Some Useful Equivalents

Equivalents of Length		
1 inch	=	2.54 cm

Equivalents of Volume		
1 fluidounce	=	29.57 mL
1 pint (16 fl. oz.)	=	473 mL
1 quart (32 fl. oz.)	=	946 mL
1 gallon, U.S. (128 fl. oz.)	=	3785 mL

Equivalents of Weight		
1 grain (gr)	=	0.065 g or 65 mg
1 pound (lb)	=	454 g
2.2 pounds	=	1 kg

Practice Problems

1. Add 0.5 kg, 50 mg, and 2.5 g. Reduce the result to grams.

2. Add 7.25 L and 875 mL. Reduce the result to milliliters.

3. Add 0.00250 kg, 1750 mg, 2.25 g, and 825,000 μg and express the answer in grams.

4. Reduce 1.256 g to micrograms, to milligrams, and to kilograms.

5. Multiply 255 mg by 380, divide the result by 0.85, and reduce the result to grams.

6. A low-strength children's/adult chewable aspirin tablet contains 81 mg of aspirin per tablet. How many tablets may be prepared from 1 kg of aspirin?

7. Adhesive tape made from fabric has a tensile strength of not less than 20.41 kg per 2.54 cm of width. Reduce these quantities to grams and millimeters.

8. A liquid contains 0.25 mg of a substance per milliliter. How many milligrams of the substance will 3.5 L contain?

9. An inhalation aerosol contains 225 mg of metaproterenol sulfate, which is sufficient for 300 inhalations. How many micrograms of metaproterenol sulfate would be contained in each inhalation?

10. A certain suppository contains the following:
    Ergotamine Tartrate   2.0 mg
    Caffeine   100.0 mg
    Cocoa Butter q.s. ad
                             2.0 g
    (a) How many milligrams of cocoa butter are required in the formula?
    (b) How many grams of caffeine would be required to make 24 such suppositories?

11. How many colchicine tablets, each containing 600 μg, may be prepared from 30 g of colchicine?

12. ℞   Codeine Sulfate
     Papaverine Hydrochloride   aa   0 | 015
     Calcium Carbonate   ad   0 | 3
     M. ft. cap. no. i D.T.D. no. xv
     Sig. Cap. i q.i.d. p.c. and h.s.

    (a) How many milligrams of codeine sulfate would be contained in each capsule?
    (b) How many grams of calcium carbonate should be used in filling the prescription?
    (c) How many milligrams of papaverine hydrochloride would be taken daily?

13. Aspirin tablets generally contain 325 mg of aspirin. How many such tablets may be prepared from 5 kg of aspirin?

14. A cold tablet contains the following amounts of active ingredients:
    Acetaminophen   325 mg
    Chlorpheniramine Maleate   2 mg
    Pseudoephedrine Hydrochloride   30 mg
    Dextromethorphan hydrochloride   15 mg
    How many tablets may be prepared if a manufacturing pharmacist has 1 kg of acetaminophen, 125 g of chlorpheniramine maleate, and unlimited quantities of the other two ingredients?

15. Norgestrel and ethinyl estradiol tablets usually available contain 0.5 mg of norgestrel and 50 μg of ethinyl estradiol. How many grams of each ingredient would be used in making 10,000 tablets?

16. ℞   Phenobarbital   0.540 g
     Hyoscine Hydrobromide   0.34   mg
     Atropine Sulfate   0.84   mg
     Lactose   ad   10.0   g
     M. Div. in caps. no. 36
     Sig. One capsule q.i.d.

    How many micrograms of hyoscine hydrobromide, milligrams of atropine sulfate, and grams of phenobarbital would be contained in each capsule of the prescription?

17. How many grams of reserpine would be required to make 25,000 tablets each containing 250 μg of reserpine?

18. ℞   Paregoric   15.0 mL
         Pectin   0.6 g
         Kaolin   22.0 g
         Alcohol   0.8 mL
         Purified Water   ad   120.0 mL
         Mix and make a suspension.
         Sig. 15 mL p.r.n. for diarrhea.

      (a) How many milliliters of paregoric would be contained in each 15-mL dose?
      (b) How many milligrams of pectin would be contained in each prescribed dose?
      (c) How many microliters of alcohol would be contained in each dose?

19. If an injectable solution contains 25 μg of a drug substance in each 0.5 mL, how many milliliters will be required to provide a patient with 0.25 mg of the drug substance?

20. ℞   Ergonovine Maleate
         200-μg tablets
         Disp. tabs. no. 16
         Sig. One tab. 4 times daily.
             How many milligrams of ergonovine maleate would the patient taking this prescription receive daily?

21. ℞   Hydrocodone Bitartrate   0.2 g
         Phenacetin   3.6 g
         Aspirin   6.0 g
         Caffeine   0.6 g
         M. ft. caps. no. 24
         Sig. One capsule t.i.d. p.r.n. for
         pain.

      (a) How many milligrams of hydrocodone bitartrate would be contained in each capsule?
      (b) What is the total weight, in milligrams, of the ingredients in each capsule?
      (c) How many milligrams of caffeine would be taken daily?

22. Digitoxin is available for parenteral pediatric use in a concentration of 0.1 mg/mL. How many milliliters would provide a dose of 40 μg?

23. ℞   Actifed Syrup   60 mL
         Robitussin Syrup   ad   120 mL
         Sig. 5 mL p.r.n. for cough.

            If a pharmacist had four 1-liter stock bottles of each of the ingredients, how many times could this prescription be filled?

24. If one 20-mL ampul contains 0.5 g of aminophylline, how many milliliters should be administered to provide a 25-mg dose of aminophylline?

25. ℞   Belladonna Tincture   10 mL
         Alurate Elixir   60 mL

Maalox Suspension   ad   120 mL
Sig. 5 mL t.i.d.

How many milliliters of Maalox Suspension would be contained in each dose?

26. An intravenous solution contains 500 μg of a drug substance in each milliliter. How many milligrams of the drug would a patient receive from the intravenous infusion of a liter of the solution?

27. If an intravenous solution containing 123 mg of a drug substance in each 250-mL bottle is to be administered at the rate of 200 μg of drug per minute, how many milliliters of the solution would be given per hour?

28. ℞   Decadron Elixir
      Benadryl Elixir   aa   20 mL
      Triple Sulfas Suspension   80 mL
      Sig. 10 mL stat., then 5 mL t.i.d.

    How many milliliters of Decadron Elixir would be taken in the initial dose of the prescription?

29. The prophylactic dose of riboflavin is 2 mg. How many micrograms of riboflavin are in a multiple vitamin capsule containing ⅕ the prophylactic dose?

30. One milligram of streptomycin sulfate contains the antibiotic activity of 650 μg of streptomycin base. How many grams of streptomycin sulfate would be the equivalent of 1 g of streptomycin base?

31. A commercial package contains thirty-six 200-mg tablets of ibuprofen. How many kilograms of ibuprofen were used in the manufacture of 1000 packages of the product?

32. If 480 mL of a certain solution contain 0.24 g of a chemical:
    (a) What is the volume of the thirtieth aliquot?
    (b) How many milligrams of the chemical will the thirtieth aliquot contain?
    (c) How many micrograms of the chemical are in this aliquot?

33. A prefilled syringe of furosemide contains 20 mg of drug in 2 mL of solution. How many micrograms of drug would be administered by an injection of 0.5 mL of the solution?

34. A vial of tobramycin sulfate contains 80 mg of drug in 2 mL of injection. How many milliliters of the injection should be administered to obtain 0.02 g of tobramycin sulfate?

35. A half-liter of D5W contains 2000 μg of added drug. How many milliliters of the fluid would contain 0.5 mg of the drug?

36. A multidose vial of sulfisoxazole diolamine contains 2 g of drug per 5 mL. How many milliliters would be used to administer 400 mg of the drug to a patient?

37. An effervescent tablet has the following formula:

Acetaminophen	325 mg
Calcium Carbonate	280 mg
Citric Acid	900 mg
Potassium Bicarbonate	300 mg
Sodium Bicarbonate	465 mg

(a) Calculate the total weight, in grams, of the above ingredients in each tablet.

(b) How many tablets could be made with a supply of 5 kg of acetaminophen?

38. A new analytic instrument is capable of detecting picogram quantities of a chemical substance. How many times more capable is this instrument than one that can detect nanogram quantities of the same chemical?

39. A pharmacist has a computer for drug information with a hard disk drive capacity of 20 megabytes. He wishes to upgrade it to a capacity of 5 gigabytes. What would be the increased capacity in megabytes?

40. ℞   Sodium Chloride   1.46 g
        Potassium Chloride   0.745 g
        Sodium Bicarbonate   1.68 g
        Sodium Sulfate   5.68 g
        PEG 3350   60.00 g
        Water   ad   4.00 L
     Sig. Drink 8 oz (240 mL) every 10 minutes until gone.
     Label: Colon Electrolyte Lavage.

    How many milligrams of total sodium and potassium salts would be contained in each dose?

41. How many grams of ethinyl estradiol are needed to prepare 2,500 tablets, each containing 50 μg of the medicinal substance?

42. The dimensions of a nicotine transdermal patch system are 4.7 cm by 4.8 cm. Express these dimensions in corresponding inches if 1 inch is equivalent to 25.4 mm.

43. If an albuterol inhaler contains 20 mg of albuterol, how many inhalation-doses can be delivered if each inhalation-dose contains 90 μg?

44. Acetaminophen, in amounts greater than 4 g per day, has been associated with liver toxicity. What is the maximum number of 325-mg tablets of acetaminophen that a person may take daily and not reach the toxic level?

45. Compazine® for injection is available in 10-mL multiple dose vials containing 5 mg/mL. How many 2-mg doses can be withdrawn from the vial?

46. The recommended dose for a nicotine patch is one 21-mg dose per day for 6 weeks, followed by 14 mg per day for 2 weeks, and then 7 mg per day for 2 more weeks. What total quantity, in grams, would a patient receive during this course of treatment?

47. Digoxin is available for parenteral use in a concentration of 0.1 mg/mL. How many milliliters are required to deliver a 40-μg dose?

4

Calculation of Doses

The *dose* of a drug is the quantitative *amount* administered or taken by a patient for the intended medicinal effect. The dose may be expressed as a *single dose,* the amount taken at one time; a *daily dose*; or a *total dose,* the amount taken during the time-course of therapy. A daily dose may be subdivided and taken in *divided doses,* two or more times per day depending on the characteristics of the drug and the illness. The schedule of dosing (e.g., *four times per day for 10 days*) is referred to as the *dosage regimen.*

Drug doses vary greatly between drug substances; some drugs have small doses, other drugs have relatively large doses. The dose of a drug is based on its biochemical and pharmacologic activity, its physical and chemical properties, the dosage form used, the route of administration, and various patient factors. The dose of a drug for a particular patient may be determined in part on the basis of the patient's age, weight, body surface area, general physical health, liver and kidney function (for drug metabolism and elimination), and the severity of the illness being treated.

The *usual adult dose* of a drug is the amount that ordinarily produces the medicinal effect intended in adults. The *usual pediatric dose* is similarly defined for the infant- or child-patient. The "usual" adult and pediatric doses of a drug serve as a guide to physicians who may select to prescribe that dose initially or vary it depending on the assessed requirements of the particular patient. The *usual dosage range* for a drug indicates the quantitative range or amounts of the drug that may be prescribed within the guidelines of usual medical practice. General dosing information for drug substances is provided in the monographs in the *United States Pharmacopeia Dispensing Information* (USP DI) as well as in the package inserts that accompany manufacturers' pharmaceutical products. Again, these sources provide the prescriber and pharmacists with guidelines of usual dosage and usual dosage range.

The dose response of individuals may vary (Fig. 4.1) and may require dosage adjustment in a given patient. For certain conditions, as in the treatment of cancer patients, drug dosing is highly specialized and individualized. Frequently, combinations of drugs are used, with the doses of each adjusted according to the patient's response. Many anticancer drugs are administered *cyclically,* usually for 21 to 28 days, with a rest period between dosing cycles to allow recovery from the toxic effects of the drugs. As noted later in this chapter, anticancer drugs are most commonly dosed on the basis of the patient's body surface area.

The *median effective dose* of a drug is the amount that produces the desired intensity of effect in 50% of the individuals tested. The *median toxic dose* of a drug is the amount that produces toxic effects in 50% of the individuals tested. Drugs intended to produce systemic effects must be absorbed or placed directly into the circulation and distributed in adequate concentrations to the body's cellular sites of action. For certain drugs, a correlation exists between drug dosage, the drug's blood serum concentration after administration, and the presentation and degree of drug effects. An average blood serum concentration of a drug can be determined. This amount represents the minimum concentration that can be expected to produce the drug's desired effects in a patient. This concentration is referred to as the *minimum effective concentration* (MEC). The base level of blood serum concentration that produces dose-related toxic effects is referred to as the *minimum toxic concentration* (MTC) of the drug.

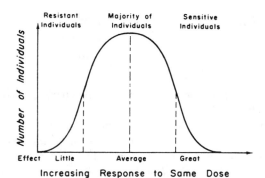

Fig. 4.1. Drug effect in a population sample.

Optimally, appropriate drug dosage should result in blood serum drug concentrations that are above the MEC and below the MTC for the period of time that drug effects are desired. As shown in Figure 4.2 for a hypothetical drug, the serum concentration of the drug reaches the MEC 2 hours after its administration and achieves a peak concentration in 4 hours, and falls below the MEC in 10 hours. If it would be desired to maintain the drug serum concentration above the MEC for a longer period of time, a second dose would be required at about an 8-hour time frame.

For certain drugs, a larger than usual initial dose may be required to achieve the desired blood drug level. This dose is referred to as the *priming* or *loading dose*. Subsequent *maintenance* doses, similar in amount to usual doses, are then administered according to the dosage regimen to sustain the desired drug blood levels or drug effects. To achieve the desired drug blood level rapidly, the loading dose may be administered as an injection or oral liquid, whereas the subsequent maintenance doses may be administered in other forms, such as tablets or capsules.

Certain biologic or immunologic products, such as vaccines, may be administered in *prophylactic doses* to protect the patient from contracting a specific disease. Other products, such as antitoxins, may be administered in *therapeutic doses* to counter a disease after exposure or its contraction. The doses of some biologic products, e.g., insulin, are expressed in *units of activity*, derived from biologic assay methods.

Most pharmaceutical products are prepared on a large scale within the pharmaceutical manufacturing industry for distribution to institutional and community pharmacies.

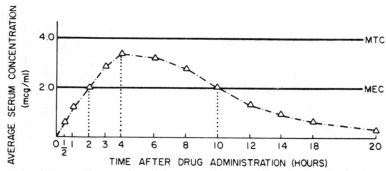

Fig. 4.2. Example of a blood level curve for a hypothetical drug as a function of the time after oral administration. MEC, minimum effective concentration; MTC, minimum toxic concentration.

These *prefabricated* products and dosage units are used in filling prescriptions and medication orders in the pharmacy. On a smaller scale, many hospital pharmacists and some community pharmacists manufacture bulk quantities of a limited number of products for use in their practices. Community and hospital pharmacists also fill prescriptions and medication orders requiring compounding; i.e., the fabrication of a pharmaceutical product from individual ingredients, carefully weighed, measured, and mixed.

Whether a pharmaceutical product is prepared on a large scale, small scale, or compounded individually in the pharmacy, drug dosage is a part of the pharmacist's calculation and, along with the prescribed dosage regimen, is vital to the health and welfare of the patient. This chapter presents dosage calculations relevant to the dispensing of prefabricated dosage forms and the preparation of compounded prescriptions. Calculations encountered in the large- and small-scale manufacture of pharmaceutical products are provided in Chapter 5, and an introduction to pharmacokinetic dosing is presented in Chapter 14.

One of the primary responsibilities of the pharmacist is to check doses specified in prescriptions based on a knowledge of the usual doses, usual dose ranges, and dosage regimens of the medicines prescribed. If an unusual dose is noted, the pharmacist is ethically bound to consult the physician to make sure that the dosage is correct.

For the patient, liquid dosage is usually measured in "household" terms, most commonly by the teaspoonful and tablespoonful. In *calculating* doses, pharmacists and physicians accept a capacity of 5 mL for the teaspoonful and 15 mL for the tablespoonful. It should be noted that the capacities of household teaspoons may vary from 3 to 7 mL and those of tablespoons may vary from 15 to 22 mL. Such factors as viscosity and surface tension of a given liquid, as well as the technique of the person measuring the liquid, can influence the actual volume held by a household spoon.

According to the *United States Pharmacopeia,* "For household purposes, an American Standard Teaspoon has been established by the American National Standards Institute as containing 4.93 ± 0.24 mL. In view of the almost universal practice of using teaspoons ordinarily available in the household for the administration of medicine, the teaspoon

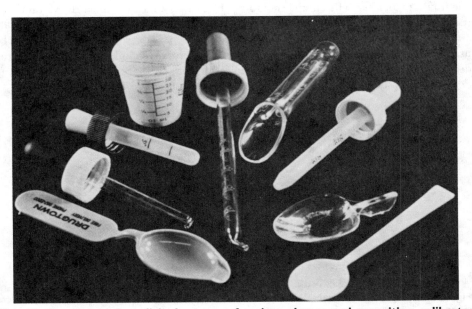

Fig. 4.3. Examples of medicinal spoons of various shapes and capacities, calibrated medicine droppers, an oral medication tube, and a disposable medication cup.

Table 4.1. Useful Approximate Equivalents

Common Measure		Metric Measure		
1 teaspoonful	=	$\frac{1}{6}$ fluidounce	=	5 mL
1 tablespoonful	=	$\frac{1}{2}$ fluidounce	=	15 mL

may be regarded as representing 5 mL. Preparations intended for administration by teaspoon should be formulated on the basis of dosage in 5-mL units. Any dropper, syringe, medicine cup, special spoon, or other device used to administer liquids should deliver 5 mL wherever a teaspoon calibration is indicated." In general, pharmaceutical manufacturers use the 5-mL teaspoon and the 15-mL tablespoon as a basis for the formulation of oral liquid preparations. Figure 4.3 presents examples of various devices used for measuring liquid medications.

Through habit and tradition, the f3-symbol (fluidram) is used by many physicians in the *Signa* portion of the prescription when indicating teaspoonful dosage. The pharmacist may interpret this symbol as a teaspoonful in dispensing prefabricated manufacturers' products called for on prescriptions and allow the patient to use the household teaspoon.

For calculating dosages, useful equivalent measures are provided in Table 4.1.

Frequently, the "drop" is used as a measure for medicines. It does not represent a definite quantity, because drops of different liquids vary greatly. In an attempt to standardize the drop as a unit of volume, the *United States Pharmacopeia* defines the official medicine dropper as being constricted at the delivery end to a round opening with an external diameter of about 3 mm. The dropper, when held vertically, delivers water in drops, each of which weighs between 45 and 55 mg. Accordingly, the official dropper is calibrated to deliver 20 drops of water per milliliter.

One should keep in mind, however, that few medicinal liquids have the same surface and flow characteristics as water, and therefore the size of drops varies materially from one liquid to another. The "drop" should not be used as a measure until the volume that it represents has been determined for each specific liquid. This determination is made by *calibrating* the dispensing dropper. The calibrated dropper is the only one that should be used for the measurement of medicine. Most manufacturers include a specially calibrated dropper along with their prepackaged medication for use by the patient in measuring dosage. Examples of specially calibrated droppers are shown in Figure 4.4.

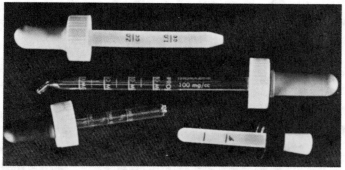

Fig. 4.4. Examples of calibrated droppers used in the administration of pediatric medications.

CALIBRATION OF DROPPERS

A dropper may be calibrated by counting the drops of a liquid as they fall into a graduate until a measurable volume is obtained. The volume of the drop is then calculated in terms of a definite unit (e.g., milliliters).

Example:

If a pharmacist counted 40 drops of a medication in filling a graduate cylinder to the 2.5-mL mark, how many drops per milliliter did the dropper deliver?

$$\frac{40 \text{ (drops)}}{x \text{ (drops)}} = \frac{2.5 \text{ (mL)}}{1 \text{ (mL)}}$$

$$x = 16 \text{ drops mL}, \textit{ answer.}$$

CALCULATIONS IN MISCELLANEOUS DOSAGE PROBLEMS

Number of Doses in a Specified Amount of Medicine.

$$\text{Number of doses} = \frac{\text{Total amount}}{\text{Size of dose}}$$

The *total* amount and the *dose* must be measured in a common denomination.

Examples:

If the dose of a drug is 200 mg, how many doses are contained in 10 g?

$$10 \text{ g} = 10{,}000 \text{ mg}$$

$$\text{Number of doses} = \frac{10{,}000 \text{ (mg)}}{200 \text{ (mg)}} = 50 \text{ doses}, \textit{ answer.}$$

Or, solving by dimensional analysis:

$$10 \text{ g} \times \frac{1000 \text{ mg}}{1 \text{ g}} \times \frac{1 \text{ dose}}{200 \text{ mg}} = 50 \text{ doses}, \textit{ answer.}$$

If 1 tablespoon is prescribed as the dose, approximately how many doses will be contained in 1 pint of the medicine?

$$\begin{aligned}
1 \text{ tablespoon} &= 15 \text{ mL} \\
1 \text{ pint} &= 473 \text{ mL}
\end{aligned}$$

$$\text{Number of doses} = \frac{473 \text{ mL}}{15 \text{ mL}} = 31.5 \text{ or } 31 \text{ doses}, \textit{ answer.}$$

If the dose of a drug is 50 μg, how many doses are contained in 0.020 g?

$$\begin{aligned}
0.020 \text{ g} &= 20 \text{ mg} \\
50 \text{ } \mu\text{g} &= 0.05 \text{ mg}
\end{aligned}$$

$$\text{Number of doses} = \frac{20 \text{ (mg)}}{0.05 \text{ (mg)}} = 400 \text{ doses}, \textit{ answer.}$$

Size of Each Dose, Given a Specified Amount of Medicine and Number of Doses it Contains.

$$\text{Size of dose} = \frac{\text{Total amount}}{\text{Number of doses}}$$

The *size of the dose* is expressed in whatever denomination is chosen for measuring the given total amount.

Examples:

How many teaspoonfuls would be prescribed in each dose of an elixir if 180 mL contained 18 doses?

$$\text{Size of dose} = \frac{180 \text{ mL}}{18} = 10 \text{ mL} = 2 \text{ teaspoonfuls, } \textit{answer.}$$

How many drops would be prescribed in each dose of a liquid medicine if 15 mL contained 60 doses? The dispensing dropper calibrates 32 drops/mL.

$$15 \text{ mL} = 15 \times 32 \text{ drops} = 480 \text{ drops}$$

$$\text{Size of dose} = \frac{480 \text{ (drops)}}{60} = 8 \text{ drops, } \textit{answer.}$$

Or, solving by dimensional analysis:

$$15 \text{ mL} \times \frac{32 \text{ drops}}{1 \text{ mL}} \times \frac{1}{60 \text{ doses}} = 8 \text{ drops/dose, } \textit{answer.}$$

Amount of a Medicine, Given Number of Doses it Contains and Size of Each Dose.
Total amount = number of doses × size of dose
It is convenient first to convert the given dose to the denomination in which the total amount is to be expressed.

Examples:

How many milliliters of a liquid medicine would provide a patient with 2 tablespoonfuls twice a day for 8 days?

Number of doses   = 16
Size of dose   = 2 tablespoonfuls or 30 mL
Total amount   = 16 × 30 mL = 480 mL, *answer.*

How many milliliters of a mixture would provide a patient with a teaspoonful dose to be taken 3 times a day for 16 days?

Number of tsp doses   = 16 × 3 = 48 tsp
Total amount   = 48 × 5 mL = 240 mL, *answer.*

How many grams of a drug will be needed to prepare 72 dosage forms if each is to contain 30 mg?

Number of doses   = 72
Size of dose   = 30 mg
Total amount   = 72 × 30 mg = 2160 mg = 2.16 g, *answer.*

It takes approximately 4 g of ointment to cover an adult patient's leg. If a physician prescribes an ointment for a patient with total leg eczema to be applied twice a day for 1 week, which of the following product sizes should be dispensed: 15 g, 30 g, or 60 g?

Number of doses   = 2 per day × 7 days = 14
Size of dose   = 4 g
Total amount   = 14 × 4 g = 56 g; thus, 60 g product size, *answer.*

Quantity of an Ingredient in Each Specified Dose, Given the Quantity in a Total Amount. If the number of doses in the total amount is known or can be quickly calculated, the following is a convenient equation.

$$\text{Quantity in each dose} = \frac{\text{Quantity in total amount}}{\text{Number of doses}}$$

The quantity of the ingredient in the total amount should first be reduced or converted to the denomination desired in the answer.

When the number of doses is not given, it is sometimes more convenient to use this proportion:

$$\frac{\text{Total amount}}{\text{Size of dose}} = \frac{\text{Quantity of ingredient in total}}{x}$$

$$x = \text{Quantity in each dose}$$

Examples:

If 0.050 g of a substance is used in preparing 125 tablets, how many micrograms are represented in each tablet?

$$0.050 \text{ g} = 50 \text{ mg} = 50,000 \text{ } \mu g$$

$$\frac{50,000 \text{ } (\mu g)}{125} = 400 \text{ } \mu g, \textit{ answer.}$$

Or, solving by dimensional analysis:

$$0.050 \text{ g} \times \frac{1,000,000 \text{ } \mu g}{1 \text{ g}} \times \frac{1}{125 \text{ tablets}} = 400 \text{ } \mu g/\text{tablet}, \textit{ answer.}$$

If a preparation contains 5 g of a drug in 500 mL, how many grams are contained in each tablespoonful dose?

$$1 \text{ tablespoonful} = 15 \text{ mL}$$

$$\frac{500 \text{ (mL)}}{15 \text{ (mL)}} = \frac{5 \text{ (g)}}{x}$$

$$x = 0.15 \text{ g}, \textit{ answer.}$$

A cough mixture contains 48 mg of hydromorphone hydrochloride in 8 fl. oz. How many milligrams of hydromorphone hydrochloride are in each 2-teaspoonful (tsp) dose?

1 fl. oz.   = 6 tsp
8 fl. oz.   = 48 tsp
48 tsp ÷ 2   = 24 doses
48 mg ÷ 24   = 2 mg, *answer.*

Or,

$$\frac{48 \text{ (tsp)}}{2 \text{ (tsp)}} = \frac{48 \text{ (mg)}}{x \text{ (mg)}}$$

$$x = 2 \text{ mg, } answer.$$

How many milligrams of codeine sulfate and of ammonium chloride will be contained in each dose of the following prescription?

R	Codeine Sulfate		0.6 g
	Ammonium Chloride		6.0 g
	Cherry Syrup	ad	120.0 mL

Sig. Teaspoonful for cough.
1 teaspoonful = 5 mL
120 ÷ 5 = 24 doses
0.6 g ÷ 24 = 0.025 g = 25 mg of codeine sulfate, *and*
6.0 g ÷ 24 = 0.25 g = 250 mg of ammonium chloride, *answers.*

Or,

$$\frac{120 \text{ (mL)}}{5 \text{ (mL)}} = \frac{0.6 \text{ (g)}}{x \text{ (g)}}$$

$$x = 0.025 \text{ g} = 25 \text{ mg of codeine sulfate, } and$$

$$\frac{120 \text{ (mL)}}{5 \text{ (mL)}} = \frac{6 \text{ (g)}}{y \text{ (g)}}$$

$$y = 0.25 \text{ g} = 250 \text{ mg of ammonium chloride, } answers.$$

Quantity of an Ingredient in a Specified Total Amount, Given the Quantity of the Ingredient in Each Specified Dose. As always, we can make a sound ratio of two amounts only by measuring them in a common denomination. When the number of doses is known or can be quickly calculated, use this equation:

Quantity in total = Quantity in dose × Number of doses

Otherwise this proportion may be used:

$$\frac{\text{Size of dose}}{\text{Total amount}} = \frac{\text{Quantity of ingredient in each dose}}{x}$$

$$x = \text{Quantity in total amount}$$

Examples:

How many grams of a drug substance are required to make 120 mL of a solution each teaspoonful of which contains 3 mg of the drug substance?

$$1 \text{ teaspoonful} = 5 \text{ mL}$$

$$\frac{5 \text{ (mL)}}{120 \text{ (mL)}} = \frac{3 \text{ (mg)}}{x \text{ (mg)}}$$

$$x = 72 \text{ mg or } 0.072 \text{ g, } answer.$$

Or, solving by dimensional analysis:

$$120 \text{ mL} \times \frac{3 \text{ mg}}{5 \text{ mL}} \times \frac{1 \text{ g}}{1000 \text{ mg}} = 0.072 \text{ g, } answer.$$

A physician ordered 250-mg capsules of tetracycline to be taken four times per day for 10 days. How many total grams of tetracycline would be prescribed?

Size of dose   = 250 mg
Number of doses   = 4 × 10 (days) = 40 doses
Quantity in total   = 250 mg × 40 = 10000 mg = 10 g, *answer.*

SPECIAL DOSING CONSIDERATIONS FOR THE PEDIATRIC AND ELDERLY PATIENT

Pediatric Patients

Pediatrics is the branch of medicine that deals with disease in children from birth through adolescence. Because of the range in age and bodily development in this patient population, the inclusive groups are defined further as follows: *neonate* (newborn), from birth to 1 month; *infant*, 1 month to 1 year; *early childhood*, 1 year through 5 years; *late childhood*, 6 years through 12 years; and, *adolescence*, 13 years through 17 years of age.[1]

Proper drug dosing of the pediatric patient depends on a number of factors, including the patient's age and weight, overall health status, the condition of such biologic functions as respiration and circulation, and the stage of development of body systems for drug metabolism (e.g., liver enzymes) and drug elimination (e.g., renal system). In the neonate, these biologic functions and systems are underdeveloped. Renal function, for example, develops over the span of the first 2 years of life. This fact is particularly important because the most commonly used drugs in neonates, infants, and young children are antimicrobial agents, which are eliminated primarily through the kidney. If the rate of drug elimination is not properly considered, drug accumulation in the body could occur, leading to drug overdosage and toxicity. Thus, the use of *pharmacokinetic* data (i.e., the rates and extent of drug absorption, distribution, metabolism, and elimination; see Chapter 14), together with individual patient drug handling characteristics and therapeutic response, provides a rational approach to pediatric drug dosage calculations.[1]

Geriatric Patients

Although the term "elderly" is subject to varying definitions with regard to chronologic age, it is clear that the functional capacities of most organ systems decline throughout adulthood and important changes in drug response occur with advancing age. *Geriatric medicine* or *geriatrics* is the field that encompasses the management of illness disability in the elderly.

Most age-related physiologic functions peak before age 30 years, with subsequent gradual linear decline.[1] Reductions in physiologic capacity and function are cumulative, becoming more profound with age. Kidney function is a major consideration in drug dosing in the elderly because reduced function results in reduced drug elimination. Renal blood flow demonstrates nearly 1% cumulative decline in most persons 60 to 70 years of age, a value that is even greater in persons 70 years of age and older.[1]

With reduced kidney function come reduced drug elimination, drug accumulation, and prolongation in the body, and possible toxic drug levels and related adverse events. Thus, dosing determinations in the elderly patient frequently include a variance from the

[1] The Merck Manual, 15th Ed., Rahway, NJ, Merck Sharp & Dohme Research Laboratories, 1987.

usual adult dose because of reduced renal clearance. As with the pediatric patient, renal clearance as well as other pharmacokinetic parameters are important in the dosing of certain drugs in the elderly patient population.

The reader is again referred to some introductory aspects of pharmacokinetic drug dosing in Chapter 14. Dosing calculations based on age, weight, and body surface area are the primary focus of the following sections of this chapter.[2]

DRUG DOSAGE BASED ON AGE

The age of the individual being treated is frequently a consideration in the determination of drug dosage, especially in the young or very old. As stated previously, newborns are abnormally sensitive to certain drugs because of the immature state of their hepatic and renal function. Elderly individuals may also respond abnormally to the usual adult dose of a drug because of impaired ability to metabolize or eliminate the drug or because of other concurrent pathologic conditions.

Before the physiologic differences between adult and pediatric patients were clarified, the latter were treated with drugs as if they were merely miniature adults. Various rules of dosage in which the pediatric dose was a fraction of the adult dose, based on relative age, were created for youngsters (e.g., *Young's rule*). Today these rules are not in general use because age alone is no longer considered a singularly valid criterion in the determination of children's dosage, especially when calculated from the *usual* adult dose, which itself provides wide clinical variations in response. Some of these rules are shown in footnote 3.

Currently, when age *is* considered in determining dosage of a potent therapeutic agent, it is used generally in conjunction with another factor, such as weight (Table 4.2).

Example:

From the data in Table 4.2, calculate the dosage range for digoxin for a 20-month-old infant weighing 6.8 kg.

---

[2] In consideration of the special problems associated with pediatric and geriatric dosing, useful sources of information have been made available to the pharmacist, such as the *Pediatric Dosage Handbook* and the *Geriatric Dosage Handbook* (Washington, DC, American Pharmaceutical Association, 1993) and *Guidelines for Administration of Intravenous Medications to Pediatric Patients* (Bethesda, MD, American Society of Hospital Pharmacists, 1988).

[3] *Young's rule*, based on age:

$$\frac{Age}{Age + 12} \times Adult\ dose = Dose\ for\ child$$

Cowling's rule:

$$\frac{Age\ at\ next\ birthday\ (in\ years) \times Adult\ dose}{24} = Dose\ for\ child$$

Fried's rule for Infants:

$$\frac{Age\ (in\ months) \times Adult\ dose}{150} = Dose\ for\ infant$$

Clark's rule, based on weight:

$$\frac{Weight\ (in\ lb) \times Adult\ dose}{150\ (average\ weight\ of\ adult\ in\ lb)} = Dose\ for\ child$$

**Table 4.2. Calculation of Pediatric Dosages
of Digoxin Based on Age and Weight**

Age	Digoxin Dose ($\mu g/kg$)
Premature	15 to 25
Full term	20 to 30
1 to 24 months	30 to 50
2 to 5 years	25 to 35
5 to 10 years	15 to 30
Over 10 years	8 to 12

$$\frac{30\ \mu g}{x\ \mu g} = \frac{1\ kg}{6.8\ kg} \qquad \frac{50\ \mu g}{x\ \mu g} = \frac{1\ kg}{6.8\ kg}$$

$$x = 204\ \mu g; \qquad x = 340\ \mu g$$

Dose range, 204 to 340 μg, *answer*.

In contrast to the preceding example of dose determination for a potent prescription drug, over-the-counter medications purchased for self-medication include labeling instructions that provide guidelines for safe and effective dosing. For pediatric use, doses generally are based on age groupings, e.g., 2 to 6 years old; 6 to 12 years old; and, over 12 years of age. For children 2 years of age or younger, the label recommendation generally states "consult your physician."

DRUG DOSAGE BASED ON BODY WEIGHT

The *usual doses* for drugs are considered generally suitable for 70-kg (154-lb) individuals. The ratio between the amount of drug administered and the size of the body influences the drug concentration at its site of action. Therefore, drug dosage may require adjustment from the usual adult dose for abnormally lean or obese patients.

The determination of drug dosage for young patients on the basis of body weight is considered more dependable than that based strictly on age. Consideration of the individual drug and the patient's pathologic and physiologic state still reigns supreme, however, and limits the clinical utility of any *general* rule, such as Clark's rule of pediatric dosage.

The dosage of a number of drug substances is based on body weight and is frequently expressed on a *milligram* (drug) *per kilogram* (body weight) or *milligram per pound* basis.

Examples:

The usual initial dose of chlorambucil is 150 $\mu g/kg$ of body weight once a day. How many milligrams should be administered to a person weighing 154 lb?

$$150\ \mu g \quad = 0.15\ mg$$
$$1\ kg \quad = 2.2\ lb$$
$$\frac{2.2\ (lb)}{154\ (lb)} = \frac{0.15\ (mg)}{x\ (mg)}$$
$$x \quad = 10.5\ mg,\ answer.$$

Or, solving by dimensional analysis:

$$\frac{150 \ \mu g}{1 \ kg} \times \frac{1 \ kg}{2.2 \ lb} \times \frac{154 \ lb}{1} \times \frac{1 \ mg}{1000 \ \mu g} = 10.5 \ mg, \ answer.$$

The usual dose of sulfisoxazole for infants over 2 months of age and children is 60 to 75 mg/ kg of body weight. What would be the usual range for a child weighing 44 lb?

1 kg	= 2.2 lb
20 kg	= 44 lb
60 mg/kg $\times$ 20 kg	= 1200 mg
75 mg/kg $\times$ 20 kg	= 1500 mg

Thus, the dosage range would be 1200 to 1500 mg, *answer.*

Table 4.3. Dosing by Body Weight

Body Weight		Total mg/day		
kilograms	pounds	0.5 mg/kg	1 mg/kg	2 mg/kg
40	88	20	40	80
50	110	25	50	100
60	132	30	60	120
70	154	35	70	140
80	176	40	80	160
90	198	45	90	180
100	220	50	100	200

Use of Dosing Tables. For some drugs dosed according to body weight or body surface area, dosing tables appear in product literature to assist the physician and pharmacist. An example is presented in Table 4.3.

Example:

Using Table 4.3 and a daily dose of 0.5 mg/kg, how many 20-mg capsules of the drug product should be dispensed to a patient weighing 176 lb if the dosage regimen calls for 15 weeks of therapy?

2 capsules/day $\times$ 7 days/week $\times$ 15 weeks = 210 capsules, *answer.*

DRUG DOSAGE BASED ON BODY SURFACE AREA

The *body surface area* (BSA) method of calculating drug doses provides results that are particularly desired and therefore widely used in two types of patient groups: (1) cancer patients receiving chemotherapy, and (2) pediatric patients of all childhood ages, with the exception of premature and full-term newborns, whose immature renal and liver functions require additional assessment in dosing.

Body Surface Area Dosage with Relation to Weight in Children. Table 4.4 shows the approximate relation between body weight and surface area of average body dimensions. It may be used in the calculation of pediatric doses based on BSA as related to weight.

By reference to Table 4.4, we find that the pediatric dose is expressed as a percentage of the adult dose, based on the relationship of the square meter area of a given weight and the average adult surface area of 1.73 m^2. Approximate doses for children may be calculated by multiplying the adult dose by this percentage.

Body Surface Area Dosage with Relation to Weight and Height in Children or Adults. For more precise calculation of doses based on BSA, one should refer to a standard *nomogram,* which includes both weight and height as factors influencing BSA. The nomo-

**Table 4.4. Approximate Relation of Surface Area and
Weights of Individuals of Average Body Dimension**

Kilograms	Pounds	Surface Area in Square Meters	Percent of Adult Dose*
2	4.4	0.15	9
3	6.6	0.20	11.5
4	8.8	0.25	14
5	11.0	0.29	16.5
6	13.2	0.33	19
7	15.4	0.37	21
8	17.6	0.40	23
9	19.8	0.43	25
10	22.0	0.46	27
15	33.0	0.63	36
20	44.0	0.83	48
25	55.0	0.95	55
30	66.0	1.08	62
35	77.0	1.20	69
40	88.0	1.30	75
45	99.0	1.40	81
50	110.0	1.51	87
55	121.0	1.58	91

* Based on average adult surface area of 1.73 square meters.
Adapted from *Techniques of Medication* by Eric W. Martin, et al., J. B.
Lippincott Co., 1969, p. 31, who adapted it from Modell's Drugs of Choice
(Mosby).

grams in Figures 4.5 and 4.6 may be used for determining BSA from weight and height.
The BSA in square meters (m^2) is indicated where a straight line drawn to connect the
height and weight of the child intersects the surface area column. In the example shown
in Figure 4.5, a child weighing 15 kg and measuring 100 cm in height has a BSA of
0.64 m^2. The dose is then calculated as follows:

If the adult dose is given,

$$\frac{\text{BSA of child (in } m^2)}{1.73 \ m^2 \text{ (average adult BSA)}} \times \frac{\text{Adult}}{\text{dose}} = \frac{\text{Approximate dose}}{\text{for child}}$$

If the dose per square millimeter is given,

$$\text{BSA of child (in } m^2) \times \text{Dose per } m^2 = \frac{\text{Approximate dose}}{\text{for child}}$$

Examples:

*If the adult dose of a drug is 75 mg, what would be the dose for a child weighing 40 lb and
measuring 32 in. in height? (Use the body surface area method.)*

$$\text{From the nomogram, the BSA} = 0.60 \ m^2$$

$$\frac{0.60 \ (m^2)}{1.73 \ (m^2)} \times 75 \ mg = 26 \ mg, \text{ answer.}$$

*The usual pediatric dose of ephedrine sulfate is stated as 25 mg/m^2. Using the nomogram,
calculate the dose for a child weighing 18 kg and measuring 82 cm in height.*

$$\text{From the nomogram, the BSA} = 0.60 \ m^2$$
$$25 \ mg \times 0.60 = 15 \ mg, \text{ answer.}$$

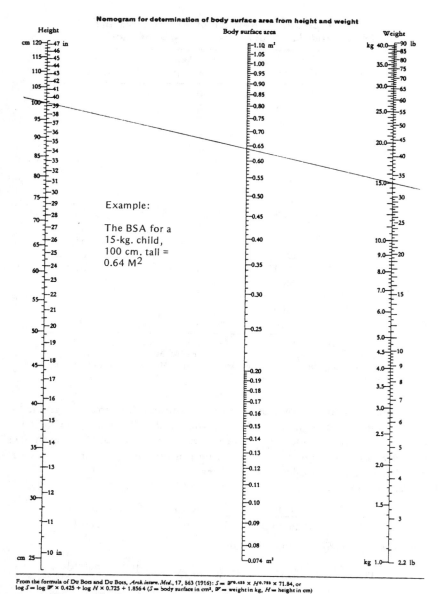

Fig. 4.5. Body surface area of children. From *Scientific Tables*, 7th Ed. Basel, J. R. Geigy, p. 538.

The nomogram in Figure 4.6 designed specifically for determining the BSA of *adults* may be used in the same manner as the one previously described. The adult dose is then calculated as follows:

$$\frac{\text{BSA of adult (m}^2)}{1.73 \text{ m}^2} \times \text{Usual adult dose} = \text{Dose for adult}$$

Examples:

If the usual adult dose of a drug is 120 mg, what would be the dose based on BSA for a person measuring 6 ft tall and weighing 200 lb?

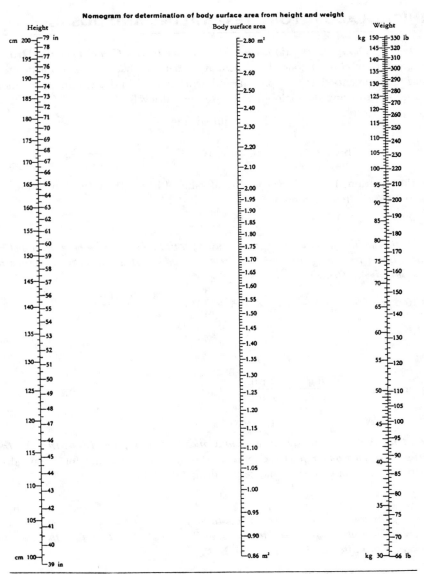

Nomogram for determination of body surface area from height and weight

Height   Body surface area   Weight

Fig. 4.6. Body surface area of adults. From *Scientific Tables*, 7th Ed. Basel, J. R. Geigy, p. 537.

$$\text{BSA (from the nomogram)} = 2.13 \text{ m}^2$$

$$\frac{2.13 \text{ m}^2}{1.73 \text{ m}^2} \times 120 \text{ mg} = 147.75 \text{ mg or } 148 \text{ mg, } answer.$$

If the dose of a drug is 5 mg/m², what would be the dose for a patient with a BSA of 1.9 m²?

$$5 \text{ mg} \times 1.9 = 9.5 \text{ mg, } answer.$$

CLINICAL LABORATORY TEST VALUES AND DOSAGE

Determining Dosage Using Equations Specific to Clinical Conditions and Drug Products. For certain clinical conditions there are equations that are useful for determining patient requirements. For example, the following is used in determining the amount of iron required to bring hemoglobin values to normal levels:

$$\text{Iron required (mg)} =$$

$$\text{body wt (lb)} \times 0.3 \times \left[100 - \frac{\text{Hb (g/dL)} \times 100}{14.8 \text{ g/dL}} \right]$$

In the equation, 14.8 g/dL is the normal value of hemoglobin (Hb) in adults and the factor 0.3 (%) is its iron content.

Example:

Using the equation for determining iron deficiency, calculate the number of milliliters of an iron dextran solution containing 50 mg/mL of iron to be administered to a 150-lb patient with a hemoglobin value of 10 g/dL.

$$\text{Iron required (mg)} = 150 \times 0.3 \times \left[100 - \frac{10 \times 100}{14.8} \right]$$

$$= 150 \times 0.3 \times 32.4$$

$$= 1458 \text{ mg}$$

$$\text{by proportion,} \quad \frac{50 \text{ mg}}{1458 \text{ mg}} = \frac{1 \text{ mL}}{\text{x mL}}$$

$$\text{x} = 29 \text{ mL, } answer.$$

Calculating Approximate Drug Serum Concentrations from Literature Data and Loading Dose Information. Experience in dosing has shown that for certain drugs, a correlation exists between dose and serum drug concentrations.[4]

Example:

In dosing the drug gentamicin in pediatric patients, for every 1 mg/kg of gentamicin administered, serum drug concentrations are expected to increase by 2.5 μg/mL. What would be the expected serum drug concentration after administration of a 2.5-mg/kg dose of gentamicin?

$$1 \text{ mg/kg} \quad = 2.5 \text{ μg/mL serum drug concentration}$$
$$2.5 \text{ mg/kg} \quad = 6.25 \text{ μg/mL serum drug concentration, } answer.$$

Practice Problems

1. If the dose of a drug is 150 μg, how many doses are contained in 0.120 g?

2. If a liquid medicine is to be taken three times daily, and if 180 mL are to be taken in 4 days, how many tablespoonfuls should be prescribed for each dose?

---

[4] Hoppe, M.M., et al.: A pediatric drug dosing and monitoring guide. Fla. J. Hosp. Pharm., 8:259, 1988; Greenspoon, J.S., Masaki, D.I., and Pastel, D.: Gentamicin dosing for the treatment of postcesarean endometritis. Hosp. Pharm., 27:861, 1992.

3. If a cough syrup contains 0.24 g of codeine in 120 mL, how many milligrams are contained in each teaspoonful dose?

4. The product Mylicon® drops contains 2 g of simethicone in a 30-mL container. How many milligrams of the drug are contained in each 0.6-mL dose?

5. Sudafed® cough syrup contains 0.09 g of dextromethorphan hydrobromide in each fluidounce. How many milligrams of this agent would be present in each teaspoonful dose?

6. The formula for Auralgan,® an otic solution is:

Antipyrine		54.0 mg
Benzocaine		14.0 mg
Glycerin, dehydrated,	ad	1.0 mL

    If a dropper delivers 20 drops/mL, how many milligrams of benzocaine would be delivered by a 3-drop dose of the solution?

7. A physician prescribes tetracycline suspension for a patient who is to take 2 teaspoonfuls four times per day for 4 days, and then 1 teaspoonful four times per day for 2 days. How many milliliters of the suspension should be dispensed to provide the quantity for the prescribed dosage regimen?

8. Digoxin injection is available in a concentration of 0.1 mg/mL. How many milliliters of the injection will provide a dose of 75 μg?

9. The usual dose of digoxin for rapid digitalization is a total of 1.0 mg, divided into two or more portions at intervals of 6 to 8 hours. How many milliliters of digoxin elixir containing 50 μg/mL would provide this dose?

10. Each milliliter of a brand of sodium fluoride drops contains 2.25 mg of fluoride ion. If the dropper supplied issues 18 drops/mL and the dose for a 3-year-old child is 3 drops, how many micrograms of fluoride ion would be administered per dose?

11. The dose of beclomethasone, an aerosolized inhalant, is 200 μg twice daily. The commercial inhaler delivers 50 μg per metered inhalation and contains 200 inhalations. How many inhalers should be dispensed to a patient if a 60-day supply is prescribed?

12. If a physician prescribed Keflex®, 250 mg q.i.d. $\times$ 10 days, how many milliliters of Keflex® suspension containing 250 mg per 5 mL should be dispensed?

13. A patient has been instructed to take 15 mL of alumina and magnesium oral suspension every other hour for four doses daily. How many days will two 12-fl. oz. bottles of the suspension last?

14. A 16-week regimen for a brand of a nicotine patch calls for a patient to wear a 15-mg patch each day for the first 12 weeks, followed by a 10-mg patch each day for the next 2 weeks, and then a 5-mg patch each day to conclude the treatment regimen. In all, how many milligrams of nicotine are administered?

15. The following regimen of oral prednisone is prescribed for a patient: 50 mg/d $\times$ 10 days; 25 mg/d $\times$ 10 days; 12.5 mg/d $\times$ 10 days; 5 mg/d $\times$ 10 weeks. How many scored 25-mg tablets and how many 5-mg tablets should be dispensed to meet the dosing requirements?

16. ℞   Codeine Phosphate   30 mg/tsp
         Robitussin® Syrup   30 mL
         Elixophylline   ad   240 mL
         Sig. 5 mL q.i.d. p.c. h.s.

    (a) If 5 mL of Robitussin® syrup contains 100 mg of guaifenesin, how many
        milligrams of the drug would be taken daily?
    (b) If a dropper delivers 20 drops/mL and the dose of codeine phosphate is
        0.5 mg/kg of body weight, how many drops of the prescription might be
        administered as a dose for a 22-lb child?

17. Lugol's Solution contains 5 g of iodine per 100 mL and its usual dose is 0.3 mL
    three times per day. How many milligrams of iodine are represented in the daily
    dose of the solution?

18. ℞   Dextromethorphan   50 mg/tsp
         Robitussin® Syrup   40 mL
         Guaifenesin Syrup   ad   120 mL
         Sig. ℥i q.i.d. a.c. & h.s.

    How many milligrams of dextromethorphan would be needed to fill the pre-
    scription?

19. Terpin Hydrate and Codeine Elixir contains 60 mg of codeine per 30 mL. How
    much additional codeine should be added to 180 mL of the elixir so that each
    teaspoonful will contain 15 mg of codeine?

20. ℞   Lincocin®   1.2 g
         Propylene Glycol   4.0 mL
         Isopropyl Alcohol 70%
         Purified Water   aa ad   60   mL
         Sig. Apply b.i.d. for acne.

    If the source of Lincocin® is an injection containing the equivalent of 300 mg
    Lincocin® per milliliter, how many milliliters of the injection should be used in
    filling the prescription?

21. How many milliliters of an injection containing 20 mg of gentamicin in each 2
    mL should be used in filling a medication order calling for 2.5 mg of gentamicin
    to be administered intramuscularly?

22. A physician ordered 1.5 mg of theophylline to be administered orally to a baby.
    How many milliliters of theophylline elixir containing 80 mg of theophylline per
    15 mL should be used in filling the medication order?

23. How many milliliters of aminophylline injection containing 250 mg of aminophyl-
    line in each 10 mL should be used in filling a medication order calling for 15 mg
    of aminophylline?

24. A physician ordered 20 mg of Demerol® and 0.3 mg of atropine sulfate to be
    administered preoperatively to a patient. Demerol® is available in a syringe contain-
    ing 25 mg/mL and atropine sulfate is in an ampul containing 0.4 mg per 0.5 mL.
    How many milliliters of each should be used in filling the medication order?

25. A solution contains 660 mg of sodium fluoride per 120 mL and has a dose of 10

drops. If the dispensing dropper calibrates 25 drops/mL, how many milligrams of sodium fluoride are contained in each dose?

26. ℞   Acetaminophen drops
        Disp. 15 mL
        Sig. 0.6 mL t.i.d.

    (a) If acetaminophen drops contain 25 grains of acetaminophen per 15-mL container, how many milligrams are there in each prescribed dose?
    (b) If the dropper calibrates 20 drops/mL, how many drops should be administered per dose?

27. Cyclosporine is an immunosuppressive agent administered before and after organ transplantation at a single daily dose of 15 mg/kg. How many milliliters of a 50-mL bottle containing 100 mg of cyclosporine per milliliter would be administered to a 140-lb kidney transplant patient?

28. The dose of gentamicin for premature and full-term neonates is 2.5 mg/kg administered every 12 hours. What would be the daily dose for a newborn weighing 5.6 lb?

29. The dose of gentamicin for patients with impaired renal function is adjusted (according to clinical laboratory tests) to assure therapeutically adequate but not excessive dosage. If the normal daily dose of the drug for adults is 3 mg/kg/day, administered in three divided doses, what would be the single (8-hour) dose for a patient weighing 165 lb and scheduled to receive only 40% of the usual dose, based on renal impairment?

30. If the cost of human growth hormone is $40/mg, what is the yearly cost of treating a 30-kg child at a dose of 0.04 mg/kg/day?

31. The dose of a drug is 500 μg/kg of body weight. How many milligrams should be given to a child weighing 55 lb?

32. The usual dosage range of dimercaprol is 2.5 to 5 mg/kg of body weight. What would be the dosage range, in grams, for a person weighing 165 lb?

33. ℞   Erythromycin Estolate   400 mg/5 mL
        Disp. 100 mL
        Sig. ———— tsp. q.i.d. until all medication is taken.

        If the dose of erythromycin estolate is given as 40 mg/kg per day,
    (a) What would be the proper dose of the medication in the Signa if the prescription is for a 44-lb child?
    (b) How many days will the medication last?

34. An intravenous infusion contains 1 g of carbenicillin in each 20 mL. How many milliliters of the infusion should be administered daily to a 154-lb patient if the dose of carbenicillin is 200 mg/kg per day?

35. The adult dose of a liquid medication is 0.1 mL/kg of body weight to be administered as a single dose. How many teaspoonfuls should be administered to a person weighing 220 lb?

36. A physician orders 2 mg of ampicillin to be added to each milliliter of a 250-mL bottle of 5% dextrose in water (D5W) for intravenous infusion.

(*a*) How many milligrams of ampicillin should be added?

(*b*) If the 250 mL of solution represents a single dose and if the dose of ampicillin is 25 mg/kg of body weight, how many pounds does the patient weigh?

37. ℞   Piperazine syrup   500 mg/5 mL
         Disp. _____ mL
         Sig. Parents: Take __ teaspoonfuls daily for 2 days.
              Child: Take __ teaspoonfuls daily for 2 days.

The dose of piperazine for adults is 3.5 g as a single daily dose for 2 consecutive days. For children, the dose is 75 mg/kg of body weight per day for 2 consecutive days. If both parents and a 66-lb child are to take the medication as directed,

(*a*) How many milliliters of piperazine syrup should be dispensed?

(*b*) How many teaspoonfuls each should the parents and the child take daily?

38. A physician desires a dose of 40 μg/kg of digoxin for an 8-lb newborn child. How many milliliters of an injection containing 0.25 mg of digoxin per milliliter should be given?

39. The dose of gentamicin sulfate is 1.7 mg/kg of body weight. How many milliliters of an injectable solution containing the equivalent of 40 mg of gentamicin per milliliter should be administered to a person weighing 198 lb?

40. The usual intramuscular dose of kanamycin sulfate is the equivalent of 7.5 mg of kanamycin per kilogram of body weight. How many milliliters of kanamycin sulfate injection containing the equivalent of 250 mg of kanamycin per milliliter should be given to a person weighing 176 lb?

41. The dose of pyrvinium pamoate is 5 mg/kg of body weight as a single dose. How many tablets, each containing 50 mg of pyrvinium pamoate, should be dispensed for a person weighing 110 lb to provide an initial dose and a second dose in 2 weeks?

42. How many chloramphenicol capsules, each containing 250 mg of chloramphenicol, are needed to provide 25 mg/kg of body weight per day for 1 week for a person weighing 154 lb?

43. A 25-lb child is to receive 4 mg of phenytoin per kilogram of body weight daily as an anticonvulsant. How many milliliters of pediatric phenytoin suspension containing 30 mg per 5 mL should the child receive?

44. The loading dose of digoxin in premature infants with a birth weight of less than 1.5 kg is 20 μg/kg administered in three *un*equally divided doses ($\frac{1}{2}$, $\frac{1}{4}$, $\frac{1}{4}$) at 8-hour intervals. What would be the initial dose for an infant weighing 1.2 kg?

45. The pediatric dose of cefadroxil is 30 mg/kg/day. If a child was given a daily dose of 2 teaspoonfuls of a pediatric suspension containing 125 mg of cefadroxil per 5 mL, what was the weight, in pounds, of the child?

46. How many milliliters of terbutaline injection containing 1 mg of terbutaline per milliliter of injection should be administered to a 6-month-old child weighing 16 pounds to achieve a subcutaneous dose of 0.01 mg/kg?

47. If a child weighing 40 lb accidentally ingested thirty-five 5-grain ferrous sulfate tablets, calculate the quantity of ferrous sulfate ingested on a milligram per kilogram basis.

48. Using Table 4.3 and a daily dose of 2 mg/kg, how many 20-mg capsules would a 176-lb patient be instructed to take per dose if the daily dose is to be taken in divided doses, q.i.d.?

49. If the daily dose of levothyroxine sodium is 5 μg/kg of body weight, what would be the weight, in pounds, of a child who was administered a daily dose of 0.1 mg?

50. How many capsules, each containing 250 mg of chloramphenicol, are needed to provide 50 mg/kg/day for 10 days for a person weighing 176 lb?

51. If the pediatric dose of dactinomycin is 15 μg/kg/day $\times$ 5 days, how many micrograms should be administered to a 40-lb child over the course of treatment?

52. If the administration of gentamicin at a dose of 1.75 mg/kg of body weight is determined to result in peak blood serum levels of 4 μg/mL, calculate the dose, in milligrams, for a 120-lb patient that may be expected to result in a blood serum gentamicin level of 4.5 μg/mL.

53. A medication order calls for tobramycin sulfate, 1 mg/kg of body weight, to be administered by IM injection to a patient weighing 220 lb. Tobramycin sulfate is available in a vial containing 80 mg per 2 mL. How many milliliters of the injection should the patient receive?

54. The usual pediatric dose of cefazolin sodium is 25 mg/kg/day divided equally into three doses. What would be the single dose, in milligrams, for a child weighing 33 lb?

55. If the recommended dose of tobramycin for a premature infant is 4 mg/kg/day, divided into two equal doses administered every 12 hours, how many milligrams of the drug should be given every 12 hours to a 2.2-lb infant?

56. If a 3-year-old child weighing 35 lb accidentally ingested twenty 5-grain aspirin tablets, how much aspirin did the child ingest on a milligram per kilogram basis?

57. How many grams of fluorouracil will a 154-lb patient receive in 5 successive days at a dosage rate of 12 mg/kg/day?

58. The initial maintenance dose of vancomycin for infants less than 1 week old is 15 mg/kg every 18 hours.
     (a) What would be the dose, in milligrams, for an infant weighing 2500 g?
     (b) How many milliliters of an injection containing 500 mg per 25 mL should be administered to obtain this dose?

59. The loading dose of chloramphenicol in neonates is 20 mg/kg of body weight.
     (a) What would be the dose for a neonate weighing 6 lb, 4 oz?
     (b) How many milliliters of an injection containing 1 g of chloramphenicol per 30 mL should be administered to obtain this dose?

60. If the daily dose of a drug is given in the literature as 8 mg/kg of body weight or 350 mg/m^2, calculate the dose on each basis for a patient weighing 150 lb and measuring 5 ft, 8 in. in height.

61. If the dose of Taxol® (paclitaxel) in the treatment of metastatic ovarian cancer is 135 mg/m^2, what would be the dose for a patient 155 cm tall and weighing 53 kg?

62.   If the adult dose of a drug is 100 mg, what would be the dose for a child with a body surface area of 0.70 m^2?

63.   If the adult dose of a drug is 25 mg, what would be the dose for a child weighing 40 lb and measuring 32 in. in height? (Use the body surface area method.)

64.   If the dose of a drug is 10 mg/m^2 per day, what would be the daily dose, in milligrams, for a child weighing 30 lb and measuring 26 in. in height?

65.   The dose of Mitomycin injection is 20 mg/m^2 per day. Using the nomogram in Figure 4.6, determine the daily dose for a patient who weighs 144 lb and measures 68 in. in height.

66.   An anticancer treatment includes methotrexate, 35 mg/m^2 of body surface area once per week for 8 weeks. How many grams of methotrexate would a 5 ft, 8 in., 150-lb patient receive during this course of therapy?

67.   If the dose of a drug is 0.8 mg/m^2 of body surface area, how many micrograms should be administered to a child whose body surface area is 0.75 m^2?

68.   If the dose of a drug is 5 mg/m^2, how many milliliters of a 0.2% w/v injection should be administered to a 3 ft, 8-in. child weighing 40 lb?

69.   The daily dose of diphenhydramine hydrochloride for a child may be determined on the basis of 5 mg/kg of body weight or on the basis of 150 mg/m^2. Calculate the dose on each basis for a child weighing 55 lb and measuring 40 in. in height.

70.   Naturally derived Taxol, an anticancer drug from the bark of the Pacific yew tree, requires the extraction of 25,000 pounds of bark for each kilogram of drug (Taxol) obtained. The drug is supplied in 5-mL ampuls containing 6 mg/mL of injection. It is administered by slow intravenous infusion over a 24-hour period at a dosage range of 110 to 250 mg/m^2 of body surface area.
      (a)   How many grams of bark are required to obtain the amount of drug in a 5-mL ampul?
      (b)   What would be the maximum daily dose of Taxol for a patient measuring 5 ft, 8 in. in height and weighing 112 lb?
      (c)   How many milliliters of the injection would supply the dose required in (b)?

5

Reducing and Enlarging Formulas

Pharmacists may have to reduce or enlarge formulas for pharmaceutical preparations in the course of their professional practice or manufacturing activities. Official formulas and most other formulas for manufacturing are based on the preparation of 1000 mL or 1000 g of product. The pharmacist may be called on to make a smaller or greater quantity and thus must reduce or enlarge the formula while maintaining the correct proportion of each ingredient.

When a formula specifies a *total amount*, we may determine how much of each ingredient is needed to obtain a desired amount by this proportion:

$$\frac{\text{Total amount specified in formula}}{\text{Total amount desired}} = \frac{\text{Quantity of each ingredient in formula}}{x}$$

$$x = \text{Quantity of each ingredient in amount desired}$$

Although all problems specifying a total amount may be solved by this proportion, it is usually more convenient—particularly if the quantities are given in the metric system—to solve them by using short cuts. Thus, given a formula for 1000 mL or 1000 g, we may divide or multiply the quantity of each ingredient by a power of 10 simply by moving the decimal point to the left or right the required number of places. Or, given a formula for the same amounts, we may reduce or enlarge it by using factors. For example, if we wish to prepare 1 gallon (3785 mL) of a formula the specified total amount of which is 1000 mL, we would multiply the quantity of each ingredient by the factor 3.785. If we are to prepare 50 g of a formula with a specified total amount of 1000 g, we would multiply the quantity of each ingredient by $\frac{1}{20}$ or 0.05 (because 50 g is $\frac{1}{20}$ or 5% of 1000 g).

Some formulas, however, do not specify a total amount, instead indicating relative quantities of ingredients or *proportional parts* to be used in obtaining any desired total amount. Such problems may be solved by this proportion:

$$\frac{\text{Total number of parts in formula}}{\text{Number of parts of each ingredient}} = \frac{\text{Total amount desired}}{x}$$

$$x = \text{Quantity of each ingredient in amount desired}$$

In solving problems that involve reducing and enlarging formulas, the following facts should be noted. First, to make a valid ratio, the total amounts compared must be expressed in a common denomination, whether in grams, fluidounces, pounds, or anything else. Consequently, if they are unlike from the start, one or the other must be reduced or converted. If, for example, the formula is given in the metric system and the required quantity is in the common system, it is generally best to convert the required quantity into the metric system. The answers may then be converted into weighable or measurable denominations in the common system or, if this is not indicated, the results may be left in the metric system.

Second, because the quantity of each ingredient is calculated separately, it does not matter if the formula includes an assortment of terms (pounds and fluidounces, grams and milliliters, and so on).

FORMULAS THAT SPECIFY AMOUNTS OF INGREDIENTS

Calculating Quantities of Ingredients when Reducing or Enlarging a Formula. Calculating the quantities of ingredients to be used when reducing or enlarging a formula for a specified total amount involves the following.

Examples:

From the following formula, calculate the quantity of each ingredient required to make 240 mL of calamine lotion.

Calamine	80 g
Zinc Oxide	80 g
Glycerin	20 g
Bentonite Magma	250 mL
Calcium Hydroxide Topical Solution, to make	1000 mL

Using the factor 0.24 (because 240 mL is 24% 1000 mL), the quantity of each ingredient is calculated as follows:

Calamine $=$ 80 $\times$ 0.24 $=$ 19.2 g
Zinc Oxide $=$ 80 $\times$ 0.24 $=$ 19.2 g
Glycerin $=$ 20 $\times$ 0.24 $=$ 4.8 mL
Bentonite Magma $=$ 250 $\times$ 0.24 $=$ 60 mL
Calcium Hydroxide Topical Solution, to make 240 mL, *answers*

Or, solving by dimensional analysis:

$$\text{Calamine } \frac{80 \text{ g}}{1000 \text{ mL}} \times \frac{240 \text{ mL}}{1} = 19.2 \text{ g}$$

$$\text{Zinc Oxide } \frac{80 \text{ g}}{1000 \text{ mL}} \times \frac{240 \text{ mL}}{1} = 19.2 \text{ g}$$

$$\text{Glycerin } \frac{20 \text{ mL}}{1000 \text{ mL}} \times \frac{240 \text{ mL}}{1} = 4.8 \text{ mL}$$

$$\text{Bentonite Magma } \frac{250 \text{ mL}}{1000 \text{ mL}} \times \frac{240 \text{ mL}}{1} = 60 \text{ mL}$$

Calcium Hydroxide Topical Solution, to make 240 mL, answers.

If, in this problem, the required amount were *60 mL,* we should *move the decimal point one place to the left and multiply by 0.6.* Or, if the required amount were *50 mL,* we would either *divide by 20, multiply by 0.05 (5%),* or *move the decimal point one place to the left and divide by 2.* If the required amount were *125 mL,* we should *multiply by the* $\frac{1}{8}$ *or 0.125* (because 125 mL is $\frac{1}{8}$ or 12.5% of 1000 mL).

From the following formula, calculate the quantity of each ingredient required to make 1 gallon of Compound Benzoin Tincture.

Benzoin	100 g
Aloe	20 g
Storax	80 g
Tolu Balsam	40 g
Alcohol, to make	1000 mL

Using the factor 3.785, the quantity of each ingredient is calculated as follows:

Benzoin	= 100 × 3.785 = 378.5 g
Aloe	= 20 × 3.785 = 75.7 g
Storax	= 80 × 3.785 = 302.8 g
Tolu Balsam	= 40 × 3.785 = 151.4 g
Alcohol, to make	3785 mL or 1 gallon, *answers.*

From the following formula, calculate the quantity of each ingredient required to make 1 lb of the ointment.

Coal Tar	50 g
Starch	250 g
Zinc Oxide	150 g
Petrolatum	550 g

Because the formula is for 1000 g, and using the factor 0.454, the quantity of each ingredient is calculated as follows:

Coal Tar	= 50 × 0.454 = 22.7 g
Starch	= 250 × 0.454 = 113.5 g
Zinc Oxide	= 150 × 0.454 = 68.1 g
Petrolatum	= 550 × 0.454 = 249.7 g
	454.0 g or 1 lb, *answers.*

From the following formula for 100 capsules, calculate the quantity of each ingredient required to make 24 capsules.

Belladonna Extract	1.0 g
Ephedrine Sulfate	1.6 g
Phenobarbital	2.0 g
Aspirin	32.0 g

Using the factor 0.24 (because 24 capsules are represented by 0.24 × 100), the quantity of each ingredient is calculated as follows:

Belladonna Extract	= 1.0 × 0.24 = 0.24 g
Ephedrine Sulfate	= 1.6 × 0.24 = 0.384 g
Phenobarbital	= 2.0 × 0.24 = 0.48 g
Aspirin	= 32.0 × 0.24 = 7.68 g

answers.

FORMULAS THAT SPECIFY PROPORTIONAL PARTS

Calculating Quantities of Ingredients in Formula Preparation with Specified Proportional Parts. If a formula gives quantities in terms of *proportional parts*, these facts should be noted:

1. When parts by weight are specified, we can convert only to weights and not to volumes, whereas when parts by volume are specified, we can convert only to volumes.
2. Just as the formula measures all quantities in a common denomination (namely, in terms of parts), so will our calculations result in a single denomination, which we will select at the outset for measuring the desired total amount.

Examples:

From the following formula, calculate the quantity of each ingredient required to make 1000 g of the ointment.

Coal Tar	5 parts
Zinc Oxide	10 parts
Hydrophilic Ointment	50 parts

Total number of parts (by weight) = 65
1000 g will contain 65 parts

$$\frac{65 \text{ (parts)}}{5 \text{ (parts)}} = \frac{1000 \text{ (g)}}{x \text{ (g)}}$$

$$x = 76.92 \text{ g of Coal Tar,}$$

and

$$\frac{65 \text{ (parts)}}{10 \text{ (parts)}} = \frac{1000 \text{ (g)}}{y \text{ (g)}}$$

$$y = 153.85 \text{ g of Zinc Oxide,}$$

and

$$\frac{65 \text{ (parts)}}{50 \text{ (parts)}} = \frac{1000 \text{ (g)}}{z \text{ (g)}}$$

$$z = 769.23 \text{ g of Hydrophilic Ointment, } \textit{answers.}$$

(Check total: 1000 g)

From the following formula, calculate the quantity, in grams, of each ingredient required to make 5 lb of the powder.

Bismuth Subcarbonate	8 parts
Kaolin	15 parts
Magnesium Oxide	2 parts

Total number of parts (by weight) = 25 parts
5 lb (454 g × 5) or 2270 g will contain 25 parts

$$\frac{25 \text{ (parts)}}{8 \text{ (parts)}} = \frac{2270 \text{ (g)}}{x \text{ (g)}}$$

$$x = 726.4 \text{ g of Bismuth Subcarbonate,}$$

and

$$\frac{25 \text{ (parts)}}{15 \text{ (parts)}} = \frac{2270 \text{ (g)}}{y \text{ (g)}}$$

$$y = 1362 \text{ g of Kaolin,}$$

and

$$\frac{25 \text{ (parts)}}{2 \text{ (parts)}} = \frac{2270 \text{ (g)}}{z \text{ (g)}}$$

z = 181.6 g of Magnesium Oxide, *answers.*

(Check total: 2270 g)

Calculating Quantities of Ingredients When Proportional Parts are Reckoned from the Formula. If the ingredients are all measured by weight, or all by volume, we may consider the sum of the weights (or volumes) when expressed in a common denomination as specifying a total number of parts.

Example:

   From the following formula, calculate the quantity of each ingredient required to make 500 g of the powder.

Boric acid	5 g
Starch	20 g
Talc	50 g

Total number of parts (by weight) = 75
500 g will contain 75 parts

$$\frac{75 \text{ (parts)}}{5 \text{ (parts)}} = \frac{500 \text{ (g)}}{x \text{ (g)}}$$

x = 33.3 g of Boric Acid,

and

$$\frac{75 \text{ (parts)}}{20 \text{ (parts)}} = \frac{500 \text{ (g)}}{y \text{ (g)}}$$

y = 133.3 g of Starch,

and

$$\frac{75 \text{ (parts)}}{50 \text{ (parts)}} = \frac{500 \text{ (g)}}{z \text{ (g)}}$$

z = 333.3 g of Talc, *answers.*

(Check total: 500 g)

Practice Problems

1. From the following formula, calculate the quantities required to make 180 mL of benzyl benzoate lotion.

Benzyl Benzoate	250 mL
Triethanolamine	5 mL
Oleic Acid	20 mL
Purified Water, to make	1000 mL

2. From the following formula, calculate the quantities required to make 5 gallons of a phenobarbital elixir.

Phenobarbital	4	g
Orange Oil	0.25	mL
Certified Red Color		q.s.
Alcohol	200	mL
Propylene Glycol	100	mL
Sorbitol Solution	600	mL
Water, to make	1000	mL

3. From the following formula, calculate the quantities required to make 5 lb of hydrophilic ointment.

Methylparaben	0.25	g
Propylparaben	0.15	g
Sodium Lauryl Sulfate	10	g
Propylene Glycol	120	g
Stearyl Alcohol	250	g
White Petrolatum	250	g
Purified Water, to make	1000	g

4. From the following formula, calculate the amount, in grams, of each ingredient required to make 1 lb of cold cream.

Cetyl Esters Wax	12.5 parts
White Wax	12.0 parts
Mineral Oil	56.0 parts
Sodium Borate	0.5 parts
Water	19.0 parts

5. A timed-release cold capsule contains the following ingredients. Calculate, in grams, the amount of each ingredient required to manufacture 100,000 capsules.

Phenindamine	24 mg
Chlorpheniramine Maleate	4 mg
Phenylpropanolamine Hydrochloride	50 mg

6. From the following formula, calculate the quantity of each ingredient present in 8 fluidounces of the antacid suspension.

Aluminum Hydroxide Compressed Gel	362.8	g
Sorbitol Solution	282	mL
Syrup	93	mL
Glycerin	25	mL
Methylparaben	0.9	g
Propylparaben	0.3	g
Flavor		q.s.
Water, to make	1000	mL

7. From the following formula, calculate the quantity of each ingredient required to make 1500 g of the powder.

Calcium Carbonate	5 parts
Magnesium Oxide	1 part
Sodium Bicarbonate	4 parts
Bismuth Subcarbonate	3 parts

8. From the following formula, calculate the number of grams of each ingredient required to make 1000 g of the ointment.

Salicylic Acid	0.5 part
Precipitated Sulfur	4.5 parts
Hydrophilic Ointment	35.0 parts

9. From the following formula, calculate the quantity of each ingredient required to make 4 liters of the lotion.

Witch Hazel	4 parts (by volume)
Glycerin	1 part " "
Boric Acid Solution	15 parts " "

10. From the following formula for ipecac syrup, calculate the amount of each ingredient needed to prepare enough syrup to fill sixty 15-mL prescription bottles.

Ipecac Fluidextract	70 mL
Glycerin	100 mL
Syrup, to make	1000 mL

11. A narcotic analgesic tablet contains 5 mg of hydrocodone bitartrate and 500 mg of aspirin. How many grams of each ingredient are needed to prepare 1000 tablets?

12. From the following formula for a progesterone vaginal suppository, calculate the amount of each ingredient needed to prepare 36 suppositories.

Progesterone	75 mg
Polyethylene Glycol 3350	1 g
Polyethylene Glycol 1000	3 g

13. From the following formula, calculate the quantity of each ingredient required to prepare 10 pints of the lotion.

Hexachlorophene	0.1 g
Cetyl Alcohol	0.5 g
Isopropyl Alcohol	70.0 g
Purified Water, to make	100.0 mL

14. An antihypertensive tablet contains the following medicinal agents. How many grams of each ingredient are required to prepare 5000 tablets?

Reserpine	100 μg
Hydralazine Hydrochloride	25 mg
Hydrochlorothiazide	15 mg

15. An estradiol transdermal system contains in each skin patch 4 mg of estradiol and 0.3 mL of alcohol. How many grams of estradiol and how many liters of alcohol would be required to manufacture a half-million patches?

16. From the following formula for an antacid tablet, calculate the quantity of each ingredient required to prepare a batch of 5000 tablets.

Magnesium Trisilicate	500 mg
Aluminum Hydroxide Dried Gel	250 mg
Mannitol	300 mg
Magnesium Stearate	10 mg

Starch   10 mg
Flavor   q.s.

17. Each 5 mL of a pediatric cough syrup is to contain the following amounts of medication. Calculate the amount of each ingredient needed to prepare a pint of the syrup.

Dextromethorphan Hydrobromide   7.5 mg
Phenylpropanolamine Hydrochloride   9.0 mg
Guaifenesin   100.0 mg
Flavored Syrup, to make   5.0 mL

18. A nasal inhaler contains 250 mg of propylhexedrine and 12.5 mg of menthol. How many grams of each ingredient would be used in preparing 5000 inhalers?

19. Each milliliter of an otic solution contains the following ingredients. Calculate the amount of each ingredient needed to manufacture one thousand 10-mL containers of the product.

Antipyrine   54 mg
Benzocaine   14 mg
Dehydrated Glycerin, to make   1 mL

20. A pediatric product is formulated to contain 100 mg of erythromycin ethylsuccinate in each dropperful (2.5 mL) of the product. How many grams of erythromycin ethylsuccinate would be required to prepare 5000 bottles, each containing 50 mL of the preparation?

21. An antacid tablet contains 80 mg of dried aluminum hydroxide gel and 20 mg of magnesium trisilicate. How many kilograms of each ingredient are required to manufacture 250,000 bottles of the product, each containing 100 tablets?

22. From the following formula for an oral electrolyte solution, calculate the amount of each ingredient required to prepare 240 mL of the solution.

Sodium   45 mEq
Potassium   20 mEq
Chloride   35 mEq
Citrate   30 mEq
Dextrose   25 g
Water ad   1000 mL

6

Density, Specific Gravity, and Specific Volume

The relative weights of equal volumes of substances are shown by their densities and their specific gravities.

DENSITY

Density is mass per unit volume of a substance, e.g., the number of grams per cubic centimeter or milliliter, the number of grains per fluidounce, the number of pounds per gallon, and so on. It is *usually* expressed as *grams per cubic centimeter (g/cc)*. Because the *gram* is defined as the mass of 1 cc of water at 4°C, the density of water is *1 g/cc*. Because the *United States Pharmacopeia* states that 1 mL may be used as the equivalent of 1 cc, for our purposes, the density of water may be expressed as *1 g/mL*. One milliliter of mercury, on the other hand, weighs 13.6 g, hence its density is *13.6 g/mL*.

Density may be calculated by dividing mass by volume. Thus, if 10 mL of sulfuric acid weigh 18 g, its density is:

$$\frac{18 \ (g)}{10 \ (mL)} = 1.8 \ g \ per \ mL$$

SPECIFIC GRAVITY

Specific gravity is a ratio, *expressed decimally,* of the weight of a substance to the weight of an equal volume of a substance chosen as a standard, both substances having the same temperature or the temperature of each being definitely known.

Water is used as the standard for the specific gravities of liquids and solids; the most useful standard for gases, which have little or no pharmaceutical significance, is hydrogen (although sometimes air is used).

Specific gravity may be calculated by dividing the weight of a given substance by the weight of an equal volume of water. Thus, if 10 mL of sulfuric acid weigh 18 g, and 10 mL of water, under similar conditions, weigh 10 g, the specific gravity of the acid is:

$$\frac{\text{Weight of 10 mL of sulfuric acid}}{\text{Weight of 10 mL of water}} = \frac{18 \ (g)}{10 \ (g)} = 1.8$$

Specific gravities can be expressed decimally to as many places as the accuracy of their determination warrants. In pharmaceutical work, this expression may be to two, three, or four decimal places. Because substances expand or contract at different rates when their temperatures change, accurate work necessitates allowing carefully for variations in the specific gravity of a substance. In the *United States Pharmacopeia,* the standard temperature for specific gravities is 25°C, except for that of alcohol, which is 15.56°C by government regulation.

DENSITY VS. SPECIFIC GRAVITY

The density of a substance is a concrete number (*1.8 g/mL* in the example), whereas specific gravity, being a ratio between like quantities, is an abstract number (*1.8* in the example). Whereas density must vary with the table of measure, specific gravity has no dimension and is therefore a constant value for each substance (when measured under controlled conditions). Thus, the density of water may be variously expressed as *1 g/mL,* or *455 gr/f℥,* or *62½ lb/cu ft,* but the specific gravity of water is always 1.

The specific gravity of a substance and its density in the metric system are numerically equal (as a result of the definition of the gram), but they are quite different when the density is expressed in the common system.

The factor *455* (rounded off from 454.57 or 454.6 gr, the weight of 1 f℥ of water at 25°C) is useful for calculating the approximate weight of a small volume of water measured in the apothecaries' system. But if *455* is used, the result should be expressed in no more than three significant figures. When quantities greater than a pint are involved, it is usually more convenient to convert them to their metric equivalent before calculating.

SPECIFIC GRAVITY OF LIQUIDS

Known Weight and Volume. Calculating the specific gravity of a liquid when its weight and volume are known involves the following.

Examples:

If 54.96 mL of an oil weigh 52.78 g, what is the specific gravity of the oil?

54.96 mL of water weigh 54.96 g

$$\text{Specific gravity of oil} = \frac{52.78 \text{ (g)}}{54.96 \text{ (g)}} = 0.9603, \text{ } answer.$$

If a pint of a certain liquid weighs 601 g, what is the specific gravity of the liquid?

1 pint = 16 fl. oz.
16 fl. oz. of water weigh 473 g

$$\text{Specific gravity of liquid} = \frac{601 \text{ (g)}}{473 \text{ (g)}} = 1.27, \text{ } answer.$$

Specific Gravity Bottle. To calculate the specific gravity of a liquid by means of a *specific gravity bottle,*[1] the container is filled and weighed first with water and then with the liquid. By subtracting the weight of the empty container from the two weights, we have the *weights of equal volumes,* even though we may not know the volumes exactly.

Example:

A specific gravity bottle weighs 23.66 g. When filled with water, it weighs 72.95 g; when filled with another liquid, it weighs 73.56 g. What is the specific gravity of the liquid?

73.56 g − 23.66 g = 49.90 g of liquid
72.95 g − 23.66 g = 49.29 g of water

---

[1] A container intended to be used as a specific gravity bottle, with a known capacity (commonly 10, 25, or 100 mL) so that the weight of water it will contain is already known, is called a *pycnometer.*

$$\text{Specific gravity of liquid} = \frac{49.90 \text{ (g)}}{49.29 \text{ (g)}} = 1.012, \text{ answer.}$$

Displacement or Plummet Method. Calculating the specific gravity of a liquid determined by the displacement or plummet method is based on the *Archimedes' principle,* which states that a body immersed in a liquid displaces an amount of the liquid equal to its own volume and suffers an apparent loss in weight equal to the weight of the displaced liquid. Thus, we can weigh a plummet when suspended in water and when suspended in a liquid the specific gravity of which is to be determined, and by subtracting these weights from the weight of the plummet in air, we get the *weights of equal volumes of the liquids* needed in our calculation.

Example:

A glass plummet weighs 12.64 g in air, 8.57 g when immersed in water, and 9.12 g when immersed in an oil. Calculate the specific gravity of the oil.

12.64 g − 9.12 g = 3.52 g of displaced oil
12.64 g − 8.57 g = 4.07 g of displaced water

$$\text{Specific gravity of oil} = \frac{3.52 \text{ (g)}}{4.07 \text{ (g)}} = 0.865, \text{ answer.}$$

SPECIFIC GRAVITY OF SOLIDS

Solids Heavier Than and Insoluble in Water. To calculate the specific gravity of a solid *heavier than* and *insoluble in water,* simply divide the weight of the solid in air by the weight of water that it displaces when immersed in it. The weight of water displaced (apparent loss of weight in water) is equal to the *weight of an equal volume of water.*

Example:

A piece of glass weighs 38.525 g in air and 23.525 g when immersed in water. What is its specific gravity?

38.525 g − 23.525 g = 15.000 g of displaced water *(weight of an equal volume of water)*

$$\text{Specific gravity of glass} = \frac{38.525 \text{ (g)}}{15.000 \text{ (g)}} = 2.568, \text{ answer.}$$

Solids Heavier Than and Soluble in Water. *The weights of equal volumes of any two substances are proportional to their specific gravities.* Therefore, given a solid heavier than and soluble in water, we may use the method just discussed, but *substituting some liquid of known specific gravity* in which the solid is insoluble.

Example:

A crystal of a chemical salt weighs 6.423 g in air and 2.873 g when immersed in an oil having a specific gravity of 0.858. What is the specific gravity of the salt?

6.423 g − 2.873 g = 3.550 g of displaced oil

$$\frac{3.550 \text{ (g of oil)}}{6.423 \text{ (g of salt)}} = \frac{0.858 \text{ (sp. gr. of oil)}}{x \text{ (sp. gr. of salt)}}$$

$$x = 1.55, \text{ answer.}$$

Solids Lighter Than and Insoluble in Water. Calculating the specific gravity of a solid *lighter than* and *insoluble in water* involves the use of a sinker, which is attached to the solid to prevent it from floating (and therefore, having no apparent weight at all). The weight of the sinker in air is of no interest to us here, but its weight when immersed in water alone must be known so that the combined weight of the solid in air and the sinker in water may be calculated. By subtracting from this weight the weight of solid and sinker when immersed in water, the weight of the water displaced by the solid (and therefore the *weight of an equal volume of water*) is calculated.

Example:

A piece of wax weighs 16.35 g in air, and a sinker weighs 32.84 g immersed in water. When they are fastened together and immersed in water, their combined weight is 29.68 g. Calculate the specific gravity of the wax.

32.84 g + 16.35 g = 49.19 g, combined weight of sinker in water and of wax in air

49.19 g − 29.68 g = 19.51 g, weight of water displaced by wax *(weight of equal volume of water)*

$$\text{Specific gravity of wax} = \frac{16.35 \ (g)}{19.51 \ (g)} = 0.838, \textit{answer.}$$

Granulated Solids Heavier Than and Insoluble in Water. To calculate the specific gravity of granulated solids heavier than and insoluble in water, a specific gravity bottle can be used with crystals, powders, and other forms of solids the volume of which cannot be directly measured. If such a substance is *insoluble in water,* we may weigh a portion of it, introduce this amount into the bottle, fill up the bottle with water, and weigh the mixture. The solid will displace a *volume of water equal to its own volume,* and the weight of this displaced water can be calculated.

Example:

A bottle weighs 50.0 g when empty and 96.8 g when filled with water. If 28.8 g of granulated metal are placed in the bottle and the bottle is filled with water, the total weight is 118.4 g. What is the specific gravity of the metal?

96.8 g − 50.0 g   = 46.8 g, weight of water filling the bottle
46.8 g + 28.8 g   = 75.6 g, combined weight of water and metal
118.4 g − 50.0 g   = 68.4 g, combined weight of water and metal in bottle
75.6 g − 68.4 g   = 7.2 g, weight of water displaced by metal
(weight of equal volume of water)

$$\text{Specific gravity of metal} = \frac{28.8 \ (g)}{7.2 \ (g)} = 4.0, \textit{answer.}$$

SPECIFIC VOLUME

The volume of a unit weight of a substance may be expressed in any convenient denominations, such as so many *cubic feet per pound* or *gallons per pound,* but more frequently as *milliliters per gram (mL/g).*

Specific volume, in pharmaceutical practice, is usually defined as an abstract number representing the ratio, *expressed decimally,* of the volume of a substance to the volume of an equal weight of another substance taken as a standard, both having the same temperature. Water is the standard for liquids and solids.

Whereas specific gravity is a comparison of weights of equal volumes, specific volume is a comparison of volumes of equal weights. Because of this relationship, specific gravity and specific volume are *reciprocals,* i.e., if they are multiplied together, the product is 1. Specific volume tells us how much greater (or smaller) in volume a mass is than the same weight of water. It may be calculated by dividing the volume of a given mass by the volume of an equal weight of water. Thus, if 25 g of glycerin measure 20 mL and 25 g of water measure 25 mL under the same conditions, the specific volume of the glycerin is:

$$\frac{\text{Volume of 25 g of glycerin}}{\text{Volume of 25 g of water}} = \frac{20 \text{ (mL)}}{25 \text{ (mL)}} = 0.8$$

Volume of a Liquid, Given the Volume of a Specified Weight. Calculating the specific volume of a liquid, given the volume of a specified weight, involves the following.

Example:

Calculate the specific volume of a syrup, 91.0 mL of which weigh 107.16 g.

107.16 g of water measure 107.16 mL

$$\text{Specific volume of syrup} = \frac{91.0 \text{ (mL)}}{107.16 \text{ (mL)}} = 0.849, \text{ answer.}$$

Specific Volume of a Liquid, Given its Specific Gravity and its Specific Gravity Given its Specific Volume. Because specific gravity and specific volume are reciprocals, a substance that is heavier than water will have a higher specific gravity and a lower specific volume, whereas a substance that is lighter than water will have a lower specific gravity and a higher specific volume. It follows, therefore, that we may determine the specific volume of a substance by dividing 1 by its specific gravity, and we may determine the specific gravity of a substance by dividing 1 by its specific volume.

Examples:

What is the specific volume of phosphoric acid having a specific gravity of 1.71?

$$\frac{1}{1.71} = 0.585, \text{ answer.}$$

If a liquid has specific volume of 1.396, what is its specific gravity?

$$\frac{1}{1.396} = 0.716, \text{ answer.}$$

Practice Problems

1. If 250 mL of alcohol weigh 203 g, what is its density?

2. A piece of copper metal weighs 53.6 g, and has a volume of 6 mL. Calculate its density.

3. If 150 mL of polyethylene glycol 400 weigh 170 g, what is its specific gravity?

4. If a liter of sorbitol solution weighs 1285 g, what is its specific gravity?

5. If 500 mL of ferric chloride solution weigh 650 g, what is its specific gravity?

6. If 380 g of cottonseed oil measure 415 mL, what is its specific gravity?

7. If 2 fluidounces of glycerin weigh 74.1 g, what is its specific gravity?

8. Five pints of hydrochloric acid weigh 2.79 kg. Calculate its specific gravity.

9. A pycnometer weighs 21.62 g. Filled with water, it weighs 46.71 g; filled with another liquid, it weighs 43.28 g. Calculate the specific gravity of the liquid.

10. A glass plummet weighs 14.35 g in air, 11.40 g when immersed in water, and 8.95 g when immersed in sulfuric acid. Calculate the specific gravity of the acid.

11. If a solid weighs 84.62 g in air and 58.48 g when immersed in water, what is its specific gravity?

12. A chemical crystal weighs 3.630 g in air and 1.820 g when immersed in an oil. If the specific gravity of the oil is 0.837, what is the specific gravity of the chemical?

13. A piece of wax weighs 42.65 g in air, and a sinker weighs 38.42 g in water. Together, they weigh 33.18 g in water. Calculate the specific gravity of the wax.

14. An insoluble powder weighs 12 g. A specific gravity bottle, weighing 21 g when empty, weighs 121 g when filled with water. When the powder is introduced into the bottle and the bottle is filled with water, the three together weigh 130 g. What is the specific gravity of the powder?

15. If 73.42 g of a liquid measure 81.5 mL, what is its specific volume?

16. If 120 g of acetone measure 150 mL, what is its specific volume?

17. The specific gravity of alcohol is 0.815. What is its specific volume?

18. If chloroform has a specific gravity of 1.476, what is its specific volume?

19. What is the specific gravity of a liquid having a specific volume of 0.825?

20. A modified Ringer's Irrigation has the following formula:

Sodium Chloride	8.6 g
Potassium Chloride	0.3 g
Calcium Chloride	0.33 g
PEG 3350	60.0 g
Water for Injection ad	1000. mL

Assuming that 980 mL of water are used in preparing the irrigation, calculate its specific gravity.

USE OF SPECIFIC GRAVITY IN CALCULATIONS OF WEIGHT AND VOLUME

The weights of equal volumes and the volumes of equal weights of liquids are proportional to their specific gravities. To calculate, therefore, the *weight of a given volume* or the *volume of a given weight* of a liquid, its specific gravity must be known.

When *specific gravity is used as a factor in a calculation, the result should contain no more significant figures than the number in the factor.*

Because of the simple relationship between the units in the metric system, such problems are solved simply and easily when only metric quantities are involved, but they become more complex when units of the common systems are used.

Weight of a Liquid with Known Volume and Specific Gravity. The *weight of any given volume* of a liquid of known specific gravity can be calculated by this proportion:

$$\frac{\text{Specific gravity of water}}{\text{Specific gravity of liquid}} = \frac{\text{Weight of equal volume of water}}{x}$$

$$x = \text{Weight of liquid}$$

From this calculation, we may derive a useful equation:

Weight of liquid $=$ Weight of equal volume of water $\times$ Specific gravity of liquid

Examples:

What is the weight of 3620 mL of alcohol with a specific gravity of 0.820?

3620 mL of water weigh 3620 g
3620 g $\times$ 0.820 $=$ 2968 g, *answer.*

What is the weight, in grams, of 2 fluidounces of a liquid having a specific gravity of 1.118?

In this type of problem, it is best to convert the given volume to its metric equivalent first and then solve the problem in the metric system.

2 $\times$ 29.57 mL $=$ 59.14 mL
59.14 mL of water weigh 59.14 g
59.14 g $\times$ 1.118 $=$ 66.12 g, *answer.*

Volume of a Liquid with Known Weight and Specific Gravity. The *volume of any given weight* of a liquid of known specific gravity can be calculated by this proportion:

$$\frac{\text{Specific gravity of liquid}}{\text{Specific gravity of water}} = \frac{\text{Volume of equal weight of water}}{x}$$

$$x = \text{Volume of liquid}$$

And the derived equation will be:

$$\text{Volume of liquid} = \frac{\text{Volume of equal weight of water}}{\text{Specific gravity of liquid}}$$

Examples:

What is the volume of 492 g of nitric acid with a specific gravity of 1.40?

492 g of water measure 492 mL

$$\frac{492 \text{ mL}}{1.40} = 351 \text{ mL, } answer.$$

What is the volume, in milliliters, of 1 lb methyl salicylate with a specific gravity of 1.185?

1 lb = 454 g
454 g of water measure 454 mL

$$\frac{454 \text{ mL}}{1.185} = 383.1 \text{ mL, } answer.$$

What is the volume, in pints, of 50 lb of glycerin having a specific gravity of 1.25?

50 lb = 454 × 50 = 22700 g
22700 g of water measure 22700 mL and 1 pint = 473 mL

$$\frac{22700 \text{ mL}}{1.25} = 18160 \text{ mL} \div 473 \text{ mL} = 38.4 \text{ pints, } answer.$$

Cost of Given Volume of Liquid by Weight. Calculating the cost of a given volume of
a liquid bought by weight involves the following.

Examples:

What is the cost of 1000 mL of glycerin, specific gravity 1.25, bought at $4.25 per pound?

1000 mL of water weigh 1000 g
Weight of 1000 mL of glycerin = 1000 g × 1.25 = 1250 g
1 lb = 454 g

$$\frac{454 \text{ (g)}}{1250 \text{ (g)}} = \frac{(\$) \ 4.25}{(\$) \ x}$$

$$x = \$11.70, \ answer.$$

*What is the cost of 2 fluidounces of cinnamon oil, specific gravity 1.055, bought at $27.00
per quarter pound?*

2 fl. oz. = 59.14 mL
59.14 mL of water weigh 59.14 g
Weight of 59.14 mL of oil = 59.14 g × 1.055 = 62.39 g
¼ lb = 113.5 g

$$\frac{113.5 \text{ (g)}}{62.39 \text{ (g)}} = \frac{(\$) \ 27.00}{(\$) \ x}$$

$$x = \$14.84, \ answer.$$

What is the cost of 1 pint of chloroform, specific gravity 1.475, bought at $10.25 per pound?

1 pint = 473 mL
473 mL of water weigh 473 g
Weight of 473 mL of chloroform = 473 g × 1.475 = 697.7 g
1 lb = 454 g

$$\frac{454 \text{ (g)}}{697.7 \text{ (g)}} = \frac{(\$) \ 10.25}{(\$) \ x}$$

$$x = \$15.75, \ answer.$$

Practice Problems

1. What is the weight of 100 mL of hydrochloric acid having a specific gravity of
   1.16?

2.   What is the weight of 300 mL of glycerin having a specific gravity of 1.25?

3.   What is the weight, in grams, of 14 mL of mercury having a specific gravity of 13.6?

4.   What is the weight, in grams, of 225 mL of sulfuric acid having a specific gravity of 1.83?

5.   What is the weight, in kilograms, of 5 liters of sulfuric acid with a specific gravity of 1.84?

6.   What is the weight, in pounds, of 5 pints of nitric acid having a specific gravity of 1.42?

7.   What is the weight, in grams, of 4 fluidounces of orange oil with a specific gravity of 0.844?

8.   Calculate the weight, in grams, of 10 pints of hydrochloric acid having a specific gravity of 1.155.

9.   What is the weight, in kilograms, of 1 gallon of sorbitol solution having a specific gravity of 1.285?

10. What is the weight, in grams, of 1 pint of a mixture of equal parts of alcohol (specific gravity 0.812) and glycerin (specific gravity 1.25)?

11. If 500 mL of mineral oil are used to prepare a liter of mineral oil emulsion, how many grams of the oil, having a specific gravity of 0.87, would be used in the preparation of 1 gallon of the emulsion?

12. What is the volume, in milliliters, of 5 lb of ether having a specific gravity of 0.71?

13. What is the volume, in milliliters, of 1 lb of benzyl benzoate having a specific gravity of 1.120?

14. What is the volume, in milliliters, of 1 kg of sulfuric acid with a specific gravity of 1.83?

15. What is the volume of 1000 g of mercury having a specific gravity of 13.6?

16. A sunscreen lotion contains 5 g of menthyl salicylate (specific gravity 1.045) per 100 mL. How many milliliters of menthyl salicylate should be used in preparing 1 gallon of the lotion?

17. What is the volume of 650 g of ferric chloride solution with a specific gravity of 1.30?

18. If ampuls of amyl nitrite inhalant each contain 0.3 mL of amyl nitrite, having a specific gravity of 0.87, how many grams of the drug would be used in preparing 4000 ampuls?

19. What is the volume, in milliliters, of a liniment containing 1 lb of chloroform (specific gravity 1.475) and 5 lb of methyl salicylate (specific gravity 1.180)?

20. If Light Mineral Oil has a specific gravity of 0.85 and Mineral Oil has a specific gravity of 0.87, what is the difference, in grams, between the weights of a pint of each oil?

21. If fifty glycerin suppositories are made from the following formula, how many

milliliters of glycerin, having a specific gravity of 1.25, would be used in the preparation of 96 suppositories?

Glycerin	91 g
Sodium Stearate	9 g
Purified Water	5 g

22. What is the volume, in pints, of 10 lb of peppermint oil having a specific gravity of 0.908?

23. The normal range of specific gravity of urine is about 1.003 to 1.030. Using 10-mL urine samples with these extremes of specific gravity, what would be the difference in weight, in milligrams, between the two samples?

24. What is the cost of 3 liters of chloroform (specific gravity 1.475) bought at $9.75 per pound?

25. What will 10 lb of glycerin (specific gravity 1.25) cost at $4.75 per pint?

26. If 250 mg of propylhexedrine, a liquid having a specific gravity of 0.85, are used in a single nasal inhaler, how many milliliters of the drug would be used in the manufacture of 1000 inhalers?

27. The formula for 1000 g of Polyethylene Glycol Ointment calls for 600 g polyethylene glycol 400. At $9.15 per pint, what is the cost of the polyethylene glycol 400, specific gravity 1.140, needed to prepare 4000 g of the ointment?

28. Glycerin, USP (specific gravity 1.25) costs $4.25 per pound. If students in a dispensing laboratory use 1 pint of glycerin in preparing compounded prescriptions, what is the cost of the glycerin used?

29. Cocoa butter (theobroma oil), which is solid at room temperature and melts at 34°C, has a specific gravity of 0.86. If a formula calls for 48 mL of theobroma oil, what would be the corresponding weight of cocoa butter to use?

30. A transdermal patch for smoking cessation contains 30 mg of liquid nicotine per patch. If nicotine has a specific gravity of 1.01, how many milliliters of the agent are required to manufacture 1 million patches?

7

Percentage and Ratio Strength Calculations

PERCENTAGE

The term *percent* and its corresponding sign (%) mean "by the hundred" or "in a hundred," and *percentage* means "rate per hundred"; so *50 percent* (or 50%) and *a percentage of 50* are equivalent expressions. A percent may also be expressed as a *ratio*, represented as a common or decimal fraction. For example, *50%* means *50 parts in 100* of the same kind, and may be expressed as $^{50}/_{100}$ or *0.50.* Percent, therefore, is simply another fraction of such frequent and familiar use that its numerator is expressed but its denominator is left understood. It should be noted that percent is always an abstract quantity, and that, as such, it may be applied to anything.

For the purposes of computation, percents are usually changed to equivalent decimal fractions. This change is made by dropping the percent sign (%) and dividing the expressed numerator by *100.* Thus, *12.5%* $= \dfrac{12.5}{100}$, or *0.125;* and *0.05%* $= \dfrac{0.05}{100}$, or *0.0005.* We must not forget that in the reverse process (changing a decimal to a percent), the decimal is multiplied by *100* and the percent sign (%) is affixed.

Percentage is an essential part of pharmaceutical calculations. The pharmacist encounters it frequently and uses it as a convenient means of expressing the concentration of a solute in a solution, the amount of active material in a drug or preparation, or the quantity of an ingredient in a mixture.

PERCENTAGE PREPARATIONS

Percentage, as it applies to solutions and other liquid preparations (mixtures, lotions, suspensions), expresses *parts per 100 parts.* Therefore, in a *true percentage solution* or *liquid preparation,* the *parts* of the percentage would represent the *grams* of solute or constituent in *100 g* of solution or liquid preparation. In general practice, however, the pharmacist most frequently encounters a different kind of percentage solution or liquid preparation, one in which the *parts* of the percentage represent *grams* of a solute or constituent in *100 mL* of solution or liquid preparation.

To avoid the possibility of any misinterpretation of the meaning of the term "percentage solution or liquid preparation," percentage concentrations are expressed as follows:

Percent weight-in-volume (w/v) expresses the number of *g* of a constituent in *100 mL* of solution or liquid preparation, and is used regardless of whether water or another liquid is the solvent or vehicle.

Percent volume-in-volume (v/v) expresses the number of *milliliters* of a constituent in *100 mL* of solution or liquid preparation.

Percent weight-in-weight (w/w) expresses the number of *grams* of a constituent in *100 g* of solution or preparation.

The term *percent* used without qualification means, for mixtures of solids and semisolids, percent weight-in-weight; for solutions or suspensions of solids in liquids, percent weight-in-volume; for solutions of liquids in liquids, percent volume-in-volume; and for solutions of gases in liquids, percent weight-in-volume. For example, a 1% solution is prepared by dissolving 1 g of a solid or 1 mL of a liquid in sufficient of the solvent to make 100 mL of the solution. In the dispensing of prescription medications, slight changes in volume owing to variations in room temperature may be disregarded.

The term *milligrams percent* (mg%) expresses the number of milligrams of a substance in 100 mL of liquid. It is used frequently to denote the concentration of a drug or natural substance in a biologic fluid, as in the blood. Thus, the statement that the concentration of nonprotein nitrogen in the blood is 30 mg% means that each 100 mL of blood contains 30 mg of nonprotein nitrogen. As noted in this chapter in the section entitled, "Expressing Clinical Laboratory Test Values," quantities of substances present in biologic fluids may also be stated in terms of milligrams per deciliter (mg/dL) of fluid.

For dilute solutions, it is convenient to express concentrations in terms of *parts per million* (ppm). The term is commonly used in designating test limits, as in the example, the limit of arsenic in zinc oxide is 6 parts per million (6 ppm) or 0.0006%.

PERCENTAGE WEIGHT-IN-VOLUME

One way of making all weight-in-volume solutions conform to the definition is to convert all common and apothecaries' weights to grams and all volumes to milliliters before expressing percentage strength (see Appendix A for intersystem conversion). Although this method is recommended in the text for ease of calculation and in keeping with contemporary practice, such a procedure is not required.

For, if 1 g in 100 mL of solution or liquid preparation is taken as the only "correct" strength of a 1% (w/v) solution, this means that 1 g of solute is contained in a volume of solution *that would weigh 100 g if, like water, the solution had a specific gravity of 1*; in other words, each milliliter of solution weighed *1 g*. Hence, to make a solution of the same strength by any system of measure, we have only to dissolve *1* weight unit of solute in sufficient solvent to make a volume that would weigh *100* of those weight units if the solution were pure water.

A solution so compounded, then, would contain not only *1 g* in every *100 mL* (the volume of *100 g* of water), but likewise approximately *4.55* grains in every fluidounce (the volume of *455 grains* of water at 25°C). Therefore, we may look on a *weight-in-volume* solution as a kind of *weight-in-weight* solution in disguise—the percentage strength based after all on a comparison of parts by weight, but the weight of the solution arbitrarily calculated from its designated volume as if it has a specific gravity of *1.00*.

Weight of Active Ingredient in a Specific Volume, Given its Percentage Weight-in-Volume. Taking water to represent any solvent or vehicle, we may prepare weight-in-volume percentage solutions or liquid preparations by the metric system if we use the following rule.

Multiply the required number of milliliters by the percentage strength, expressed as a decimal, to obtain the number of grams of solute or constituent in the solution or liquid preparation. *The volume, in milliliters, represents the weight in grams of the solution or liquid preparation as if it were pure water.*

Volume (mL) (representing grams) $\times$ % (expressed as a decimal) $=$ g of solute or constituent

Examples:

How many grams of dextrose are required to prepare 4000 mL of a 5% solution?

4000 mL represent 4000 g of solution

5% = 0.05
4000 g × 0.05 = 200 g, *answer.*

Or, solving by dimensional analysis:

$$\frac{5 \text{ g}}{100 \text{ ml}} \times 4000 \text{ ml} = 200 \text{ g, } answer.$$

How many grams of potassium permanganate should be used in compounding the following prescription?

℞   Potassium Permanganate   0.02%
       Purified Water   ad   250.0
       Sig. As directed.
   250 mL represent 250 g of solution
            0.02% = 0.0002
   250 g × 0.0002 = 0.05 g, *answer.*

How many grams of aminobenzoic acid should be used in preparing 8 fluidounces of a 5% solution in 70% alcohol?

   8 fl. oz. = 8 × 29.57 mL = 236.56 mL
   236.56 mL represents 236.56 g of solution
   5% = 0.05
   236.56 g × 0.05 = 11.83 g, *answer.*

Percentage Weight-in-Volume of Solution, Given Weight of Solute or Constituent and Volume of Solution or Liquid Preparation. To calculate the percentage weight-in-volume of a solution or liquid preparation, given the weight of the solute or constituent and the volume of the solution or liquid preparation, it should be remembered that the volume, in milliliters, of the solution represents the weight, in grams, of the solution or liquid preparation as if it were pure water.

Example:

   What is the percentage strength (w/v) of a solution of urea, if 80 mL contain 12 g?

   80 mL of water weigh 80 g

$$\frac{80 \text{ (g)}}{12 \text{ (g)}} = \frac{100 \text{ (\%)}}{x \text{ (\%)}}$$

$$x = 15\%, answer.$$

Volume of Solution or Liquid Preparation, Given Percentage Strength Weight-in-Volume and Weight of Solute. Calculating the volume of a solution or liquid preparation, given its percentage strength weight-in-volume and the weight of the solute or constituent, involves the following.

Example:

   How many milliliters of a 3% solution can be made from 27 g of ephedrine sulfate?

$$\frac{3 \text{ (\%)}}{100 \text{ (\%)}} = \frac{27 \text{ (g)}}{x \text{ (g)}}$$

$$x = 900 \text{ g, weight of the solution if it were water}$$

   Volume (in mL) = 900 mL, *answer.*

PERCENTAGE VOLUME-IN-VOLUME

Liquids are usually measured by volume, and the percentage strength indicates the number of parts by volume of the active ingredient contained in the total volume of the solution or liquid preparation considered as 100 parts by volume. If there is any possibility of misinterpretation, this kind of percentage should be specified: e.g., *10% (v/v)*.

Volume of Active Ingredient in a Specific Volume, Given Percentage Strength Volume-in-Volume. Calculating the volume of the active ingredient in a specified volume of a solution or liquid preparation, given its percentage strength volume-in-volume, involves the following.

Example:

How many milliliters of liquefied phenol should be used in compounding the following prescription?

   R   Liquefied Phenol   2.5%
         Calamine Lotion   ad   240.0 mL
         Sig. For external use.

Volume (mL) × % (expressed as a decimal) = milliliters of active ingredient
240 mL × 0.025 = 6 mL, *answer.*

Or, solving by dimensional analysis:

$$\frac{2.5 \text{ mL}}{100 \text{ mL}} \times 240 \text{ ml} = 6 \text{ mL}, \textit{ answer.}$$

Percentage Volume-in-Volume of Solution or Liquid Preparation, Given Volume of Active Ingredient and Volume of Solution. To determine the percentage volume-in-volume of a solution or liquid preparation, given the volume of active ingredient and the volume of the solution or liquid preparation, the required volumes may have to be calculated from given weights and specific gravities.

Example:

In preparing 250 mL of a certain lotion, a pharmacist used 4 mL of liquefied phenol. What was the percentage (v/v) of liquefied phenol in the lotion?

$$\frac{250 \text{ (mL)}}{4 \text{ (mL)}} = \frac{100 \text{ (\%)}}{x \text{ (\%)}}$$

$$x = 1.6\%, \textit{ answer.}$$

What is the percentage strength (v/v) of a solution of 800 g of a liquid with a specific gravity of 0.800 in enough water to make 4000 mL?

800 g of water measure 800 mL
800 mL ÷ 0.800 = 1000 mL of active ingredient

$$\frac{4000 \text{ (mL)}}{1000 \text{ (mL)}} = \frac{100 \text{ (\%)}}{x \text{ (\%)}}$$

$$x = 25\%, \textit{ answer.}$$

Or, solving by dimensional analysis:

$$\frac{800 \text{ mL}}{0.800} \times \frac{1}{4000 \text{ mL}} \times 100\% = 25\%, \textit{ answer.}$$

Volume of Solution or Liquid Preparation, Given Volume of Active Ingredient and its Percentage Strength (v/v). Calculating the volume of a solution or liquid preparation, given the volume of the active ingredient and its percentage strength (v/v), may require first determining the volume of the active ingredient from its weight and specific gravity.

Examples:

Peppermint spirit contains 10% (v/v) of peppermint oil. What volume of the spirit will contain 75 mL of peppermint oil?

$$\frac{10 \text{ (\%)}}{100 \text{ (\%)}} = \frac{75 \text{ (mL)}}{x \text{ (mL)}}$$

$$x = 750 \text{ mL, } \textit{answer.}$$

Chloroform liniment contains 30% (v/v) of chloroform. How many milliliters of chloroform liniment can be prepared from 1 lb of chloroform (sp. gr. 1.475)?

1 lb = <u>454 g</u>
454 g of water measure <u>454 mL</u>
454 mL ÷ <u>1.475</u> = 308 mL of chloroform

$$\frac{30 \text{ (\%)}}{100 \text{ (\%)}} = \frac{308 \text{ (mL)}}{x \text{ (mL)}}$$

$$x = 1027 \text{ or } 1030 \text{ mL, } \textit{answer.}$$

Or, solving by dimensional analysis:

$$\frac{1 \text{ lb}}{30\%} \times \frac{454 \text{ g}}{1 \text{ lb}} \times \frac{1 \text{ mL}}{1 \text{ g}} \times \frac{1}{1.475} \times 100\% = 1026 \text{ or } 1030 \text{ mL, } \textit{answer.}$$

PERCENTAGE WEIGHT-IN-WEIGHT

Percentage weight-in-weight (*true percentage* or *percentage by weight*) indicates the number of parts by weight of active ingredient contained in the total weight of the solution or mixture considered as 100 parts by weight.

Liquids are not customarily measured by weight. Therefore, a weight-in-weight solution or liquid preparation of a solid or a liquid in a liquid should be so designated: e.g., *10% (w/w).*

Weight of Active Ingredient in a Specific Weight of Solution or Liquid Preparation, Given its Weight-in-Weight Percentage Strength. Calculating this value in a specified weight of the solution or liquid preparation involves the following.

Examples:

How many grams of phenol should be used to prepare 240 g of a 5% (w/w) solution in water?

Weight of solution (g) × % (expressed as a decimal) = g of solute
240 g × 0.05 = 12 g, *answer.*

How many grams of a drug substance are required to make 120 mL of a 20% (w/w) solution having a specific gravity of 1.15?

120 mL of water weigh 120 g
120 g × 1.15 = 138 g, weight of 120 mL of solution
138 g × 0.20 = 27.6 g plus enough water to make 120 mL, *answer*.

Or, solving by dimensional analysis:

$$120 \text{ mL} \times \frac{1.15 \text{ g}}{1 \text{ mL}} \times \frac{20\%}{100\%} = 27.6 \text{ g, } \textit{answer}.$$

Weight of Either Active Ingredient or Diluent, Given Weight of the Other and Percentage Strength (w/w) of Solution. Calculating these values involves the following. The weights of active ingredient and diluent are proportional to their percentages.

Example:

How many grams of a drug substance should be dissolved in 240 mL of water to make a 4% (w/w) solution?

100% − 4% = 96% (by weight) of water
240 mL of water weigh 240 g

$$\frac{96 \ (\%)}{4 \ (\%)} = \frac{240 \ (\text{g})}{\text{x} \ (\text{g})}$$

$$\text{x} = 10 \text{ g, } \textit{answer}.$$

It is usually impossible to prepare a specified *volume* of a solution or liquid preparation of given weight-in-weight percentage strength, because the volume displaced by the active ingredient cannot be known in advance. If an excess is acceptable, we may make a volume somewhat more than that specified by taking the given volume to refer to the solvent or vehicle and from this quantity calculating the weight of the solvent or vehicle (the specific gravity of the solvent or vehicle must be known). Using this weight, we may follow the method just described to calculate the corresponding weight of the active ingredient needed.

Example:

How should you prepare 100 mL of a 2% (w/w) solution of a drug substance in a solvent having a specific gravity of 1.25?

100 mL of water weigh 100 g
100 g × 1.25 = 125 g, weight of 100 mL of solvent
100% − 2% = 98% (by weight) of solvent

$$\frac{98 \ (\%)}{2 \ (\%)} = \frac{125 \ (\text{g})}{\text{x} \ (\text{g})}$$

$$\text{x} = 2.55 \text{ g}$$

Therefore, dissolve 2.55 g of drug substance in 125 g (or 100 mL) of solvent, *answer*.

Percentage Strength (w/w) of Solution, Given Weight of Active Ingredient and Weight of Solution. If the weight of the finished solution or liquid preparation is not given when calculating its percentage strength, other data must be supplied from which it may be calculated: the weights of both ingredients, for instance, or the volume and specific gravity of the solution or liquid preparation.

Examples:

If 1500 g of a solution contain 75 g of a drug substance, what is the percentage strength (w/w) of the solution?

$$\frac{1500 \text{ (g)}}{75 \text{ (g)}} = \frac{100 \text{ (\%)}}{x \text{ (\%)}}$$

$$x = 5\%, \text{ answer.}$$

Or, solving by dimensional analysis:

$$\frac{75 \text{ g}}{1500 \text{ g}} \times 100\% = 5\%, \text{ answer.}$$

If 5 g of boric acid are dissolved in 100 mL of water, what is the percentage strength (w/w) of the solution?

100 mL of water weigh 100 g
100 g + 5 g = 105 g, weight of solution

$$\frac{105 \text{ (g)}}{5 \text{ (g)}} = \frac{100 \text{ (\%)}}{x \text{ (\%)}}$$

$$x = 4.76\%, \text{ answer.}$$

If 1000 mL of syrup with a specific gravity of 1.313 contain 850 g of sucrose, what is its percentage strength (w/w)?

1000 mL of water weigh 1000 g
1000 g × 1.313 = 1313 g, weight of 1000 mL of syrup

$$\frac{1313 \text{ (g)}}{850 \text{ (g)}} = \frac{100 \text{ (\%)}}{x \text{ (\%)}}$$

$$x = 64.7\%, \text{ answer.}$$

Weight of Solution or Liquid Preparation, Given Weight of its Active Ingredient and Percentage Strength (w/w). Calculating the weight of a solution or liquid preparation, given the weight of its active ingredient and its percentage strength (w/w) involves the following.

Example:

What weight of a 5% (w/w) solution can be prepared from 2 g of active ingredient?

$$\frac{5 \text{ (\%)}}{100 \text{ (\%)}} = \frac{2 \text{ (g)}}{x \text{ (g)}}$$

$$x = 40 \text{ g, answer.}$$

Weight-in-Weight Mixtures of Solids and Semisolids

Solids and semisolids are usually measured by weight, and the percentage strength of a mixture of solids indicates the number of parts by weight of the active ingredient contained in the total weight of the mixture considered as *100 parts* by weight.

Amount of Active Ingredient in a Specified Weight of a Solid/Semisolid Mixture, Given its Percentage Strength (w/w). Calculating this amount involves the following.

Examples:

How many milligrams of hydrocortisone should be used in compounding the following prescription?

R̶   Hydrocortisone   1/8%
         Hydrophilic Ointment   ad   10.0 g
         Sig. Apply.

⅛% = 0.125%
10 g × 0.00125 = 0.0125 g or 12.5 mg, *answer.*

How many grams of benzocaine should be used in compounding the following prescription?

R̶   Benzocaine   2%
         Polyethylene Glycol Base   ad   2.0
         Make 24 such suppositories
         Sig. Insert one as directed.

2 g × 24 = 48 g, total weight of mixture
48 g × 0.02 = 0.96 g, *answer.*

Or, solving by dimensional analysis:

$$24 \text{ supp.} \times \frac{2.0 \text{ g}}{1 \text{ supp.}} \times \frac{2\%}{100\%} = 0.96 \text{ g, } answer.$$

USE OF PERCENT IN COMPENDIAL STANDARDS

Percent is used in the *United States Pharmacopeia* to express the degree of tolerance permitted in the purity of single chemical entities and in the labeled quantities of ingredients in dosage forms. For instance, according to the USP, "Aspirin contains not less than 99.5% and not more than 100.5% of $C_9H_8O_4$ (pure chemical aspirin) calculated on a dried basis." Further, "Aspirin Tablets contain not less than 90.0% and not more than 110.0% of the labeled amount of $C_9H_8O_4$." Although dosage forms are formulated with the intent to provide 100% of the quantity of each ingredient declared on the label, some tolerance is permitted to allow for analytic error, unavoidable variations in manufacturing and compounding, and for deterioration to an extent considered insignificant under practical conditions.

Problem Solving. To solve problems involving the use of percent in compendial standards, observe the following.

Example:

If ibuprofen tablets are permitted to contain not less than 90% and not more than 110% of the labeled amount of ibuprofen, what would be the permissible range in content of the drug, expressed in milligrams, for ibuprofen tablets labeled 200 mg each?

$$90\% \text{ of } 200 \text{ mg} \quad = \quad 180 \text{ mg}$$
$$110\% \text{ of } 200 \text{ mg} \quad = \quad 220 \text{ mg}$$
$$\text{range} \quad = \quad 180 \text{ mg to } 220 \text{ mg, } answer.$$

RATIO STRENGTH

The concentration of weak solutions or liquid preparations is frequently expressed in terms of ratio strength. Because all percentages are a ratio of parts per hundred, ratio strength is merely another way of expressing the percentage strength of solutions or liquid preparations (and, less frequently, of mixtures of solids). For example, *5% means 5 parts per 100* or *5:100*. Although *5 parts per 100* designates a ratio strength, it is customary to translate this designation into a ratio, the first figure of which is *1*; thus, *5:100 = 1:20*.

When a ratio strength, for example, *1:1000*, is used to designate a concentration, it is to be interpreted as follows:

For solids in liquids = 1 g of solute or constituent in *1000* mL of solution or liquid preparation.
For liquids in liquids = 1 mL of constituent in *1000 mL* of solution or liquid preparation.
For solids in solids = 1 g of constituent in *1000 g* of mixture.

The ratio and percentage strengths of any solution or mixture of solids are proportional, and either is easily converted to the other by the use of proportion.

Ratio Strength Given Percentage Strength. To calculate this value, observe the following.

Example:

Express 0.02% as a ratio strength.

$$\frac{0.02 \ (\%)}{100 \ (\%)} = \frac{1 \ (\text{part})}{x \ (\text{parts})}$$

$$x = 5000$$

$$\text{Ratio strength} = 1:5000, \ answer.$$

Percentage Strength Given Ratio Strength. To calculate this value, observe the following.

Example:

Express 1:4000 as a percentage strength.

$$\frac{4000 \ (\text{parts})}{1 \ (\text{part})} = \frac{100 \ (\%)}{x \ (\%)}$$

$$x = 0.025\%, \ answer.$$

NOTE: To change ratio strength to percent strength, it is sometimes convenient to "convert" the last two zeros in a ratio strength to a percent sign (%), change the remaining ratio to a common fraction, and then to a decimal fraction in expressing percent.

Examples:

$$1:100 = \frac{1}{1}\% = 1\%$$
$$1:200 = \frac{1}{2}\% = 0.5\%$$
$$3:500 = \frac{3}{5}\% = 0.6\%$$
$$1:2500 = \frac{1}{25}\% = 0.04\%$$
$$1:10,000 = \frac{1}{100}\% = 0.01\%$$

Ratio Strength of Solution or Liquid Preparation, Given Weight of Solute in a Specified Volume. Calculating the ratio strength of a solution or liquid preparation, given the weight of solute or constituent in a specified volume of solution or liquid preparation involves the following.

Examples:

A *certain injectable contains 2 mg of a drug per milliliter of solution. What is the ratio strength (w/v) of the solution?*

$$2 \text{ mg} = 0.002 \text{ g}$$

$$\frac{0.002 \text{ (g)}}{1 \text{ (g)}} = \frac{1 \text{ (mL)}}{x \text{ (mL)}}$$

$$x = 500 \text{ mL}$$

Ratio strength $= 1:500$, *answer.*

What is the ratio strength (w/v) of a solution made by dissolving five tablets, each containing 2.25 g of sodium chloride, in enough water to make 1800 mL?

$$2.25 \text{ g} \times 5 = 11.25 \text{ g of sodium chloride}$$

$$\frac{11.25 \text{ (g)}}{1 \text{ (g)}} = \frac{1800 \text{ (mL)}}{x \text{ (mL)}}$$

$$x = 160 \text{ mL}$$

Ratio strength $= 1:160$, *answer.*

Problems Involving Ratio Strength. In solving problems in which the calculations are based on ratio strength, it is sometimes convenient to translate the problem into one based on percentage strength and to solve it according to the rules and methods discussed under percentage preparations.

Examples:

How many grams of potassium permanganate should be used in preparing 500 mL of a 1:2500 solution?

$$1:2500 = 0.04\%$$
$$500 \text{ (g)} \times 0.0004 = 0.2 \text{ g, *answer.*}$$

Or,

1:2500 means 1 g in 2500 mL of solution

$$\frac{2500 \text{ (mL)}}{500 \text{ (mL)}} = \frac{1 \text{ (g)}}{x \text{ (g)}}$$

$$x = 0.2 \text{ g, *answer.*}$$

How many milligrams of gentian violet should be used in preparing the following solution?

R Gentian Violet Solution   500 mL
     1:10,000
    Sig. Instill as directed.

$$1:10,000 = 0.01\%$$
$$500 \text{ (g)} \times 0.0001 = 0.050 \text{ g or 50 mg, } answer.$$

Or,

1:10,000 means 1 g of 10,000 mL of solution

$$\frac{10,000 \text{ (mL)}}{500 \text{ (mL)}} = \frac{1 \text{ (g)}}{x \text{ (g)}}$$

$$x = 0.050 \text{ g or 50 mg, } answer.$$

How many milligrams of hexachlorophene should be used in compounding the following prescription?

R Hexachlorophene   1:400
   Hydrophilic Ointment ad 10 g
   Sig. Apply.

1:400 = 0.25%
10 (g) × 0.0025 = 0.025 g or 25 mg, *answer.*
Or,

1:400 means 1 g in 400 g of ointment

$$\frac{400 \text{ (g)}}{10 \text{ (g)}} = \frac{1 \text{ (g)}}{x \text{ (g)}}$$

$$x = 0.025 \text{ g or 25 mg, } answer.$$

SIMPLE CONVERSIONS OF CONCENTRATION TO "mg/mL"

Occasionally, pharmacists, particularly those practicing in patient care settings, need to *convert rapidly* product concentrations expressed as percentage strength, ratio strength, or as grams per liter (as in IV infusions) *to milligrams per milliliter* (mg/mL). These conversions may be made quickly by using simple techniques. Some suggestions follow.

To convert **product percentage strengths to mg/mL**, multiply the percentage strength, expressed as a whole number, by 10.

Example:

Convert 4% (w/v) to mg/mL.

   4 × 10   = 40 mg/mL, *answer.*
   Proof or alternate method: 4% (w/v) = 4 g/100 mL
               = 4000 mg/100 mL
               = 40 mg/mL

To convert **product ratio strengths to mg/mL**, divide the ratio strength by 1000.

Example:

Convert 1 : 10000 (w/v) to mg/mL.

$$10000 \div 1000 \qquad\qquad\qquad = 1 \text{ mg/10 mL, } \textit{answer.}$$

Proof or alternate method: 1 : 10000 (w/v)   = 1 g/10000 mL
                                              = 1000 mg/10000 mL
                                              = 1 mg/10 mL

To convert **product strengths expressed as grams per liter (g/L) to mg/mL,** convert the numerator to milligrams and divide by the number of milliliters in the denominator.

Example:

Convert a product concentration of 1 g per 250 mL to mg/mL.

$$1000 \div 250 \qquad\qquad\qquad = 4 \text{ mg/mL, } \textit{answer.}$$

Proof or alternate method: 1 g/250 mL   = 1000 mg/250 mL = 4 mg/mL

EXPRESSING CLINICAL LABORATORY TEST VALUES

It is common practice in assessing health status to analyze biologic fluids, especially blood and urine, for specific chemical content. The clinical laboratory tests used, known as "chemistries," analyze samples for such chemicals as glucose, cholesterol, total lipids, creatinine, blood urea nitrogen, bilirubin, potassium, sodium, calcium, carbon dioxide, and other substances, including drugs following their administration. Blood chemistries are performed on plasma (the fluid part of the blood) or serum (the watery portion of clotted blood). Depending on the laboratory equipment used as well as patient factors (such as age and gender), the "usual" amount of each chemical substance varies, with no single "normal" value, but rather a common range. For example, the common amount of glucose in serum is 60 to 110 mg/dL, and the normal range of creatinine in the blood serum of adults is 0.7 to 1.5 mg/dL.

The unit of measurement for cholesterol levels changed recently from a reading in milligrams per deciliter to the international system of units that uses millimoles per liter of blood plasma. For example, a cholesterol reading of 180 (mg/dL) is now recorded as 4.65 millimoles per liter (mmol/L).

The pharmacist needs to understand both the quantitative aspects of clinical laboratory values as well as their clinical significance. "Abnormal" levels may reflect clinical problems requiring further evaluation and treatment.

Problems Involving Clinical Laboratory Test Values. To solve problems expressing clinical laboratory test values, observe the following.

Examples:

If a patient is determined to have a serum cholesterol level of 200 mg/dL, (a) what is the equivalent value expressed in terms of milligrams percent, and (b) how many milligrams of cholesterol would be present in a 10-mL sample of the patient's serum?

(a) 200 mg/dL = 200 mg/100 mL = 200 mg%, *answer.*

(b) $\dfrac{200 \text{ (mg)}}{x \text{ (mg)}} = \dfrac{100 \text{ (mL)}}{10 \text{ (mL)}}$

$$x = 20 \text{ mg, } \textit{answer.}$$

If a patient is determined to have a serum cholesterol level of 200 mg/dL, what is the equivalent value expressed in terms of millimoles (mmol) per liter?

$$
\begin{aligned}
\text{m.w. of cholesterol} &= 387 \\
\text{1 mmol cholesterol} &= 387 \text{ mg} \\
200 \text{ mg/dL} &= 2000 \text{ mg/L}
\end{aligned}
$$

$$
\frac{387 \text{ (mg)}}{2000 \text{ (mg)}} = \frac{1 \text{ (millimole)}}{x \text{ (millimoles)}}
$$

$$
x = 5.17 \text{ mmol/L, } answer.
$$

PARTS PER MILLION (PPM)

The strength of very dilute solutions is commonly expressed in terms of *parts per million (ppm)*; i.e., the number of parts of the agent per 1 million parts of the whole. For example, fluoridated drinking water, used to reduce dental caries, often contains 1 part of fluoride per million parts of drinking water (1 : 1,000,000). Content in parts per million also may be used to describe the quantities of trace impurities in chemical samples and trace elements in biologic samples.

Depending on the physical forms of the trace substituent and the final product, a concentration expressed in ppm could, in theory, be calculated on a weight-in-volume, volume-in-volume, or weight-in-weight basis. For all practical purposes, however, the unit-terms of the solute and solution are generally considered like units (i.e., the same type of "parts").

Equivalent Values of Percent Strength, Ratio Strength, and Parts per Million. The ppm concentration of a substance may be expressed in quantitatively equivalent values of percent strength or ratio strength.

Example:

Express 5 ppm of iron in water in percent strength and ratio strength.

$$
\begin{aligned}
5 \text{ ppm} = 5 \text{ parts in 1,000,000 parts} &= 1 : 200,000, \text{ ratio strength, } answer, \\
&= 0.0005\%, \text{ percent strength, } answer.
\end{aligned}
$$

Using Parts per Million. To use ppm in calculations, observe the following.

Example:

The concentration of a drug additive in an animal feed is 12.5 ppm. How many milligrams of the drug should be used in preparing 5.2 kg of feed?

12.5 ppm = 12.5 g (drug) in 1,000,000 g (feed)

Thus,

$$
\frac{1,000,000 \text{ g}}{12.5 \text{ g}} = \frac{5,200 \text{ g}}{x \text{ g}}
$$

$$
x = 0.065 \text{ g} = 65 \text{ mg, } answer.
$$

Practice Problems

1. ℞   Antipyrine   5%
         Glycerin   ad   60.0
         Sig. Five drops in right ear.

   How many grams of antipyrine should be used in preparing the prescription?

2. ℞   Sol. Ephedrine Sulfate
            ½%   30 mL
            Sig. For the nose.

How many milligrams of ephedrine sulfate should be used in preparing the prescription?

3. ℞   Resin of Podophyllum   25%
            Compound Benzoin
            Tincture   ad   30.0
            Sig. Apply to papillomas t.i.d.

How many grams of resin of podophyllum should be used in preparing the prescription?

4. How many milligrams of a certified red color should be used in preparing 5 liters of a 0.01% solution?

5. ℞   Potassium Iodide Solution (10%)
            Ephedrine Sulfate
            Solution (3%)   aa   15.0 mL
            Sig. Five drops in water as directed.

How many grams each of potassium iodide and ephedrine sulfate should be used in preparing the prescription?

6. How many milligrams of methylparaben are needed to prepare 8 fluidounces of a solution containing 0.12% (w/v) of methylparaben?

7. If a pharmacist dissolves the contents of eight capsules, each containing 250 mg of clindamycin hydrochloride, into a sufficient amount of Ionax® Astringent Liquid to prepare 120 mL of solution, what is the percentage strength (w/v) of clindamycin hydrochloride in the prescription?

8. If 50 mL of a 7.5% (w/v) sodium bicarbonate injection are added to 500 mL of a 5% dextrose injection, what is the percentage strength (w/v) of sodium bicarbonate in the product?

9. A formula for a mouth rinse contains ⅒% (w/v) of zinc chloride. How many grams of zinc chloride should be used in preparing 25 liters of the mouth rinse?

10. Mellaril-S® Suspension contains 25 mg of thioridazine per 5 mL of suspension. What is the percentage strength (w/v) of thioridazine in the suspension?

11. An injection contains 50 mg of pentobarbital sodium in each milliliter of solution. What is the percentage strength (w/v) of the solution?

12. If 425 g of sucrose are dissolved in enough water to make 500 mL, what is the percentage strength (w/v) of the solution?

13. An ear drop formula contains 54 mg of antipyrine and 14 mg of benzocaine in each milliliter of solution. Calculate the percentage strength (w/v) of each ingredient in the formula.

14. How many liters of 2% (w/v) iodine tincture can be made from 123 g of iodine?

15. How many milliliters of 0.9% (w/v) sodium chloride solution can be made from 1 lb of sodium chloride?

16. How many milliliters of a 0.9% (w/v) solution of sodium chloride can be prepared from 50 tablets, each containing 2.25 g of sodium chloride?

17. If an intravenous injection contains 20% (w/v) of mannitol, how many milliliters of the injection should be administered to provide a patient with 100 g of mannitol?

18. An inhalant aerosol contains 0.25% (w/v) of isoproterenol hydrochloride. If each depression of the aerosol valve delivers 0.12 mg of the drug, how many doses are contained in a 15-mL aerosol package?

19. The intravenous dose of mannitol is 1.5 g/kg of body weight, administered as a 15% (w/v) solution. How many milliliters of the solution should be administered to a 150-lb patient?

20. If a physician orders a 25 mg "test dose" of sodium thiopental for a patient before anesthesia, how many milliliters of a 2.5% (w/v) solution of sodium thiopental should be used?

21. A prefilled syringe contains 50 mg of lidocaine hydrochloride per 5 mL of injection. Express the percentage concentration of lidocaine in the injection.

22. A blood volume expansion solution contains 6% (w/v) of hetastarch and 0.9% (w/v) of sodium chloride. How many grams of each agent would be present in 250 mL of the solution?

23. A pharmacist adds 10 mL of a 20% (w/v) solution of potassium iodide to 500 mL of D5W for parenteral infusion. What is the percentage strength of potassium iodide in the infusion solution?

24. If a dry powder mixture of the antibiotic amoxicillin is diluted with water to 80 mL to prepare a prescription containing 125 mg of amoxicillin per 5 mL, (a) how many grams of amoxicillin are in the dry mixture, and (b) what is the percentage strength of amoxicillin in the filled prescription?

25. If 10 mL of a nitroglycerin injection (5 mg of nitroglycerin per milliliter) are added to make a liter of intravenous fluid, what is the percentage (w/v) of nitroglycerin in the final product?

26. How many grams of pilocarpine nitrate are required to prepare 30 mL of an ophthalmic solution containing 0.25% of the drug?

27. How many milliliters of resorcinol monoacetate should be used to prepare 1 pint of a 15% (v/v) lotion?

28. A sunscreen lotion contains 5% (v/v) of menthyl salicylate. How many milliliters of menthyl salicylate should be used in preparing 5 pints of the lotion?

29. Peppermint Spirit contains 10% (v/v) of peppermint oil. How many milliliters of peppermint oil should be used in preparing 1 gallon of the spirit?

30. What is the percentage strength (v/v) if 225 g of a liquid having a specific gravity of 0.8 are added to enough water to make 1.5 liters of the solution?

31. How many liters of a mouth wash can be prepared from 100 mL of cinnamon flavor if its concentration is to be 0.5% (v/v)?

32. A lotion vehicle contains 15% (v/v) of glycerin. How many liters of glycerin should be used in preparing 5 gallons of the lotion?

33. One gallon of a certain lotion contains 946 mL of benzyl benzoate. Calculate the percentage (v/v) of benzyl benzoate in the lotion.

34. The formula for 1 liter of an elixir contains 0.25 mL of a flavoring oil. What is the percentage (v/v) of the flavoring oil in the elixir?

35. A liniment contains 15% (v/v) of methyl salicylate. How many milliliters of the liniment can be made from 1 pint of methyl salicylate?

36. A dermatologic lotion contains 1.25 mL of liquefied phenol in 500 mL. Calculate the percentage (v/v) of liquefied phenol in the lotion.

37. How many grams of sucrose must be dissolved in 475 mL of water to make a 65% (w/w) solution?

38. How many grams of tannic acid must be dissolved in 320 mL of glycerin having a specific gravity of 1.25 to make a 20% (w/w) solution?

39. How many grams of a drug substance should be dissolved in 1800 mL of water to make a 10% (w/w) solution?

40. What is the percentage strength (w/w) of a solution made by dissolving 62.5 g of potassium chloride in 187.5 mL of water?

41. If 500 g of dextrose are dissolved in 600 mL of water with a resultant final volume of 1 liter, what is the percentage strength of dextrose in the solution on a w/w basis?

42. If a pharmacist adds 6 g of hydrocortisone to 120 g of a 5% (w/w) hydrocortisone cream, what is the resultant percentage strength of hydrocortisone in the product?

43. If 1 g of a drug is dissolved in 2.5 mL of glycerin, specific gravity 1.25, what is the percentage strength (w/w) of the drug in the resultant solution?

44. Nitro-Bid® Ointment contains 2% (w/w) of nitroglycerin. If each inch of the ointment squeezed from the tube contains 15 mg of nitroglycerin, (a) how many grams would each inch of ointment weigh, and (b) how many 1-in. doses of ointment may be delivered from a 15-g tube of ointment?

45. One pound of a fungicidal ointment contains 9.08 g of undecylenic acid. Calculate the percentage (w/w) of undecylenic acid in the ointment.

46. How many grams each of resorcinol and hexachlorophene should be used in preparing 5 lb of an acne ointment that is to contain 2% of resorcinol and 0.25% of hexachlorophene?

47. ℞ Iodochlorhydroxyquin   0.9 g
       Hydrocortisone   0.15 g
       Cream Base   ad   30.0 g
       Sig. Apply.

What is the percentage strength (w/w) each of iodochlorhydroxyquin and hydrocortisone in the prescription?

48. How many milligrams of procaine hydrochloride should be used in preparing 120 suppositories each weighing 2 g and containing ¼% of procaine hydrochloride?

49. If a topical cream contains 1.8% (w/w) of hydrocortisone, how many milligrams of hydrocortisone should be used in preparing 15 g of the cream?

50. A topical cream contains 0.2% (w/w) of nitrofurazone. How many grams of nitrofurazone are in 120 g of the cream?

51. You are directed to mix 30 g of Whitfield's Ointment (containing 6% of salicylic acid) and 60 g of Lassar's Paste with Salicylic Acid (containing 2% of salicylic acid) with enough white petrolatum to make 120 g. What is the percentage (w/w) of salicylic acid in the finished product?

52. ℞   Salicylic Acid   20 g
         Whitfield's Ointment   60 g
         White Petrolatum   ad   300 g
         Sig. Apply as directed.

     If Whitfield's Ointment contains 6% of salicylic acid, calculate the percentage (w/w) of salicylic acid in the prescription.

53. A pharmacist incorporates 6 g of coal tar into 120 g of a 5% coal tar ointment. Calculate the percentage (w/w) of coal tar in the finished product.

54. If 198 g of dextrose are dissolved in 1000 mL of water, what is the percentage strength (w/w) of the solution?

55. Express each of the following as a percentage strength:
     (a) 1:1500   (d) 1:400
     (b) 1:10,000   (e) 1:3300
     (c) 1:250   (f) 1:4000

56. Express each of the following as a ratio strength:
     (a) 0.125%   (d) 0.6%
     (b) 2.5%   (e) ⅓%
     (c) 0.80%   (f) ½₀%

57. Express each of the following concentrations as a ratio strength:
     (a) 2 mg of active ingredient in 2 mL of solution
     (b) 0.275 mg of active ingredient in 5 mL of solution
     (c) 2 g of active ingredient in 250 mL of solution
     (d) 1 mg of active ingredient in 0.5 mL of solution

58. A vaginal foam contains 0.01% (w/v) of dienestrol. Express this concentration as a ratio strength.

59. A tetracycline syrup is preserved with 0.08% (w/v) of methylparaben, 0.02% (w/v) of propylparaben, and 0.10% (w/v) of sodium metabisulfite. Express these concentrations as ratio strengths.

60. An ophthalmic solution of naphazoline hydrochloride is stabilized with 0.0006% (w/v) of sodium carbonate and preserved with 0.002% (w/v) of phenylmercuric nitrate. Express these concentrations as ratio strengths.

61. An injection contains 0.50% (w/v) of lidocaine hydrochloride and 1:200,000 (w/v) of epinephrine. Express the concentration of lidocaine hydrochloride as a ratio strength and that of epinephrine as a percentage.

62. A sample of white petrolatum contains 10 mg of tocopherol per kilogram as a preservative. Express the amount of tocopherol as a ratio strength.

63. Calcium Hydroxide Topical Solution contains 170 mg of calcium hydroxide per 100 mL at 15°C. Express this concentration as a ratio strength.

64. Dibucaine hydrochloride solution is used for spinal anesthesia in a concentration of 1:1500 (w/v). How many milligrams of dibucaine hydrochloride are contained in a 20-mL vial of the solution?

65. ℞   Potassium Permanganate   0.2 g
           Tablets
           Disp. #100
           Sig. Two tablets in 4 pt of water and use as directed.

    Express the concentration, as a ratio strength, of the solution prepared according to the directions given in the prescription.

66. ℞   Menthol   1:500
           Hexachlorophene   1:800
           Hydrophilic Ointment Base   ad   30 g
           Sig. Apply to hands.

    How many milligrams each of menthol and hexachlorophene should be used in compounding the prescription?

67. Hepatitis B Immume Globulin is preserved with 1:10,000 (w/v) of thimerosal. If the dose of the injection is 0.06 mL/kg of body weight, how many micrograms of thimerosal would be contained in the dose for a 150-lb patient?

68. Hepatitis B Virus Vaccine Inactivated is inactivated with 1:4000 (w/v) of formalin. Express this ratio strength as a percentage strength.

69. Midazolam® Injection contains 5 mg of drug per milliliter of injection. Calculate the ratio strength of the injection.

70. If a 5% (w/v) benzoyl peroxide lotion is diluted with an equal volume of water, what is the resultant ratio strength of the diluted lotion?

71. If a liquid vitamin preparation contains 0.16 μg of vitamin B_{12} per 5 mL, what is the ratio strength of the preparation?

72. For bladder and urethral irrigation, it is recommended to dilute a 1:750 (w/v) solution of benzalkonium chloride with sterile water in a ratio of 3 parts of the benzalkonium chloride solution to 77 parts of sterile water. What is the ratio strength of benzalkonium chloride in the resultant solution?

73. A skin test for fire ant allergy involves the intradermal skin prick of 0.05 mL of a 1:1,000,000 (w/v) dilution of fire ant extract. How many micrograms of extract would be administered in this manner?

74. In acute hypersensitivity reactions, 0.5 mL of a 1:1000 (w/v) solution of epinephrine may be administered subcutaneously or intramuscularly. Calculate the milligrams of epinephrine given.

75. Echothiophate iodide solution is available in four strengths: 1.5 mg/5 mL, 3.0 mg/

5 mL, 6.25 mg/5 mL, and 12.5 mg/5 mL. Express each concentration as a percentage strength (w/v).

76. Triamcinolone acetonide ointment is available in three strengths: 0.025%, 0.1%, and 0.5%. Express these concentrations in terms of milligrams of triamcinolone acetonide per gram of ointment.

77. What is the percent concentration of cholesterol in a patient's blood serum if the cholesterol level is determined to be 260 mg%?

78. A patient is determined to have 0.8 mg of glucose in each milliliter of blood. Express the concentration of glucose in the blood as milligrams percent.

79. Express a patient's protein-bound iodine level of 7.7 μg/dL in terms of milligrams percent.

80. A topical solution contains 2% (w/v) of erythromycin. Express the concentration of erythromycin in terms of milligrams per milliliter (mg/mL).

81. If potassium iodide tablets are permitted to contain not less than 94% and not more than 106% of the labeled amount of potassium iodide, what would be the permissible range, in milligrams, for potassium iodide tablets labeled 300 mg each?

82. Hexachlorophene Liquid Soap is required to contain, in each 100 g, not less than 225 mg and not more than 260 mg of hexachlorophene. Express these amounts of hexachlorophene as a percentage concentration range.

83. If a serum sample is determined to contain 270 mg/dL of cholesterol, what is the concentration of cholesterol (m.w. = 386) in terms of millimoles per liter?

84. Cholesterol readings of 190 mg/dL are considered in the "good" range. Express this value of cholesterol (m.w. = 386) in terms of millimoles per liter.

85. If a patient has a serum cholesterol (m.w. = 386) of 4.40 mmol/L, what is the corresponding value in milligrams per deciliter?

86. Complete the following table, comparing serum cholesterol (m.w. 386) levels expressed equivalently in milligrams per deciliter and in millimoles per liter:

mg/dL	mmol/L
Good:	Good:
170	(a)
(b)	4.91
Borderline:	Borderline:
(c)	5.69
240	(d)
High:	High:
(e)	6.46

87. A glucose meter shows that a patient's blood contains 125 mg% of glucose. Express this value as mg/mL.

88. Total serum cholesterol includes LDL-cholesterol and HDL-cholesterol. If a patient has a HDL-cholesterol level of 65 mg/dL and a total cholesterol of 5.43 mmol/L, what is the LDL-cholesterol value in milligrams per deciliter?

89. Federal rules prohibit transportation workers from performing safety-sensitive functions when breath alcohol is 0.04% or greater. Express this value on a milligram per deciliter basis.

90. A blood level of alcohol of 80 mg/dL is considered to diminish driving performance. Express this value in terms of percentage.

91. The average blood alcohol concentration in fatal intoxication is about 400 mg/dL. Express this concentration in terms of percentage.

92. Purified water contains not more than 10 ppm of total solids. Express this concentration as a percentage.

93. How many grams of sodium fluoride should be added to 100,000 liters of drinking water containing 0.6 ppm of sodium fluoride to provide a recommended concentration of 1.75 ppm?

94. If a city water supply has a limit of 250 ppm of nitrate ion, what is the maximum amount of nitrate ion, in grams, that may be present in a 10,000-gallon reservoir?

95. If a commercially available insulin preparation contains 1 ppm of proinsulin, how many micrograms of proinsulin would be contained in a 10-mL vial of insulin?

8 Dilution and Concentration

In Chapter 7, we considered problems arising from the quantitative relationship between specific ingredients and the pharmaceutical preparation as a whole.

Problems of a slightly different character arise when pharmaceutical preparations are *diluted* (by the addition of diluent, or by admixture with solutions or mixtures of lower strength) or are *concentrated* (by the addition of active ingredient, or by admixture with solutions or mixtures of greater strength, or by evaporation of the diluent).

Such problems sometimes seem complicated and difficult. But the complication proves to be nothing more than a series of steps required in the calculation, and the difficulty usually vanishes as each step, in itself, proves to be a simple matter.

Often a problem can be solved in several ways. The best way is not necessarily the shortest: the best way is the one that clearly is understood and that leads to the correct answer.

These two rules, wherever they may be applied, greatly simplify the calculation:

1. *When ratio strengths are given, convert them to percentage strengths before setting up a proportion.* It is more troublesome to calculate with a ratio like $1/10:1/500$ than with the equivalent *10(%):0.2(%).*

2. *Whenever proportional parts enter into a calculation, reduce them to lowest terms.* Instead of calculating with a ratio like *75 (parts):25 (parts),* simplify it to *3 (parts):1 (part).*

RELATIONSHIP BETWEEN STRENGTH AND TOTAL QUANTITY

If a mixture of a given percentage or ratio strength is diluted to twice its original quantity, its active ingredient will be contained in twice as many parts of the whole, and its strength therefore will be reduced by one-half. Contrariwise, if a mixture is concentrated by evaporation to one-half its original quantity, the active ingredient (assuming that none was lost by evaporation) will be contained in one-half as many parts of the whole, and the strength will be doubled. So, if 50 mL of a solution containing 10 g of active ingredient with a strength of 20% or 1:5 (w/v) are diluted to 100 mL, the original volume is doubled, but the original strength is now reduced by one-half to 10% or 1:10 (w/v). If, by evaporation of the solvent, the volume of the solution is reduced to 25 mL or one-half the original quantity, the 10 g of the active ingredient will indicate a strength of 40% or 1:2.5 (w/v).

If, then, *the amount of active ingredient remains constant, any change in the quantity of a solution or mixture of solids is inversely proportional to the percentage or ratio strength;* i.e., the percentage or ratio strength decreases as the quantity increases, and conversely.

This relationship is generally true for all mixtures except volume-in-volume and weight-in-volume solutions containing components that contract when mixed together.

Problems in this section generally may be solved by (1) inverse proportion, (2) the equation: (quantity) × (concentration) = (quantity) × (concentration), or (3) determining the quantity of active constituent (solute) needed and then calculating the quantity of the available solution (usually concentrated or stock solution), which will provide the needed amount of constituent.

DILUTION AND CONCENTRATION OF LIQUIDS

Determination of Percentage or Ratio Strength. Calculating the percentage or ratio strength of a solution made by diluting or concentrating (by evaporation) a solution of given quantity and strength involves the following.

Examples:

If 500 mL of a 15% (v/v) solution of methyl salicylate in alcohol are diluted to 1500 mL, what will be the percentage strength (v/v)?

$$\frac{1500 \ (mL)}{500 \ (mL)} = \frac{15 \ (\%)}{x \ (\%)}$$

$$x \ = \ 5\%, \ answer.$$

Or,

$$
\begin{aligned}
\text{(quantity)} \times \text{(concentration)} &= \text{(quantity)} \times \text{(concentration)} \\
500 \ (mL) \times 15 \ (\%) &= 1500 \ (mL) \times x \ (\%) \\
x &= 5\%, \ answer.
\end{aligned}
$$

Or,

500 mL of 15% (v/v) solution contain 75 mL of methyl salicylate (active ingredient)

$$\frac{1500 \ (mL)}{75 \ (mL)} = \frac{100 \ (\%)}{x \ (\%)}$$

$$x \ = \ 5\%, \ answer.$$

If 50 mL of a 1:20 (w/v) solution of aluminum acetate are diluted to 1000 mL, what is the ratio strength (w/v)?

$$1:20 \ = \ 5\%$$

$$\frac{1000 \ (mL)}{50 \ (mL)} = \frac{5 \ (\%)}{x \ (\%)}$$

$$x \ = \ 0.25\% \ = \ 1:400, \ answer.$$

Or,

$$\frac{1000 \ (mL)}{50 \ (mL)} = \frac{^{1}/_{20}}{x}$$

$$x \ = \ \frac{1}{400} \ = \ 1:400, \ answer.$$

Or,

$$50 \ (mL) \times 5 \ (\%) \ = \ 1000 \ (mL) \times (\%)$$

$$x \ = \ 0.25\% \ = \ 1:400, \ answer.$$

Or,

50 mL of a 1:20 solution contain 2.5 g of aluminum acetate

$$\frac{2.5 \ (g)}{1 \ (g)} = \frac{1000 \ (mL)}{x \ (mL)}$$

$$x \ = \ 400 \ mL$$

$$Ratio \ strength \ = \ 1:400, \ answer.$$

If a syrup containing 65% (w/v) of sucrose is evaporated to 85% of its volume, what percent (w/v) of sucrose will it contain?

Any convenient amount of the syrup, e.g., 100 mL, may be used in the calculation. If we evaporate 100 mL of the syrup to 85% of its volume, we will have 85 mL.

$$\frac{85 \; (mL)}{100 \; (mL)} = \frac{65 \; (\%)}{x \; (\%)}$$

$$x = 76.47\% \text{ or } 76\%, \textit{answer.}$$

Determining Amount of Solution of a Desired Strength. Calculating the amount of solution of desired strength that can be made by diluting or concentrating (by evaporation) a specified quantity of a solution of given strength involves the following.

Examples:

How many grams of 10% (w/w) ammonia solution can be made from 1800 g of 28% (w/w) strong ammonia solution?

$$\frac{10 \; (\%)}{28 \; (\%)} = \frac{1800 \; (g)}{x \; (g)}$$

$$x = 5040 \text{ g}, \textit{answer.}$$

Or,

$$1800 \; (g) \times 28 \; (\%) = x \; (g) \times 10\%$$

$$x = 5040 \text{ g}, \textit{answer.}$$

Or,

1800 g of 28% ammonia water contain 504 g of ammonia (100%)

$$\frac{10 \; (\%)}{100 \; (\%)} = \frac{504 \; (g)}{x \; (g)}$$

$$x = 5040 \text{ g}, \textit{answer.}$$

How many milliliters of a 1:5000 (w/v) solution of phenylmercuric acetate can be made from 125 mL of a 0.2% solution?

$$1:5000 = 0.02\%$$

$$\frac{0.02 \; (\%)}{0.2 \; (\%)} = \frac{125 \; (mL)}{x \; (mL)}$$

$$x = 1250 \text{ mL}, \textit{answer.}$$

Or,

$$0.2\% = 1:500$$

$$\frac{1/5000}{1/500} = \frac{125 \; (mL)}{x \; (mL)}$$

$$x = 1250 \text{ mL}, \textit{answer.}$$

Or,

125 mL of a 0.2% solution contain 0.25 g of phenylmercuric acetate

$$\frac{1\ (g)}{0.25\ (g)} = \frac{5000\ (mL)}{x\ (mL)}$$

$$x = 1250\ mL,\ answer.$$

Or,

$$125\ (mL) \times 0.2\ (\%) = x\ (mL) \times 0.02\ (\%)$$

$$x = 1250\ mL,\ answer.$$

If 1 gallon of a 30% (w/v) solution is to be evaporated so that the solution will have a strength of 50% (w/v), what will be its volume in milliliters?

$$1\ gallon = 3785\ mL$$

$$\frac{50\ (\%)}{30\ (\%)} = \frac{3785\ (mL)}{x\ (mL)}$$

$$x = 2271\ mL,\ answer.$$

STOCK SOLUTIONS

Stock solutions are solutions of known concentration that are frequently prepared by the pharmacist for convenience in dispensing. They are usually strong solutions from which weaker ones may be made conveniently. When correctly prepared, these solutions enable the pharmacist to obtain small quantities of medicinal substances that are to be dispensed in solution.

Stock solutions are invariably prepared on a weight-in-volume basis, and their concentration is expressed as a ratio strength or, less frequently, as a percentage strength.

Amount of Solution Needed to Prepare Desired Solution. Calculating the amount of a solution of given strength that must be used to prepare a solution of desired amount and strength involves the following.

Examples:

How many milliliters of a 1:400 (w/v) stock solution should be used to make 4 liters of a 1:2000 (w/v) solution?

4 liters = 4000 mL
1:400 = 0.25%   1:2000 = 0.05%

$$\frac{0.25\ (\%)}{0.05\ (\%)} = \frac{4000\ (mL)}{x\ (mL)}$$

$$x = 800\ mL,\ answer.$$

Or,

$$\frac{\frac{1}{400}}{\frac{1}{2000}} = \frac{4000\ (mL)}{x\ (mL)}$$

$$x = 800\ mL,\ answer.$$

Or,

4000 mL of a 1:2000 (w/v) solution require 2 g of active constituent (solute), thus:

$$\frac{1\ (g)}{2\ (g)} = \frac{400\ (mL)}{x\ (mL)}$$

$$x = 800\ mL,\ answer.$$

How many milliliters of a 1:400 (w/v) stock solution should be used in preparing 1 gallon of a 1:2000 (w/v) solution?

1 gallon = 3785 mL
1:400 = 0.25%   1:2000 = 0.05%

$$\frac{0.25\ (\%)}{0.05\ (\%)} = \frac{3785\ (mL)}{x\ (mL)}$$

$$x = 757\ mL,\ answer.$$

Or,

1 gallon of a 1:2000 (w/v) solution requires 1.89 g of active constituent, thus:

$$\frac{1.89\ (g)}{1\ (g)} = \frac{x\ (mL)}{400\ (mL)}$$

$$x = 756\ mL,\ answer.$$

How many milliliters of a 1% stock solution of a certified red dye should be used in preparing 4000 mL of a mouth wash that is to contain 1:20,000 (w/v) of the certified red dye as a coloring agent?

$$1:20,000 = 0.005\%$$

$$\frac{1\ (\%)}{0.005\ (\%)} = \frac{4000\ (mL)}{x\ (mL)}$$

$$x = 20\ mL,\ answer.$$

Check:

1% stock solution contains		1:20,000 solution contains
20 (mL) × 0.01 →	0.2 g certified red dye	← 4000 (mL) × 0.00005

Or,

4000 mL of a 1:20,000 (w/v) solution require 0.2 g of certified red dye, thus:

$$\frac{1\ (g)}{0.2\ (g)} = \frac{100\ (mL)}{x\ (mL)}$$

$$x = 20\ mL,\ answer.$$

How many milliliters of a 1:16 solution of sodium hypochlorite should be used in preparing 5000 mL of a 0.5% solution of sodium hypochlorite for irrigation?

$$1:16 = 6.25\%$$

$$\frac{6.25\ (\%)}{0.5\ (\%)} = \frac{5000\ (mL)}{x\ (mL)}$$

$$x = 400\ mL,\ answer.$$

Or,

5000 mL of a 0.5% (w/v) solution require 25 g of sodium hypochlorite, thus:

$$\frac{25\ (g)}{1\ (g)} = \frac{x\ (mL)}{16\ (mL)}$$

$$x = 400\ mL,\ \textit{answer}.$$

How many milliliters of a 1:50 stock solution of ephedrine sulfate should be used in compounding the following prescription?

R Ephedrine Sulfate 0.25%
  Rose Water ad 30.0 mL
  Sig. For the nose.

$$1:50 = 2\%$$

$$\frac{2\ (\%)}{0.25\ (\%)} = \frac{30\ (mL)}{x\ (mL)}$$

$$x = 3.75\ mL,\ \textit{answer}.$$

Or,

30 (g) × 0.0025 = 0.075 g of ephedrine sulfate needed

1:50 means 1 g in 50 mL of stock solution

$$\frac{1\ (g)}{0.075\ (g)} = \frac{50\ (mL)}{x\ (mL)}$$

$$x = 3.75\ mL,\ \textit{answer}.$$

Determining Quantity of Active Ingredient in Specified Amount of Solution Given Strength of Diluted Portion. From the strength of the diluted portion, we may calculate the *quantity of active ingredient* that the undiluted portion must have contained, and then by proportion, we may calculate how much active ingredient must be present in any other amount of the stock solution.

Examples:

How much silver nitrate should be used in preparing 50 mL of a solution such that 5 mL diluted to 500 mL will yield a 1:1000 solution?

1:1000 means 1 g of silver nitrate in 1000 mL of solution

$$\frac{1000\ (mL)}{500\ (mL)} = \frac{1\ (g)}{x\ (g)}$$

$$x = 0.5\ g\ of\ silver\ nitrate\ in\ 500\ mL\ of$$
diluted solution (1:1000), which
is *also* the amount in 5 mL of the
stronger (stock) solution,

and,

$$\frac{5\ (mL)}{50\ (mL)} = \frac{0.5\ (g)}{y\ (g)}$$

$$y = 5\ g,\ \textit{answer}.$$

The accompanying diagrammatic sketch should prove helpful in solving the problem.

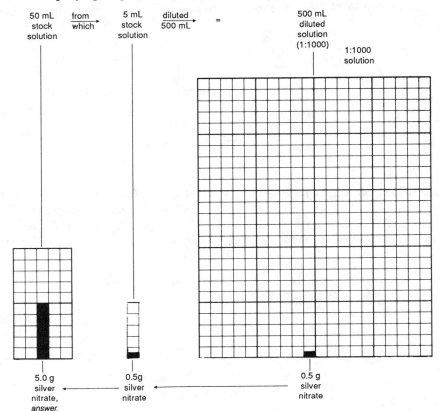

How many grams of sodium chloride should be used in preparing 500 mL of a stock solution such that 50 mL diluted to 1000 mL will yield a "$\frac{1}{3}$ normal saline" (0.3% w/v) for irrigation?

1000 (mL) × 0.003 = 3 g of sodium chloride in 1000 mL of "$\frac{1}{3}$ normal saline" (0.3% w/v), which is *also* the amount in 50 mL of the *stronger* (stock) solution to be prepared.

and,

$$\frac{50 \text{ (mL)}}{500 \text{ (mL)}} = \frac{3 \text{ (g)}}{x \text{ (g)}}$$

$$x = 30 \text{ g, } answer.$$

How many milliliters of a 17% (w/v) concentrate of benzalkonium chloride should be used in preparing 300 mL of a stock solution such that 15 mL diluted to 1 liter will yield a 1 : 5000 solution?

1 liter = 1000 mL
1 : 5000 means 1 g of benzalkonium chloride in 5000 mL of solution

$$\frac{5000 \text{ (mL)}}{1000 \text{ (mL)}} = \frac{1 \text{ (g)}}{x \text{ (g)}}$$

x = 0.2 g of benzalkonium chloride in 1000 mL of *diluted* solution (1:5000), which is *also* the amount in 15 mL of the *stronger* (stock) solution to be prepared.

and,

$$\frac{15\ (mL)}{300\ (mL)} = \frac{0.2\ (g)}{y\ (g)}$$

$$y = 4\ g\ of\ benzalkonium\ chloride\ needed$$

Because a 17% (w/v) concentrate contains 17 g per 100 mL then,

$$\frac{17\ (g)}{4\ (g)} = \frac{100\ (mL)}{z\ (mL)}$$

$$z = 23.5\ mL,\ answer.$$

Amount of Diluent Needed for Preparing Solution of Specified Lower Strength. When given the quantity and strength of a solution, we may determine how much diluent should be added to reduce its strength as desired by first calculating the quantity of weaker solution that can be made and then subtracting from this the original quantity.

Examples:

How many milliliters of water should be added to 300 mL of a 1:750 (w/v) solution of benzalkonium chloride to make a 1:2500 (w/v) solution?

1:750 = 0.133%   1:2500 = 0.04%

$$\frac{0.04\ (\%)}{0.133\ (\%)} = \frac{300\ (mL)}{x\ (mL)}$$

$$x = 997.5\ or\ 1000\ mL\ of\ 0.04\%$$

$$(w/v)\ solution\ to\ be\ prepared$$

The difference between the volume of *diluted* (weaker) solution prepared and the volume of *stronger* solution used represents the volume of water (diluent) to be used.

1000 mL − 300 mL = 700 mL, *answer.*

Or,

300 mL of a 1:750 (w/v) solution contain 0.4 g of benzalkonium chloride

$$\frac{1\ (g)}{0.4\ (g)} = \frac{2500\ (mL)}{x\ (mL)}$$

$$x = 1000\ mL$$

$$1000\ mL - 300\ mL = 700\ mL,\ answer.$$

How many milliliters of water should be added to a pint of a 5% (w/v) solution of boric acid to make a 2% (w/v) solution?

$$1\ pint = 473\ mL$$

$$\frac{2\ (\%)}{5\ (\%)} = \frac{473\ (mL)}{x\ (mL)}$$

$$x = 1182.5\ mL$$

and,

$$1182.5\ mL - 473\ mL = 709.5\ mL,\ answer.$$

If we are not given the strength of the original solution, but the quantity of active ingredient it contains, the simplest procedure is to calculate directly what must be the amount of solution of the strength desired if it contains this quantity of active ingredient. Then, by subtracting the given original amount, we may determine the required amount of diluent.

Example:

How many milliliters of water should be added to 375 mL of a solution containing 0.5 g of *benzalkonium chloride to make a 1:5000 solution?*

1:5000 means 1 g in 5000 mL of solution

$$\frac{1 \text{ (g)}}{0.5 \text{ (g)}} = \frac{5000 \text{ (mL)}}{x \text{ (mL)}}$$

$$x = 2500 \text{ mL of } 1:5000 \text{ (w/v)}$$
$$\text{solution containing } 0.5 \text{ g}$$
$$\text{of benzalkonium chloride}$$

and,

$$2500 \text{ mL} - 375 \text{ mL} = 2125 \text{ mL}, \textit{answer.}$$

DILUTION OF ALCOHOL

Because of a noticeable contraction in volume when alcohol and water are mixed, we cannot calculate the precise volume of water needed to dilute alcohol to a desired *volume-in-volume* strength. On the basis of the strength of alcohol desired, however, we may "qs" with water to the appropriate volume. Also, because the contraction of the liquids does not affect the *weights* of the components, the *weight of water* (and from this, the *volume*) needed to dilute alcohol to a desired *weight-in-weight* strength may be calculated.

Miscellaneous Problems.

Examples:

How much water should be mixed with 5000 mL of 85% (v/v) alcohol to make 50% (v/v) *alcohol?*

$$\frac{50 \text{ (\%)}}{85 \text{ (\%)}} = \frac{5000 \text{ (mL)}}{x \text{ (mL)}}$$

$$x = 8500 \text{ mL}$$

Therefore, use 5000 mL of 85% (v/v) alcohol and enough water to make 8500 mL, *answer.*

How many milliliters of 95% (v/v) alcohol and how much water should be used in compounding the following prescription?

Ꝑ	Boric Acid	1.0 g
	Alcohol 70%	30.0 mL
	Sig. Ear drops.	

$$\frac{95 \text{ (\%)}}{70 \text{ (\%)}} = \frac{30 \text{ (mL)}}{x \text{ (mL)}}$$

$$x = 22 \text{ mL}$$

Therefore, use 22 mL of 95% (v/v) alcohol and enough water to make 30 mL, *answer.*

How much water should be added to 4000 g of 90% (w/w) alcohol to make 40% (w/w) alcohol?

$$\frac{40\ (\%)}{90\ (\%)} = \frac{4000\ (g)}{x\ (g)}$$

x = 9000 g, weight of 40% (w/w) alcohol equivalent to 4000 g of 90% (w/w) alcohol

9000 g − 4000 g = 5000 g or 5000 mL, *answer.*

DILUTION OF ACIDS

The strength of an official undiluted (*concentrated*) acid is expressed as percentage weight-in-weight. For example, Hydrochloric Acid, NF, contains not less than 36.5% and not more than 38.0%, by weight, of HCl. But the strength of an official *diluted* acid is expressed as percentage weight-in-volume. For example, Diluted Hydrochloric Acid, NF, contains, in each 100 mL, not less than 9.5 g and not more than 10.5 g of HCl.

It is necessary, therefore, to consider the specific gravity of concentrated acids in calculating the volume to be used in preparing a desired quantity of a diluted acid.

Calculating Volume of Concentrated Acid Needed for Desired Quantity of Diluted Acid.

Examples:

How many milliliters of 37% (w/w) hydrochloric acid having a specific gravity of 1.20 are required to make 100 mL of diluted hydrochloric acid 10% (w/v)?

1000 g × 0.10 = 100 g of HCl (100%) in 1000 mL of 10% (w/v) acid

$$\frac{37\ (\%)}{100\ (\%)} = \frac{100\ (g)}{x\ (g)}$$

$$x = 270\ g\ of\ 37\%\ acid$$

270 g of water measure 270 mL

$$270\ (mL) \div 1.20 = 225\ mL,\ answer.$$

How many milliliters of 85% (w/w) phosphoric acid having a specific gravity of 1.71 should be used in preparing 1 gallon of ¼% (w/v) phosphoric acid solution to be used for bladder irrigation?

1 gallon = 3785 mL
3785 (g) × 0.0025 = 9.46 g of H_3PO_4 (100%) in 3785 mL (1 gallon) of ¼% (w/v) solution

$$\frac{85\ (\%)}{100\ (\%)} = \frac{9.46\ (g)}{x\ (g)}$$

$$x = 11.13\ g\ of\ 85\%\ phosphoric\ acid$$

11.13 g of water measure 11.13 mL

$$11.13\ (mL) \div 1.71 = 6.5\ mL,\ answer.$$

DILUTION AND CONCENTRATION OF SOLIDS

Miscellaneous Problems.

Examples:

   How many grams of opium containing 15% (w/w) of morphine and how many grams of lactose should be used to prepare 150 g of opium containing 10% (w/w) of morphine?

$$\frac{15\ (\%)}{10\ (\%)} = \frac{150\ (g)}{x\ (g)}$$

$$x = 100\ g\ of\ 15\%\ opium,\ and$$

$$150\ g\ -\ 100\ g = 50\ g\ of\ lactose,\ answers.$$

   If some moist crude drug contains 7.2% (w/w) of active ingredient and 21.6% of water, what will be the percentage (w/w) of active ingredient after the drug is dried?

100 g of moist drug would contain 21.6 g of water and would therefore weigh 78.4 g after drying

$$\frac{78.4\ (g)}{100\ (g)} = \frac{7.2\ (\%)}{x\ (\%)}$$

$$x = 9.2\%,\ answer.$$

   How many grams of 20% benzocaine ointment and how many grams of ointment base (diluent) should be used in preparing 5 lb of 2.5% benzocaine ointment?

5 lb = 454 g × 5 = 2270 g

$$\frac{20\ (\%)}{2.5\ (\%)} = \frac{2270\ (g)}{x\ (g)}$$

$$x = 283.75\ or\ 284\ g\ of\ 20\%\ ointment,\ and$$

$$2270\ g\ -\ 284\ g = 1986\ g\ of\ ointment\ base,\ answers.$$

Or,

5 lb = 454 g × 5 = 2270 g

2270 g × 2.5% = 56.75 g of benzocaine needed

$$\frac{20\ (g)}{56.75\ (g)} = \frac{100\ (g)}{x\ (g)}$$

$$x = 283.75\ or\ 284\ g\ of\ 20\%\ ointment\ needed$$

$$2270\ g\ -\ 284\ g = 1986\ g\ of\ ointment\ base\ needed,\ answer.$$

   How many grams of coal tar should be added to 3200 g of 5% coal tar ointment to prepare an ointment containing 20% of coal tar?

3200 g × 0.05   = 160 g of coal tar in 3200 g of 5% ointment
3200 g − 160 g   = 3040 g of base (diluent) in 3200 g of 5% ointment

In the 20% ointment, the diluent will represent 80% of the total weight

$$\frac{80\ (\%)}{20\ (\%)} = \frac{3040\ (g)}{x\ (g)}$$

$$x = 760\ g\ of\ coal\ tar\ in\ the\ 20\%\ ointment$$

Because the 5% ointment already contains 160 g of coal tar,

760 g − 160 g = 600 g, *answer.*

A simpler method of solving this problem can be used if we mentally translate it to read:

How many grams of coal tar should be added to 3200 g of coal tar ointment containing 95% diluent to prepare an ointment containing 80% diluent?

$$\frac{80\ (\%)}{95\ (\%)} = \frac{3200\ (g)}{x\ (g)}$$

x = 3800 g of ointment containing 80% diluent and 20% coal tar

3800 g − 3200 g = 600 g, *answer.*

NOTE: For another simple method, using alligation alternate (see subsequent section in this chapter).

How many milliliters of water should be added to 150 g of anhydrous lanolin to prepare lanolin containing 25% of water?

100% − 25% = 75% anhydrous lanolin in (hydrous) lanolin

$$\frac{75\ (\%)}{100\ (\%)} = \frac{150\ (g)}{x\ (g)}$$

x = 200 g of (hydrous) lanolin

200 g − 150 g = 50 g or mL of water, *answer.*

A more direct solution:

$$\frac{75\ (\%)}{25\ (\%)} = \frac{150\ (g)}{x\ (g)}$$

x = 50 g or mL of water, *answer.*

TRITURATIONS

Triturations are dilutions of potent medicinal substances. They were at one time official and were prepared by *diluting one part by weight of the finely powdered lactose.* They are, therefore, *10%* or *1:10 (w/w)* mixtures.

These dilutions offer a means of obtaining conveniently and accurately small quantities of potent drugs for compounding purposes. Although no longer official as such, triturations exemplify a method for the calculation and use of dilutions of solid medicinal substances in compounding and manufacturing procedures.

NOTE: The term "trituration" as used in this context should not be confused with the like term *trituration*, which is the pharmaceutical *process* of reducing substances to fine particles through grinding in a mortar and pestle.

Quantity of Trituration Required to Obtain Given Amount of Medicinal Substance. Calculating this quantity involves the following.

Examples:

How many grams of a 1:10 trituration are required to obtain 25 mg of drug?

10 g of trituration contain 1 g of drug

25 mg = 0.025 g

$$\frac{1\ (g)}{0.025\ (g)} = \frac{10\ (g)}{x\ (g)}$$

x = 0.25 g, *answer.*

How many milligrams of a 1:10 dilution of colchicine should be used by a manufacturing pharmacist in preparing 100 capsules for a clinical drug study if each capsule is to contain 0.5 mg of colchicine?

0.5 mg × 100 = 50 mg of colchicine needed
10 mg of dilution contain 1 mg of colchicine

$$\frac{1 \ (mg)}{50 \ (mg)} = \frac{10 \ (mg)}{x \ (mg)}$$

x = 500 mg, *answer.*

ALLIGATION

Alligation is an arithmetical method of solving problems that involve the mixing of solutions or mixtures of solids possessing different percentage strengths.

Alligation Medial

Alligation medial is a method by which the "weighted average" percentage strength of a mixture of two or more substances of known quantity and concentration may be quickly calculated. The percentage strength, expressed as a whole number, of each component of the mixture is multiplied by its corresponding quantity, and the sum of the products is divided by the sum of the quantities to give the percentage strength of the mixture, provided, of course, that the quantities have been expressed in a common denomination, whether of weight or of volume.

Determining Percentage Strength of a Mixture. Calculating the percentage strength of a mixture that has been made by mixing two or more components of given percentage strengths involves the following.

Examples:

What is the percentage (v/v) of alcohol in a mixture of 3000 mL of 40% (v/v) alcohol, 1000 mL of 60% (v/v) alcohol, and 1000 ml of 70% (v/v) alcohol (assume no contraction of volume)?

40 ×	3000 =	120000
60 ×	1000 =	60000
70 ×	1000 =	70000
Totals:	5000	250000

250000 ÷ 5000 = 50%, *answer.*

What is the percentage of zinc oxide in an ointment prepared by mixing 200 g of 10% ointment, 50 g of 20% ointment, and 100 g of 5% ointment?

10 ×	200 =	2000
20 ×	50 =	1000
5 ×	100 =	500
Totals:	350	3500

3500 ÷ 350 = 10%, *answer.*

In some problems the addition of a solvent or vehicle must be considered. It is generally best to consider the diluent as of zero percentage strength, as in the following problem.

Example:

What is the percentage (v/v) of alcohol in a mixture containing 500 mL of terpin hydrate elixir {40% (v/v) alcohol}, 400 mL of theophylline sodium glycinate elixir {21% (v/v) alcohol}, and sufficient simple syrup to make 1000 mL?

$$
\begin{array}{rrrr}
40 \times & 500 = & 20000 \\
21 \times & 400 = & 8400 \\
0 \times & \underline{100} = & \underline{0} \\
\text{Totals:} & 1000 & 28400 \\
28400 \div & 1000 = & 28.4\%, \textit{answer.}
\end{array}
$$

Alligation Alternate

Alligation alternate is a method by which we may calculate the number of parts of two or more components of a given strength when they are to be mixed to prepare a mixture of desired strength. A final proportion permits us to translate relative parts to any specific denomination.

The strength of a mixture must lie somewhere between the strengths of its components, i.e., the mixture must be somewhat stronger than its weakest component and somewhat weaker than its strongest. As indicated previously, the strength of the mixture is always a "weighted" average, i.e., it lies nearer to that of its weaker or stronger components depending on the relative amounts involved.

This "weighted" average can be found by means of an extremely simple scheme, as illustrated in the subsequent diagram.

Determining Relative Amounts of Components for Desired Mixture. Finding the relative amounts of components of different strengths for use in making a mixture of required strength involves the following.

Example:

In what proportion should alcohols of 95% and 50% strengths be mixed to make 70% alcohol?

Note that the difference between the *strength of the stronger component* (95%) and the *desired strength* (70%) indicates the *number of parts of the weaker* to be used (25 parts), and the difference between the *desired strength* (70%) and the *strength of the weaker component* (50%) indicates the *number of parts of the stronger* to be used (20 parts).

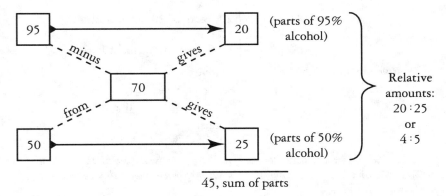

45, sum of parts

The mathematical validity of this relationship can be demonstrated.

Percent given	*Percent desired*	*Proportional parts required*
a		x
	c	
b		y

Given these data, the ratio of x to y may be derived algebraically as follows:

$$ax + by = c(x + y)$$
$$ax + by = cx + cy$$
$$ax - cx = cy - by$$
$$x(a - c) = y(c - b)$$

$$\frac{x}{y} = \frac{c - b}{a - c}$$

Given a = 95%, b = 50%, and c = 70%, we may therefore solve the problems as follows:

$$.95x + .50y = .70(x + y)$$

Or, $$95x + 50y = 70x + 70y$$
$$95x - 70x = 70y - 50y$$
$$x(95 - 70) = y(70 - 50)$$

$$\frac{x}{y} = \frac{70 - 50}{95 - 70} = \frac{20}{25} = \frac{4 \ (parts)}{5 \ (parts)}, \ answer.$$

The result can be shown to be correct by *alligation medial*:

$$95 \times 4 = 380$$
$$50 \times \underline{5} = \underline{250}$$
$$Totals: \ 9 \quad 630$$
$$630 \div 9 = 70\%$$

The customary layout of *alligation alternate*, used in the subsequent examples, is a convenient simplification of the preceding diagram.

Examples:

In what proportion should 20% benzocaine ointment be mixed with an ointment base to produce a 2.5% benzocaine ointment?

20%		2.5 parts of 20% ointment
	2.5%	
0%		17.5 parts of ointment base

Relative amounts: 2.5 : 17.5, or 1 : 7, *answer.*

Check: 20 ×   1 =   20
             0 ×   7 =   0
Totals: 8   20
        20 ÷   8 = 2.5%

A hospital pharmacist wants to use three lots of ichthammol ointment containing, respectively, 50%, 20%, and 5% of ichthammol. In what proportion should they be mixed to prepare a 10% ichthammol ointment?

The two lots containing *more* (50% and 20%) than the desired percentage may be separately linked to the lot containing *less* (5%) than the desired percentage:

50%		5 parts of 50% ointment
20%		5 parts of 20% ointment
	10%	
5%		10 + 40 = 50 parts of 5% ointment

Relative amounts: 5 : 5 : 50, or 1 : 1 : 10, *answer.*

Check: 50 ×   1 =   50
        20 ×   1 =   20
          5 × 10 =   50
Totals: 12   120
     120 ÷ 12 =   10%

Other answers are possible, of course, for the two stronger lots may be mixed first in any proportions desired, yielding a mixture that may then be mixed with the weakest lot in a proportion giving the desired strength.

In what proportions may a manufacturing pharmacist mix 20%, 15%, 5%, and 3% zinc oxide ointments to produce a 10% ointment?

Each of the weaker lots is paired with one of the stronger to give the desired strength, and because we may pair them in two ways, we may get two sets of correct answers.

20%		7 parts of 20% ointment
15%		5 parts of 15% ointment
	10%	
5%		5 parts of 5% ointment
3%		10 parts of 3% ointment

Relative amounts: 7 : 5 : 5 : 10, *answer.*

Check: 20 ×   7 = 140
        15 ×   5 =   75
          5 ×   5 =   25
          3 × 10 =   30
Totals: 27   270
     270 ÷ 27 =   10%

Or,

$$\begin{bmatrix} 20\% & & & \text{5 parts of 20\% ointment} \\ \begin{bmatrix} 15\% \\ 5\% \end{bmatrix} & 10\% & & \text{7 parts of 15\% ointment} \\ & & & \text{10 parts of 5\% ointment} \\ 3\% & & & \text{5 parts of 3\% ointment} \end{bmatrix}$$

Relative amounts: 5:7:10:5, *answer.*

Check: 20 ×   5 =   100
         15 ×   7 =   105
          5 ×   10 =   50
          3 ×   5 =   15
    Totals: 27   270

         270 ÷   27 =   10%

How many milliliters of 50% (w/v) dextrose solution and how many milliliters of 5% (w/v) dextrose solution are required to prepare 4500 mL of a 10% (w/v) solution?

$$\begin{matrix} 50\% & & \text{5 parts of 50\% solution} \\ & 10\% & \\ 5\% & & \text{40 parts of 5\% solution} \end{matrix}$$

Relative amounts 5:40, or 1:8, with a total of 9 parts

$$\frac{9 \text{ (parts)}}{1 \text{ (part)}} = \frac{4500 \text{ (mL)}}{x \text{ (mL)}}$$

$$x = 500 \text{ mL of 50\% solution, } and$$

$$\frac{9 \text{ (parts)}}{8 \text{ (parts)}} = \frac{4500 \text{ (mL)}}{y \text{ (mL)}}$$

$$y = 4000 \text{ mL of 5\% solution, } answers.$$

How many milliliters each of 2% iodine tincture and 7% strong iodine tincture should be used in preparing 1 gallon of a tincture containing 3.5% of iodine?

1 gallon = 3785 mL

$$\begin{matrix} 2\% & & \text{3.5 parts of 2\% tincture} \\ & 3.5\% & \\ 7\% & & \text{1.5 parts of 7\% tincture} \end{matrix}$$

Relative amounts: 3.5:1.5, or 7:3, with a total of 10 parts

$$\frac{10 \text{ (parts)}}{7 \text{ (parts)}} = \frac{3785 \text{ (mL)}}{x \text{ (mL)}}$$

$$x = 2650 \text{ mL of 2\% iodine tincture, } and$$

$$\frac{10 \text{ (parts}}{3 \text{ (parts)}} = \frac{3785 \text{ (mL)}}{y \text{ (mL)}}$$

$$y = 1135 \text{ mL of 7\% strong iodine tincture,}$$
answers.

Quantity of One Component to Mix with Another to Obtain Desired Preparation Strength. Calculating the quantity of a component of given strength that should be mixed with a specified quantity of another component of given strength to make a preparation of desired strength involves the following.

Examples:

How many grams of 2.5% hydrocortisone cream should be mixed with 360 g of 0.25% cream to make a 1% hydrocortisone cream?

$$
\begin{array}{c|c|c}
2.5\% & & 0.75 \text{ part of 2.5\% cream} \\
& 1\% & \\
0.25\% & & 1.5 \text{ parts of 0.25\% cream}
\end{array}
$$

Relative amounts: 0.75 : 1.5, or 1 : 2

$$\frac{2 \ (parts)}{1 \ (part)} = \frac{360 \ (g)}{x \ (g)}$$

$$x = 180 \text{ g, } \textit{answer.}$$

Alternate (algebraic) solution of the same problem:

$$2.5(x) + 0.25(360) = 1(360 + x)$$

$$2.5x + 90 = 360 + x$$

$$1.5x = 270$$

$$x = 180 \text{ g, } \textit{answer.}$$

How many grams of white petrolatum should be mixed with 250 g of 5% and 750 g of 15% sulfur ointments to prepare a 10% ointment?

$$
\begin{array}{rrr}
5 \times & 250 = & 1250 \\
15 \times & \underline{750} = & \underline{11250} \\
\text{Totals:} & 1000 & 12500
\end{array}
$$

12500 ÷ 1000 = 12.5% of sulfur in 1000 g of a mixture of 5% and 15% ointments

$$
\begin{array}{c|c|c}
12.5\% & & 10 \text{ parts of 12.5\% mixture} \\
& 10\% & \\
0\% & & 2.5 \text{ parts of white petrolatum}
\end{array}
$$

Relative amounts: 10 : 2.5, or 4 : 1

$$\frac{4 \ (parts)}{1 \ (part)} = \frac{1000 \ (g)}{x \ (g)}$$

$$x = 250 \text{ g, } \textit{answer.}$$

$$
\begin{array}{lrrr}
\text{Check:} & 12.5 \times & 1000 = & 12500 \\
& 0 \times & \underline{250} = & \underline{0} \\
& \text{Totals:} & 1250 & 12500 \\
& 12500 \div & 1250 = & 10\%
\end{array}
$$

Amount of Active Ingredient to Increase Mixture Strength. Calculating the amount of active ingredient that must be added to increase the strength of a mixture of given quantity and strength involves the following.

Example:

How many grams of coal tar should be added to 3200 g of 5% coal tar ointment to prepare an ointment containing 20% of coal tar?

Coal tar (active ingredient) = 100%

$$
\begin{array}{c|c|c}
100\% & & \text{15 parts of 100\% coal tar} \\
 & 20\% & \\
5\% & & \text{80 parts of 5\% ointment}
\end{array}
$$

Relative amounts: 15:80, or 3:16

$$
\frac{16 \text{ (parts)}}{3 \text{ (parts)}} = \frac{3200 \text{ (g)}}{x \text{ (g)}}
$$

$$
x = 600 \text{ g}, \text{ answer.}
$$

Check: $\begin{array}{rcl} 100 \times & 600 = & 60000 \\ 5 \times & \underline{3200} = & \underline{16000} \\ \text{Totals:} & 3800 & 76000 \\ 76000 \div & 3800 = & 20\% \end{array}$

Compare the solution of this problem by use of alligation alternate with other methods on pages 127 and 128.

SPECIFIC GRAVITY OF MIXTURES

The methods of alligation medial and alligation alternate may be used in solving problems involving the specific gravities of different quantities of liquids of known specific gravities provided no change in volume occurs when the liquids are mixed and that they are measured in a common denomination of *volume.*

Example:

What is the specific gravity of a mixture of 1000 mL of syrup with a specific gravity of 1.300, 400 mL of glycerin with a specific gravity of 1.250, and 1000 mL of an elixir with a specific gravity of 0.950?

$$
\begin{array}{rcl}
1.300 \times 1000 &=& 1300 \\
1.250 \times 400 &=& 500 \\
0.950 \times \underline{1000} &=& \underline{950} \\
\text{Totals:} 2400 & & 2750
\end{array}
$$

$$
2750 \div 2400 = 1.146, \text{ answer.}
$$

Amounts of Ingredients of Known Specific Gravities to Use in Making a Mixture of Desired Specific Gravity. Calculating the relative or specific amounts of ingredients of given specific gravities required to make a mixture of desired specific gravity involves the following.

Examples:

In what proportion must glycerin with a specific gravity of 1.25 and water be mixed to prepare a liquid having a specific gravity of 1.10?

$$
\begin{array}{c|c|c}
1.25 & & 0.10 \text{ parts of glycerin} \\
& 1.10 & \\
1.00 & & 0.15 \text{ parts of water}
\end{array}
$$

Relative amounts: 0.10:0.15, or 2:3, *answer.*

How many milliliters of each of two liquids with specific gravities of 0.950 and 0.875 should be used to prepare 1500 mL of a liquid having a specific gravity of 0.925?

$$
\begin{array}{c|c|l}
0.950 & & 0.050, \text{ or } 50 \text{ parts of liquid with specific} \\
& & \quad \text{gravity of } 0.950 \\
& 0.925 & \\
0.875 & & 0.025, \text{ or } 25 \text{ parts of liquid with specific} \\
& & \quad \text{gravity of } 0.875
\end{array}
$$

Relative amounts: 50:25, or 2:1, with a total of 3 parts

$$\frac{3 \text{ (parts)}}{2 \text{ (parts)}} = \frac{1500 \text{ (mL)}}{x \text{ (mL)}}$$

$$x = 1000 \text{ mL of liquid with specific gravity of } 0.950, \textit{ and}$$

$$\frac{3 \text{ (parts)}}{1 \text{ (part)}} = \frac{1500 \text{ (mL)}}{y \text{ (mL)}}$$

$$y = 500 \text{ mL of liquid with specific gravity of } 0.875, \textit{ answers}$$

Practice Problems

1. If 250 mL of a 1:800 (v/v) solution are diluted to 1000 mL, what will be the ratio strength (v/v)?

2. Aluminum acetate topical solution contains 5% (w/v) of aluminum acetate. When 100 mL are diluted to a liter, what will be the ratio strength (w/v)?

3. If 400 mL of a 20% (w/v) solution are diluted to 2 liters, what will be the percentage strength (w/v)?

4. If a 0.067% (w/v) methylbenzethonium chloride lotion is diluted with an equal volume of water, what will be the ratio strength (w/v) of the dilution?

5. In preparing a solution for a wet dressing, two 0.3-g tablets of potassium permanganate are dissolved in 1 gallon of purified water. What will be the percentage strength (w/v) of the solution?

6. If 150 mL of a 17% (w/v) concentrate of benzalkonium chloride are diluted to 5 gallons, what will be the ratio strength (w/v) of the dilution?

7. What is the strength of a sodium chloride solution obtained by evaporating 800 g of a 10% (w/w) solution to 250 g?

8. If one Domeboro® effervescent tablet dissolved in 1 pint of water makes a solution equivalent to a 1:40 (w/v) dilution, what would be the expected ratio strength if four tablets were dissolved in 1 quart of water?

9. If two tablespoonfuls of povidone iodine solution (10% w/v) are diluted to 1 quart with purified water, what is the ratio strength of the dilution?

10. How many milliliters of a 1:50 (w/v) boric acid solution can be prepared from 500 mL of a 5% (w/v) boric acid solution?

11. How many milliliters of water must be added to 250 mL of a 25% (w/v) stock solution of sodium chloride to prepare a 0.9% (w/v) sodium chloride solution?

12. How many milliliters of a 1:50 (w/v) stock solution of a chemical should be used to prepare 1 liter of a 1:4000 (w/v) solution?

13. A certain product contains benzalkonium chloride in a concentration of 1:5000 (w/v). How many milliliters of a 17% solution of benzalkonium chloride should be used in preparing 4 liters of the product?

14. How many milliliters of a 10% stock solution of a chemical are needed to prepare 120 mL of a solution containing 10 mg of the chemical per milliliter?

15. How many milliliters of water should be added to 1 gallon of 70% isopropyl alcohol to prepare a 30% solution for soaking sponges?

16. How many milliliters of water for injection must be added to 10 liters of a 50% (w/v) dextrose injection to reduce the concentration to 30% (w/v)?

17. The formula for a buffer solution contains 1.24% (w/v) of boric acid. How many milliliters of a 5% (w/v) boric acid solution should be used to obtain the boric acid needed in preparing 1 liter of the buffer solution?

18.
Menthol	0.1%
Hexachlorophene	0.1%
Glycerin	10.0%
Alcohol 70%, to make	500 mL

    Label: Menthol and Hexachlorophene Lotion.

    How many milliliters of a 5% (w/v) solution of menthol in alcohol should be used to obtain the amount of menthol needed in preparing the lotion?

19. ℞   Gentian Violet Solution   500 mL
            1:100,000
          Sig. Mouth wash.

    How many milliliters of ½% solution of gentian violet should be used in preparing the prescription?

20. How many milliliters of Burow's Solution (containing 5% w/v of aluminum acetate) should be used in preparing 2 liters of a 1:800 (w/v) solution to be used as a wet dressing?

21. How many milliliters of a solution containing 0.275 mg of histamine phosphate per milliliter should be used in preparing 15 mL of a 1:10000 histamine phosphate solution?

22. If a pharmacist adds 3 g of hydrocortisone to 60 g of a 5% (w/w) hydrocortisone cream, what is the final percentage strength of hydrocortisone in the product?

23. A physician prescribes an ophthalmic suspension to contain 100 mg of cortisone acetate in 8 mL of normal saline solution. The pharmacist has on hand a 2.5%

suspension of cortisone acetate in normal saline solution. How many milliliters of this and how many milliliters of normal saline solution should be used in preparing the prescribed suspension?

24. The formula for a mouth wash calls for 0.05% by volume of methyl salicylate. How many milliliters of a 10% (v/v) stock solution of methyl salicylate in alcohol will be needed to prepare 1 gallon of the mouth wash?

25. ℞   Benzalkonium Chloride Solution   240 mL
         Make a solution such that 10 mL diluted
             to a liter equals a 1:5000 solution.
         Sig. 10 mL diluted to a liter for external use.

How many milliliters of a 17% solution of benzalkonium chloride should be used in preparing the prescription?

26. How many milliliters of water should be added to 100 mL of a 1:125 (w/v) solution to make a solution such that 25 mL diluted to 100 mL will yield a 1:4000 dilution?

27. How many milliliters of a 0.1% (w/v) thimerosal topical solution should be used to prepare 500 mL of a 1:5000 solution for irrigation?

28. If 20 mL of a 2% (w/v) solution are diluted with water to 8 pints, what is the ratio strength (w/v) of the dilution?

29. How many milliliters of water should be added to a liter of 1:3000 (w/v) solution to make a 1:8000 (w/v) solution?

30. ℞   Zephiran Chloride Solution (17% w/v)   50 mL
         Purified Water, to make   250 mL
         Sig. One (1) tsp. diluted to a pint with
              water for topical use.

Calculate the ratio strength of zephiran chloride in the dilution.

31. How many milliliters of water should be added to 2500 mL of 83% (v/v) alcohol to prepare 50% (v/v) alcohol?

32. How many milliliters of water should be mixed with 1200 g of 65% (w/w) alcohol to make 45% (w/w) alcohol?

33. How many milliliters of a syrup containing 85% (w/v) of sucrose should be mixed with 150 mL of a syrup containing 60% (w/v) of sucrose to make a syrup containing 80% (w/v) of sucrose?

34. ℞   Castor Oil   5.0 mL
         Euresol   15.0 mL
         Alcohol 85%   ad   240.0 mL
         Sig. For the scalp.

How many milliliters each of 95% (v/v) alcohol and water should be used in preparing the prescription?

35. How many milliliters of 95% (w/w) sulfuric acid having a specific gravity of 1.820 should be used in preparing 2 liters of 10% (w/v) acid?

36. A pharmacist mixes 100 mL of 38% (w/w) hydrochloric acid with enough purified

water to make 360 mL. If the specific gravity of hydrochloric acid is 1.20, calculate the percentage strength (w/v) of the resulting dilution.

37. How many milliliters of 28% (w/w) strong ammonia solution having a specific gravity of 0.89 should be used in preparing 2000 mL of 10% (w/w) ammonia solution with a specific gravity of 0.96?

38. How many milliliters of a 70% (w/w) sorbitol solution, specific gravity 1.30, should be used in preparing 1 gallon of a 10% (w/v) solution?

39. In using isoproterenol hydrochloride solution (1:5000 w/v), 1 mL of the solution is diluted to 10 mL with sodium chloride injection before intravenous administration. What is the percentage concentration of the diluted solution?

40. A 1:750 (w/v) solution of benzalkonium chloride diluted with purified water in a ratio of 3 parts of the benzalkonium solution and 77 parts of purified water is recommended for bladder and urethral irrigation. What is the ratio strength of benzalkonium chloride in the final dilution?

41. In filling a medication order for 500 mL of diluted phosphoric acid, a pharmacist used 50 mL of 85% phosphoric acid with a specific gravity of 1.71. What was the percentage strength (w/v) of the finished product?

42. An insect venom concentrate for immunotherapy contains 100 μg/mL. How many milliliters of water should be added to 1.2 mL of the venom concentrate to yield a 1:100,000 dilution?

43. How many grams of a 2.5% (w/w) benzocaine ointment can be prepared by diluting 1 lb of a 20% (w/w) benzocaine ointment with white petrolatum?

44. How many grams of salicylic acid should be added to 75 g of a polyethylene glycol ointment to prepare an ointment containing 6% (w/w) of salicylic acid?

45. ℞   Zinc Oxide
     Calamine   aa   2 g
     Petrolatum   60 g
     Sig. Apply.

   If the prescription was filled as written, and then the prescriber wished to change the concentration of zinc oxide to 10% (w/w), (a) how many additional grams of zinc oxide should be added, and (b) how many grams of a 20% (w/w) zinc oxide ointment could be added to change the strength to 10% (w/w) of zinc oxide?

46. ℞   Hydrocortisone Acetate Ointment   10 g
         0.25%
     Sig. Apply to the eye.

   How many grams of 2.5% ophthalmic hydrocortisone acetate ointment and how many grams of ophthalmic base (diluent) should be used in preparing the prescription?

47. How many grams of zinc oxide should be added to 3400 g of a 10% zinc oxide ointment to prepare a product containing 15% of zinc oxide?

48. How many grams of petrolatum (diluent) should be added to 250 g of a 25% ichthammol ointment to make a 5% ointment?

49. ℞   Zinc Oxide   1.5
          Hydrophilic Petrolatum   2.5
          Purified Water   5.0
          Hydrophilic Ointment   ad   30.0
          Sig. Apply to affected areas.

     How much zinc oxide should be added to the product to make an ointment containing 10% of zinc oxide?

50. ℞   Coal Tar   5%
          Lassar's Paste   ad   50.0
          Sig. Apply as directed.

     In compounding, a pharmacist added 2.5 g of coal tar to 50 g of Lassar's Paste. Calculate the percentage concentration of coal tar in the finished product.

51. A vaginal douche powder concentrate contains 2% (w/w) of active ingredient. What would be the percentage concentration (w/v) of the resultant solution after a 5-g packet of powder is dissolved in enough water to make 1 quart of solution?

52. If one tablespoonful of a 0.2% (w/v) solution of phenylmercuric acetate is diluted to 1 quart with water, what would be the percentage concentration (w/v) of the resulting solution?

53. How many milliliters of a 10% (w/v) stock solution of a chemical should be used in preparing 120 mL of a prescription, so a 1:2500 (w/v) solution results when the patient adds 2 tablespoonfuls of the medication to 1 pint of water?

54. How many milligrams of sodium fluoride are needed to prepare 100 mL of a sodium fluoride stock solution such that a solution containing 2 ppm of sodium fluoride results when 0.5 mL is diluted to 250 mL with water?

55. How many grams of coal tar should be added to 925 g of zinc oxide paste to prepare an ointment containing 6% of coal tar?

56. A prescription calls for 0.005 g of morphine sulfate. How many milligrams of a 1:10 trituration should be used to obtain the morphine sulfate?

57. ℞   Codeine Sulfate   10 mg
          Acetylsalicylic Acid   0.3 g
          Ft. pulv. tal. no. 20
          Sig. One b.i.d.

     How many grams of a 1:10 trituration of codeine sulfate should be used in preparing the prescription?

58. Four equal amounts of belladonna extract, containing 1.15%, 1.30%, 1.35%, and 1.20% of alkaloids, respectively, were mixed. What was the percentage strength of the mixture?

59. What is the percentage of alcohol in a mixture containing 1500 mL of witch hazel (14% alcohol), 2000 mL of glycerin, and 5000 mL of 50% alcohol?

60. A pharmacist mixes 200 g of 10% ichthammol ointment, 450 g of 5% ichthammol ointment, and 1000 g of petrolatum (diluent). What is the percentage of ichthammol in the finished product?

61.   Coal Tar Solution   80 mL (85% alcohol)
      Glycerin   160 mL
      Alcohol   500 mL (95% alcohol)
      Boric Acid Solution   ad   1000 mL
      Label: Medicated lotion.

      Calculate the percentage of alcohol in the lotion.

62.   A drug is commercially available in capsules each containing 12.5 mg of drug and 37.5 mg of diluent. How many milligrams of additional diluent must be added to the contents of one capsule to make a dilution containing 0.5 mg of drug in each 100 mg of powder?

63.   A hospital pharmacist constitutes a vial containing 1 g of aziocillin sodium to 10 mL with sterile water for injection. This solution is then diluted by adding it to 100 mL of 5% dextrose injection for administration by infusion. What is the concentration, in milligrams per milliliter (mg/mL), of aziocillin sodium in the infusion solution?

64.   Calculate the percentage of alcohol in a lotion containing 2 liters of witch hazel (14% of alcohol), 1 liter of alcohol (95%), and enough boric acid solution to make 5 liters.

65.   In what proportion should 95% alcohol be mixed with 30% alcohol to make 70% alcohol?

66.   In what proportion should 10% and 2% coal tar ointments be mixed to prepare a 5% ointment?

67.   In what proportion should a 20% zinc oxide ointment be mixed with white petrolatum (diluent) to produce a 3% zinc oxide ointment?

68.   In what proportion should 30% and 1.5% hydrogen peroxide solutions be mixed to prepare a 3% hydrogen peroxide solution.

69.   The solvent for the extraction of a vegetable drug is 70% alcohol. In what proportion may 95%, 60%, and 50% alcohol be mixed to prepare a solvent of the desired concentration?

70.   What is the percentage of iodine in a mixture of 3 liters of a 7% (w/v) iodine topical solution, 10 pints of a 2% (w/v) solution, and 2270 mL of a 3.5% (w/v) solution?

71.   A manufacturing pharmacist has four lots of ichthammol ointment, containing 50%, 25%, 10%, and 5% of ichthammol. How many grams of each may be used to prepare 4800 g of a 20% ichthammol ointment?

72.   How many milliliters of a 2.5% (w/v) thiamylal sodium solution and how many milliliters of 0.9% (w/v) sodium chloride injection should be used to prepare 500 mL of a 0.3% (w/v) thiamylal sodium solution?

73.   How many milliliters of a 2% (w/v) solution of lidocaine hydrochloride should be used in preparing 500 mL of a solution containing 4 mg of lidocaine hydrochloride per milliliter of solution?

74.   Dopamine hydrochloride solution is available in 5-mL ampuls containing 40 mg of dopamine hydrochloride per milliliter. The solution must be diluted before administration. If a physician wishes to use sodium chloride injection as the diluent

and wants a dilution containing 0.04% (w/v) of dopamine hydrochloride, how many milliliters of sodium chloride injection should be added to 5 mL of the solution?

75. A solution of benzalkonium chloride is available in a concentration of $1:750$ (w/v). How many milliliters of purified water should be added to 30 mL of the solution to prepare a $1:5000$ benzalkonium chloride solution for use as a wet dressing to the skin?

76. If an antibiotic injection contains 5% (w/v) of the drug, how many milliliters of diluent should be added to 5 mL of the injection to prepare a concentration of 5 mg of the antibiotic per milliliter?

77. A vial of kanamycin sulfate injection contains 500 mg per 2 mL. If 1.6 mL of the injection are diluted to 200 mL with sodium chloride injection, how many milliliters of the dilution should be administered daily to a child weighing 22 lb if the daily dose is 15 mg/kg of body weight?

78. How many milliliters each of phenytoin sodium suspensions containing 30 mg per 5 mL and 125 mg per 5 mL should be used in preparing 480 mL of a suspension containing 10 mg of phenytoin sodium per milliliter?

79. If anhydrous lanolin absorbs twice its weight of water, how many milliliters of additional water will be absorbed by 4000 g of hydrous lanolin containing 25% of water?

80. A disinfectant concentrate for surgical instruments contains 6.5% (w/v) of a quaternary ammonium compound. What is the percentage strength of a solution resulting from the addition of 60 mL of the concentrate to 1 gallon of water?

81. ℞   Zephiran Chloride Solution (17% w/v)   q.s.
        Purified Water, to make   480 mL
        Sig. One (1) tbsp. diluted to 1 gallon with water
            (to make a $1:10,000$ dilution).

    How many milliliters of zephiran chloride solution should be used in preparing the prescription?

82. You have on hand 800 g of a 5% coal tar ointment and 1200 g of a 10% coal tar ointment.
    (a) If the two ointments are mixed, what is the concentration of coal tar in the finished product?
    (b) How many grams of coal tar should be added to the product to obtain an ointment containing 15% of coal tar?

83. What is the specific gravity of a mixture containing 1000 mL of water, 500 mL of glycerin having a specific gravity of 1.25, and 1500 mL of alcohol having a specific gravity of 0.81? (Assume no contraction occurs when the liquids are mixed.)

84. If a pharmacist mixed 1 pint of propylene glycol having a specific gravity of 1.20 with 500 mL of water, how many milliliters additional of propylene glycol should be added to change the specific gravity to 1.15?

85. How many milliliters of a syrup having a specific gravity of 1.350 should be mixed

with 3000 mL of a syrup having a specific gravity of 1.250 to obtain a product having a specific gravity of 1.310?

86. How many grams of sorbitol solution having a specific gravity of 1.285 and how many grams (milliliters) of water should be used in preparing 500 g of a sorbitol solution having a specific gravity of 1.225?

9

Isotonic Solutions

When a solvent passes through a semipermeable membrane from a dilute solution into a more concentrated one, with the result that the concentrations become equalized, the phenomenon is known as *osmosis*. The pressure responsible for this phenomenon is called *osmotic pressure*, and it proves to be caused by and to vary with the solute.

If the solute is a nonelectrolyte, its solution will contain only molecules, and the osmotic pressure of the solution will vary only with the concentration of the solute. If the solute is an electrolyte, its solution will contain ions, and the osmotic pressure of the solution will vary not only with the concentration, but also with the degree of dissociation of the solute. Therefore, substances that dissociate have a relatively greater number of particles in solution and should exert a greater osmotic pressure than could undissociated molecules.

Like osmotic pressure, the other colligative properties of solutions, namely, vapor pressure, boiling point, and freezing point, depend on the number of particles in solution. These properties, therefore, are related, and a change in any one of them will be attended by corresponding changes in the others.

Two solutions that have the same osmotic pressure are termed *isosmotic*. Many solutions intended to be mixed with body fluids are designed to have the same osmotic pressure for greater comfort, efficacy, and safety. A solution having the same osmotic pressure as a specific body fluid is said to be *isotonic* (meaning of equal tone) with that body fluid.

Solutions of lower osmotic pressure than that of a body fluid are *hypotonic*, whereas those having a higher osmotic pressure are *hypertonic*. Blood and the fluids of the eye, nose, and bowel are of principal concern to the pharmacist in the manufacture and use of preparations to be mixed with these biologic fluids, which include *ophthalmic* (eye), *nasal* (nose), *parenteral* (by injection) and some *enema* (rectal) preparations.

PREPARATION OF ISOTONIC SOLUTIONS

The calculations involved in preparing isotonic solutions may be made in terms of data relating to the colligative properties of solutions. Theoretically, any one of these properties may be used as a basis for determining tonicity. Practically and most conveniently, a comparison of freezing points is used for this purpose. It is generally accepted that $-0.52°C$ is the freezing point of both blood serum and lacrimal fluid.

When one gram molecular weight of any nonelectrolyte, i.e., a substance with negligible dissociation, such as boric acid, is dissolved in 1000 g of water, the freezing point of the solution is about 1.86°C below the freezing point of pure water. By simple proportion, therefore, we may calculate the weight of any nonelectrolyte that should be dissolved in each 1000 g of water if the solution is to be isotonic with body fluids.

Boric acid, for example, has a molecular weight of 61.8, and hence (in theory) 61.8 g in 1000 g of water should produce a freezing point of $-1.86°C$. Therefore:

$$\frac{1.86\ (°C)}{0.52\ (°C)} = \frac{61.8\ (g)}{x\ (g)}$$
$$x = 17.3\ g$$

In short, 17.3 g of boric acid in 1000 g of water, having a weight-in-volume strength of approximately 1.73%, should make a solution isotonic with lacrimal fluid.

With electrolytes, the problem is not so simple. Because osmotic pressure depends more on the number than on the kind of particles, substances that dissociate have a tonic effect that increases with the degree of dissociation; the greater the dissociation, the smaller the quantity required to produce any given osmotic pressure. If we assume that sodium chloride in weak solutions is about 80% dissociated, then each 100 molecules yield 180 particles, or 1.8 times as many particles as are yielded by 100 molecules of a nonelectrolyte. This dissociation factor, commonly symbolized by the letter i, must be included in the proportion when we seek to determine the strength of an isotonic solution of sodium chloride (m.w. 58.5):

$$\frac{1.86 \ (^\circ C) \times 1.8}{0.52 \ (^\circ C)} = \frac{58.5 \ (g)}{x \ (g)}$$
$$x = 9.09 \ g$$

Hence, 9.09 g of sodium chloride in 1000 g of water should make a solution isotonic with blood or lacrimal fluid. Actually, a 0.90% (w/v) sodium chloride solution is considered isotonic with body fluids.

Simple isotonic solutions may then be calculated by using this formula:

$$\frac{0.52 \times \text{molecular weight}}{1.86 \times \text{dissociation } (i)} = \text{g of solute per 1000 g of water}$$

The value of i for many a medicinal salt has not been experimentally determined. Some salts (such as zinc sulfate, with only some 40% dissociation and an i value therefore of 1.4) are exceptional, but most medicinal salts approximate the dissociation of sodium chloride in weak solutions. If the number of ions is known, we may use the following values, lacking better information:

Nonelectrolytes and substances of slight dissociation : 1.0
Substances that dissociate into 2 ions: 1.8
Substances that dissociate into 3 ions: 2.6
Substances that dissociate into 4 ions: 3.4
Substances that dissociate into 5 ions: 4.2

A special problem arises when a prescription directs us to make a solution isotonic by adding the proper amount of some substance other than the active ingredient or ingredients. Given a 0.5% (w/v) solution of sodium chloride, we may easily calculate that 0.9 g − 0.5 g = 0.4 g of additional sodium chloride that should be contained in each 100 mL if the solution is to be made isotonic with a body fluid. But how much sodium chloride should be used in preparing 100 mL of a 1% (w/v) solution of atropine sulfate, which is to be made isotonic with lacrimal fluid? The answer depends on *how much sodium chloride is in effect represented by the atropine sulfate.*

The relative tonic effect of two substances, i.e., the quantity of one that is the equivalent in tonic effects to a given quantity of the other, may be calculated if the quantity of one having a certain effect in a specified quantity of solvent is divided by the quantity of the other having the same effect in the same quantity of solvent. For example, we calculated that 17.3 g of boric acid per 1000 g of water and 9.09 g of sodium chloride per 1000 g of water are both instrumental in making an aqueous solution isotonic with lacrimal fluid. If, however, 17.3 g of boric acid are equivalent in tonicity to 9.09 g of sodium chloride, then 1 g of boric acid must be the equivalent of 9.09 g ÷ 17.3 g or 0.52 g of sodium

Table 9.1. Sodium Chloride Equivalents (E Values)

Substance	Molecular Weight	Ions	i	Sodium Chloride Equivalent
Antazoline phosphate	363	2	1.8	0.16
Antipyrine	188	1	1.0	0.17
Atropine sulfate.H_2O	695	3	2.6	0.12
Benoxinate hydrochloride	345	2	1.8	0.17
Benzalkonium chloride	360	2	1.8	0.16
Benzyl alcohol	108	1	1.0	0.30
Boric acid	61.8	1	1.0	0.52
Chloramphenicol	323	1	1.0	0.10
Chlorobutanol	177	1	1.0	0.24
Chlortetracycline hydrochloride	515	2	1.8	0.11
Cocaine hydrochloride	340	2	1.8	0.16
Cromolyn sodium	512	2	1.8	0.11
Cyclopentolate hydrochloride	328	2	1.8	0.18
Demecarium bromide	717	3	2.6	0.12
Dextrose (anhydrous)	180	1	1.0	0.18
Dextrose.H_2O	198	1	1.0	0.16
Dipivefrin hydrochloride	388	2	1.8	0.15
Ephedrine hydrochloride	202	2	1.8	0.29
Ephedrine sulfate	429	3	2.6	0.23
Epinephrine bitartrate	333	2	1.8	0.18
Epinephryl borate	209	1	1.0	0.16
Eucatropine hydrochloride	328	2	1.8	0.18
Fluorescein sodium	376	3	2.6	0.31
Glycerin	92	1	1.0	0.34
Homatropine hydrobromide	356	2	1.8	0.17
Hydroxyamphetamine hydrobromide	232	2	1.8	0.25
Idoxuridine	354	1	1.0	0.09
Lidocaine hydrochloride	289	2	1.8	0.22
Mannitol	182	1	1.0	0.18
Morphine sulfate.$5H_2O$	759	3	2.6	0.11
Naphazoline hydrochloride	247	2	1.8	0.27
Oxymetazoline hydrochloride	297	2	1.8	0.20
Oxytetracycline hydrochloride	497	2	1.8	0.12
Phenacaine hydrochloride	353	2	1.8	0.20
Phenobarbital sodium	254	2	1.8	0.24
Phenylephrine hydrochloride	204	2	1.8	0.32
Physostigmine salicylate	413	2	1.8	0.16
Physostigmine sulfate	649	3	2.6	0.13
Pilocarpine hydrochloride	245	2	1.8	0.24
Pilocarpine nitrate	271	2	1.8	0.23
Potassium biphosphate	136	2	1.8	0.43
Potassium chloride	74.5	2	1.8	0.76
Potassium iodide	166	2	1.8	0.34
Potassium nitrate	101	2	1.8	0.58
Potassium penicillin G	372	2	1.8	0.18
Procaine hydrochloride	273	2	1.8	0.21
Proparacaine hydrochloride	331	2	1.8	0.18
Scopolamine hydrobromide.$3H_2O$	438	2	1.8	0.12
Silver nitrate	170	2	1.8	0.33
Sodium bicarbonate	84	2	1.8	0.65
Sodium borate.$10H_2O$	381	5	4.2	0.42
Sodium carbonate	106	3	2.6	0.80
Sodium carbonate.H_2O	124	3	2.6	0.68
Sodium chloride	58	2	1.8	1.00
Sodium citrate.$2H_2O$	294	4	3.4	0.38

Table 9.1. *(continued)*

Substance	Molecular Weight	Ions	i	Sodium Chloride Equivalent
Sodium iodide	150	2	1.8	0.39
Sodium lactate	112	2	1.8	0.52
Sodium phosphate, dibasic, anhydrous	142	3	2.6	0.53
Sodium phosphate, dibasic.$7H_2O$	268	3	2.6	0.29
Sodium phosphate, monobasic, anhydrous	120	2	1.8	0.49
Sodium phosphate, monobasic.H_2O	138	2	1.8	0.42
Tetracaine hydrochloride	301	2	1.8	0.18
Tetracycline hydrochloride	481	2	1.8	0.12
Tetrahydrozoline hydrochloride	237	2	1.8	0.25
Timolol maleate	432	2	1.8	0.14
Tobramycin	468	1	1.0	0.07
Tropicamide	284	1	1.0	0.11
Urea	60	1	1.0	0.59
Zinc chloride	136	3	2.6	0.62
Zinc sulfate.$7H_2O$	288	2	1.4	0.15

chloride. Similarly, 1 g of sodium chloride must be the "tonicic equivalent" of 17.3 g ÷ 9.09 g or 1.90 g of boric acid.

We have seen that one quantity of any substance should in theory have a constant tonic effect if dissolved in 1000 g of water: 1 g molecular weight of the substance divided by its *i* or dissociation value. Hence, the relative quantity of sodium chloride that is the tonicic equivalent of a quantity of boric acid may be calculated by these ratios:

$$\frac{58.5 \div 1.8}{61.8 \div 1.0} \text{ or } \frac{58.5 \times 1.0}{61.8 \times 1.8}$$

and we may formulate a convenient rule: *quantities of two substances that are tonicic equivalents are proportional to the molecular weights of each multiplied by the* i *value of the other.*

To return to the problem involving 1 g of atropine sulfate in 100 mL of solution:

Molecular weight of sodium chloride   = 58.5; *i* = 1.8
Molecular weight of atropine sulfate   = 695; *i* = 2.6

$$\frac{695 \times 1.8}{58.5 \times 2.6} = \frac{1 \text{ (g)}}{x \text{ (g)}}$$

x = 0.12 g of sodium chloride represented by 1 g of atropine sulfate

Because a solution isotonic with lacrimal fluid should contain the equivalent of 0.90 g of sodium chloride in each 100 mL of solution, the difference to be added must be 0.90 g − 0.12 g = 0.78 g of sodium chloride.

Table 9.1 gives the *sodium chloride equivalents* (E values) of each of the substances listed. These values were calculated according to the rule stated previously. If the number of grams of a substance included in a prescription is multiplied by its sodium chloride equivalent, the amount of sodium chloride represented by that substance is determined.

The procedure for the *calculation of isotonic solutions with sodium chloride equivalents* may be outlined as follows:

Step 1. Calculate the amount (in grams) of sodium chloride represented by the ingredients in the prescription. Multiply the amount (in grams) of each substance by its sodium chloride equivalent.

Step 2. Calculate the amount (in grams) of sodium chloride, alone, that would be contained in an isotonic solution of the volume specified in the prescription, namely, *the amount of sodium chloride in a 0.9% solution of the specified volume.* (Such a solution would contain 0.009 g/mL.)

Step 3. Subtract the amount of sodium chloride represented by the ingredients in the prescription (Step 1) from the amount of sodium chloride, alone, that would be represented in the specific volume of an isotonic solution (Step 2). The answer represents the amount (in grams) of sodium chloride to be added to make the solution isotonic.

Step 4. If an agent other than sodium chloride, such as boric acid, dextrose, sodium, or potassium nitrate, is to be used to make a solution isotonic, divide the amount of sodium chloride (Step 3) by the sodium chloride equivalent of the other substance.

Calculating the Dissociation (i) Factor of an Electrolyte.

Examples:

Zinc sulfate is a 2-ion electrolyte, dissociating 40% in a certain concentration. Calculate its dissociation (i) factor.

On the basis of 40% dissociation, 100 particles of zinc sulfate will yield:

$$\begin{array}{l} 40 \text{ zinc ions} \\ 40 \text{ sulfate ions} \\ \underline{60} \text{ undissociated particles} \\ \text{or } 140 \text{ particles} \end{array}$$

Because 140 particles represent 1.4 times as many particles as were present before dissociation, the dissociation (i) factor is 1.4, *answer.*

Zinc chloride is a 3-ion electrolyte, dissociating 80% in a certain concentration. Calculate its dissociation (i) *factor.*

On the basis of 80% dissociation, 100 particles of zinc chloride will yield:

$$\begin{array}{l} 80 \text{ zinc ions} \\ 80 \text{ chloride ions} \\ 80 \text{ chloride ions} \\ \underline{20} \text{ undissociated particles} \\ \text{or } 260 \text{ particles} \end{array}$$

Because 260 particles represent 2.6 times as many particles as were present before dissociation, the dissociation (i) factor is 2.6, *answer.*

Calculating the Sodium Chloride Equivalent of a Substance. Remember that the sodium chloride equivalent of a substance may be calculated as follows:

$$\frac{\begin{array}{c} \text{molecular weight} \\ \text{of sodium chloride} \end{array}}{\begin{array}{c} i \text{ factor} \\ \text{of sodium chloride} \end{array}} \times \frac{\begin{array}{c} i \text{ factor} \\ \text{of the substance} \end{array}}{\begin{array}{c} \text{molecular weight} \\ \text{of the substance} \end{array}} = \begin{array}{c} \text{sodium chloride} \\ \text{equivalent} \end{array}$$

Example:

Papaverine hydrochloride (m.w. 376) is a 2-ion electrolyte, dissociating 80% in a given concentration. Calculate its sodium chloride equivalent.

Because papaverine hydrochloride is a 2-ion electrolyte, dissociating 80%, its i factor is 1.8.

$$\frac{58.5}{1.8} \times \frac{1.8}{376} = 0.156, \text{ or } 0.16, \text{ } answer.$$

Calculating the Amount of Tonicic Agent Required.

Examples:

How many grams of sodium chloride should be used in compounding the following prescription?

℞	Pilocarpine Nitrate		0.3 g
	Sodium Chloride		q.s.
	Purified Water	ad	30.0 mL
	Make isoton. sol.		
	Sig. For the eye.		

Step 1. 0.23 × 0.3 g = 0.069 g of sodium chloride represented by the pilocarpine nitrate
Step 2. 30 × 0.009 = 0.270 g of sodium chloride in 30 mL of an isotonic sodium chloride solution
Step 3. 0.270 g (from Step 2)
  − 0.069 g (from Step 1)
    0.201 g of sodium chloride to be used, *answer.*

How many grams of boric acid should be used in compounding the following prescription?

℞	Phenacaine Hydrochloride		1%
	Chlorobutanol		½%
	Boric Acid		q.s.
	Purified Water	ad	60.0
	Make isoton. sol.		
	Sig. One drop in each eye.		

The prescription calls for 0.6 g of phenacaine hydrochloride and 0.3 g of chlorobutanol.

Step 1. 0.20 × 0.6 g = 0.120 g of sodium chloride represented by phenacaine hydrochloride
  0.24 × 0.3 g = 0.072 g of sodium chloride represented by chlorobutanol
  Total: 0.192 g of sodium chloride represented by both ingredients
Step 2. 60 × 0.009 = 0.540 g of sodium chloride in 60 mL of an isotonic sodium chloride solution
Step 3. 0.540 g (from Step 2)
  − 0.192 g (from Step 1)
    0.348 g of sodium chloride required to make the solution isotonic

But because the prescription calls for boric acid:
Step 4. 0.348 g ÷ 0.52 (sodium chloride equivalent of boric acid) = 0.669 g of boric acid to be used, *answer.*

How many grams of potassium nitrate could be used to make the following prescription isotonic?

℞	Sol. Silver Nitrate	60.0
	1:500 w/v	
	Make isoton. sol.	
	Sig. For eye use.	

The prescription contains 0.120 g of silver nitrate.

Step 1. 0.33 × 0.120 g = 0.040 g of sodium chloride represented by silver nitrate
Step 2.   60 × 0.009   = 0.540 g of sodium chloride in 60 mL of an isotonic sodium
      chloride solution
Step 3. 0.540 g (from step 2)
      − 0.040 g (from step 1)
      0.500 g of sodium chloride required to make solution isotonic

Because, in this solution, sodium chloride is incompatible with silver nitrate, the tonic agent of choice is potassium nitrate. Therefore,
Step 4. 0.500 g ÷ 0.58 (sodium chloride equivalent of potassium nitrate) = 0.862 g of potassium nitrate to be used, *answer.*

How many grams of sodium chloride should be used in compounding the following prescription?

℞	Ingredient X		0.5
	Sodium Chloride		q.s.
	Purified Water	ad	50.0
	Make isoton. sol.		
	Sig. Eye drops.		

Let us assume that Ingredient X is a new substance for which no sodium chloride equivalent is to be found in Table 9.1, and that its molecular weight is 295 and its *i* factor is 2.4. The sodium chloride equivalent of Ingredient X may be calculated as follows:

$$\frac{58.5}{1.8} \times \frac{2.4}{295} = 0.26, \text{ the sodium chloride equivalent for Ingredient X}$$

Then,
Step 1. 0.26 × 0.5 g = 0.130 g of sodium chloride represented by Ingredient X
Step 2. 50 × 0.009 = 0.450 g of sodium chloride in 50 mL of an isotonic sodium
      chloride solution
Step 3. 0.450 g (from Step 2)
      − 0.130 g (from Step 1)
      0.320 g of sodium chloride to be used, *answer.*

Use of Freezing Point Data in Isotonicity Calculations

Freezing point data (ΔT_f) may be used in isotonicity calculations when the agent has a tonicic effect and does not penetrate the biologic membranes in question (e.g., red blood cells). As stated previously, the freezing point of both blood and lacrimal fluid is −0.52°C. Thus, a pharmaceutical solution that has a freezing point of −0.52°C is considered isotonic.

Representative data on freezing point depression by medicinal and pharmaceutical substances are presented in Table 9.2. Although these data are for solution strengths of 1% ($\Delta T_f^{1\%}$), data for other solution strengths and for many additional agents may be found in physical pharmacy textbooks and in the literature.

Freezing point depression data may be used in isotonicity calculations as shown by the following.

Example:

How many milligrams each of sodium chloride and dibucaine hydrochloride are required to prepare 30 mL of a 1% solution of dibucaine hydrochloride isotonic with tears?

To make this solution isotonic, the freezing point must be lowered to −0.52. From

Table 9.2. Freezing Point Data For Select Agents

Agent	Freezing Point Depression, 1% Solutions ($\Delta T_f^{1\%}$)
Atropine sulfate	0.07
Boric acid	0.29
Butacaine sulfate	0.12
Chloramphenicol	0.06
Chlorobutanol	0.14
Dextrose	0.09
Dibucaine hydrochloride	0.08
Ephedrine sulfate	0.13
Epinephrine bitartrate	0.10
Ethylmorphine hydrochloride	0.09
Glycerin	0.20
Homatropine hydrobromide	0.11
Lincomycin	0.09
Morphine sulfate	0.08
Naphazoline hydrochloride	0.16
Physostigmine salicylate	0.09
Pilocarpine nitrate	0.14
Sodium bisulfite	0.36
Sodium chloride	0.58
Sulfacetamide sodium	0.14
Zinc sulfate	0.09

Table 9.2, it is determined that a 1% solution of dibucaine hydrochloride has a freezing point lowering of 0.08°. Thus, sufficient sodium chloride must be added to lower the freezing point an additional 0.44° (0.52° − 0.08°).

Also from Table 9.2, it is determined that a 1% solution of sodium chloride lowers the freezing point by 0.58°. By proportion:

$$\frac{1\% \text{ (NaCl)}}{x\% \text{ (NaCl)}} = \frac{0.58°}{0.44°}$$

$$x = 0.76\% \text{ (the concentration of sodium chloride needed to lower the freezing point by } 0.44°, \text{ required to make the solution isotonic)}$$

Thus, to make 30 mL of solution,

30 mL × 1% = 0.3 g = 300 mg dibucaine hydrochloride, and

30 mL × 0.76% = 0.228 g = 228 mg sodium chloride, *answers.*

NOTE: Should a prescription call for more than one medicinal and/or pharmaceutic ingredient, the sum of the freezing points is subtracted from the required value in determining the additional lowering required by the agent used to provide isotonicity.

Practice Problems

1. Isotonic Sodium Chloride Solution contains 0.9% of sodium chloride. If the sodium chloride equivalent of boric acid is 0.52, what is the percentage strength of an isotonic solution of boric acid?

2. Sodium chloride is a 2-ion electrolyte, dissociating 90% in a certain concentration. Calculate (a) its dissociation factor, and (b) the freezing point of a molal solution.

3. A solution of anhydrous dextrose (m.w. 180) contains 25 g in 500 mL of water. Calculate the freezing point of the solution.

4. Procaine hydrochloride (m.w. 273) is a 2-ion electrolyte, dissociating 80% in a certain concentration.
    (a) Calculate its dissociation factor.
    (b) Calculate its sodium chloride equivalent.
    (c) Calculate the freezing point of a molal solution of procaine hydrochloride.

5. The freezing point of a molal solution of a nonelectrolyte is −1.86°C. What is the freezing point of a 0.1% solution of zinc chloride (m.w. 136), dissociating 80%?[1]

6. The freezing point of a 5% solution of boric acid is −1.55°C. How many grams of boric acid should be used in preparing 1000 mL of an isotonic solution?

7. ℞ Ephedrine Sulfate   0.3 g
        Sodium Chloride   q.s.
        Purified Water   ad   30. mL
        Make isoton. sol.
        Sig. Use as directed.

    How many milligrams of sodium chloride should be used in compounding the prescription?

8. ℞ Dipivefrin Hydrochloride   ½%
        Scopolamine Hydrobromide   ⅓%
        Sodium Chloride   q.s.
        Purified Water   ad   30.0
        Make isoton. sol.
        Sig. Use in the eye.

    How many grams of sodium chloride should be used in compounding the prescription?

9. ℞ Zinc Sulfate   0.06
        Boric Acid   q.s.
        Purified Water   ad   30.0
        Make isoton. sol.
        Sig. Drop in eyes.

    How many grams of boric acid should be used in compounding the prescription?

10. ℞ Atropine Sulfate   1%
        Boric Acid   q.s.
        Purified Water   ad   30.0
        Make isoton. sol.
        Sig. One drop in each eye.

---

[1] For lack of more definite information, the student must assume that the volume of the molal solution is approximately 1 liter.

How many grams of boric acid should be used in compounding the prescription? Use the freezing point depression method.

11.   Dextrose, anhydrous 2.5%
Sodium Chloride q.s.
Sterile Water for Injection ad 1000 mL
Label: Isotonic Dextrose and Saline Solution.
How many grams of sodium chloride should be used in preparing the solution?

12.   ℞   Sol. Silver Nitrate 0.5%   15.0
Make isoton. sol.
Sig. For the eyes.

How many grams of potassium nitrate could be used to make the prescription isotonic?

13.   ℞   Cocaine Hydrochloride   0.150
Sodium Chloride   q.s.
Purified Water   ad   15.0
Make isoton. sol.
Sig. One drop in left eye.

How many grams of sodium chloride should be used in compounding the prescription?

14.   ℞   Cocaine Hydrochloride   0.6
Eucatropine Hydrochloride   0.6
Chlorobutanol   0.1
Sodium Chloride   q.s.
Purified Water   ad   30.0
Make isoton. sol.
Sig. For the eye.

How many grams of sodium chloride should be used in compounding the prescription?

15.   ℞   Tetracaine Hydrochloride   0.1
Zinc Sulfate   0.05
Boric Acid   q.s.
Purified Water   ad   30.0
Make isoton. sol.
Sig. Drop in eye.

How many grams of boric acid should be used in compounding the prescription?

16.   ℞   Sol. Homatropine Hydrobromide 1%   15.0
Make isoton. sol. with boric acid.
Sig. For the eye.

How many grams of boric acid should be used in compounding the prescription?

17. ℞   Procaine Hydrochloride   1%
          Sodium Chloride   q.s.
          Sterile Water for Injection   ad   100.0
          Make isoton. sol.
          Sig. For injection.

How many grams of sodium chloride should be used in compounding the prescription?

18. ℞   Phenylephrine Hydrochloride   1.0
          Chlorobutanol   0.5
          Sodium Chloride   q.s.
          Purified Water   ad   15.0
          Make isoton. sol.
          Sig. Use as directed.

How many milliliters of an 0.9% solution of sodium chloride should be used in compounding the prescription?

19. ℞   Oxymetazoline Hydrochloride   ½%
          Boric Acid Solution   q.s.
          Purified Water   ad   15.0
          Make isoton. sol.
          Sig. For the nose, as decongestant.

How many milliliters of a 5% solution of boric acid should be used in compounding the prescription?

20. ℞   Ephedrine Hydrochloride   0.5
          Chlorobutanol   0.25
          Dextrose   q.s.
          Rose Water   ad   50.0
          Make isoton. sol.
          Sig. Nose drops.

How many grams of dextrose should be used in compounding the prescription?

21. ℞   Naphazoline Hydrochloride   1.0%
          Sodium Chloride   q.s.
          Purified Water   ad   30. mL
          Make isoton. sol.
          Sig. Use as directed in the eye.

How many grams of sodium chloride should be used in compounding the prescription? Use the freezing point depression method.

22. ℞   Oxytetracycline Hydrochloride   0.050
          Chlorobutanol   0.1
          Sodium Chloride   q.s.
          Purified Water   ad   30.0
          Make isoton. sol.
          Sig. Eye drops.

How many milligrams of sodium chloride should be used in compounding the prescription?

23.   ℞   Tetracaine Hydrochloride   0.5%
             Sol. Epinephrine Bitartrate 1 : 1000   10.0
             Boric Acid   q.s.
             Purified Water   ad   30.0
             Make isoton. sol.
             Sig. Eye drops.

   The solution of epinephrine bitartrate (1 : 1000) is already isotonic. How many grams of boric acid should be used in compounding the prescription?

24.   Monobasic Sodium Phosphate, anhydrous   5.6 g
             Dibasic Sodium Phosphate, anhydrous   2.84 g
             Sodium Chloride   q.s.
             Purified Water   ad   1000 mL
             Label: Isotonic Buffer Solution, pH 6.5.

How many grams of sodium chloride should be used in preparing the solution?

25.   How many grams of anhydrous dextrose should be used in preparing 1 liter of a ½% isotonic ephedrine sulfate nasal spray?

26.   ℞   Ephedrine Sulfate   1%
             Chlorobutanol   ½%
             Purified Water   ad   100.0
             Make isoton. sol. and buffer to pH 6.5
             Sig. Nose drops.

   You have on hand an isotonic buffered solution, pH 6.5. How many milliliters of purified water and how many milliliters of the buffered solution should be used in compounding the prescription?

27.   ℞   Oxytetracycline Hydrochloride   0.5%
             Tetracaine Hydrochloride Sol. 2%   15.0 mL
             Sodium Chloride   q.s.
             Purified Water   ad   30.0 mL
             Make isoton. sol.
             Sig. For the eye.

   The 2% solution of tetracaine hydrochloride is already isotonic. How many milliliters of an 0.9% solution of sodium chloride should be used in compounding the prescription?

28. Determine if the following commercial products are hypotonic, isotonic, or hypertonic:
     (a) An ophthalmic solution containing 40 mg/mL of cromolyn sodium and 0.01% of benzalkonium chloride in purified water.
     (b) A parenteral infusion containing 20% (w/v) of mannitol.
     (c) A 500-mL large volume parenteral containing D5W (5%, w/v, of anhydrous dextrose in sterile water for injection).
     (d) A Fleet® Brand Enema containing 19 g of sodium biphosphate (monobasic) and 7 g of sodium phosphate (dibasic) in 118 mL of aqueous solution.

10

Electrolyte Solutions: Milliequivalents, Millimoles, and Milliosmoles

As noted in Chapter 9, the molecules of chemical compounds in solution may remain intact, or they may dissociate into particles known as *ions,* which carry an electric charge. Substances that are not dissociated in solution are called *nonelectrolytes*, and those with varying degrees of dissociation are called *electrolytes*. Urea and dextrose are examples of nonelectrolytes in body water; sodium chloride in body fluids is an example of an electrolyte.

Sodium chloride in solution provides Na^+ and Cl^- ions, which carry electric charges. If electrodes carrying a weak current are placed in the solution, the ions move in a direction opposite to the charges. Na^+ ions move to the negative electrode (*cathode*) and are called *cations*. Cl^- ions move to the positive electrode (*anode*) and are called *anions*.

Electrolyte ions in the blood plasma include the cations Na^+, K^+, Ca^{++}, and Mg^{++} and the anions Cl^-, HCO_3^-, HPO_4^-, SO_4^-, organic acids$^-$, and protein$^-$. Electrolytes in body fluids play an important role in maintaining the acid-base balance in the body. They play a part, too, in controlling body water volumes, and they also help to regulate body metabolism.

Electrolyte preparations are used for the treatment of disturbances of the electrolyte and fluid balance in the body. In clinical practice, they are provided in the form of oral solutions and syrups; as dry granules intended to be dissolved in water or juice to make an oral solution; as oral tablets and capsules; and, when necessary, as intravenous infusions.

The concentration of the liquid preparations, like the concentration of body electrolytes, was commonly expressed in terms of different units, such as grams per 100 mL, volumes percent, and milligrams percent (mg%). The latter term refers to the number of milligrams per 100 mL and represents the older concept of measuring electrolytes in units of weight or *physical units*. This concept, however, does not take into consideration chemical equivalence and, consequently, does not indicate the measurement of the chemical combining power of the electrolyte in solution. More significantly, it does not give any direct information as to the number of ions or the charges that they carry. Because the chemical combining power depends not only on the number of particles in solution but also on the total number of ionic charges, the valence of the ions in solution must be considered to make the measurement meaningful.

A *chemical unit*, the *milliequivalent* (mEq), is now used almost exclusively in the United States by clinicians, physicians, pharmacists, and manufacturers to express the concentration of electrolytes in solution.[1] This unit of measure is related to the total number of ionic charges in solution, and it takes note of the valence of the ions. In other words, it is a unit of measurement of the amount of *chemical activity* of an electrolyte.

Under normal conditions, blood plasma contains 155 mEq of cations and an equal

---

[1] In the International System (SI), which is used in European countries and in many others throughout the world, molar concentrations [as millimoles per liter (mmol/L) or micromoles per liter (μmol/L)] are used to express most clinical laboratory values, including those of electrolytes.

Table 10.1. Values for Some Important Ions

Ion	Formula	Valence	Atomic or Formula Weight	Milliequivalent Weight (mg)
Aluminum	Al^{+++}	3	27	9
Ammonium	NH_4^+	1	18	18
Calcium	Ca^{++}	2	40	20
Ferric	Fe^{+++}	3	56	18.7
Ferrous	Fe^{++}	2	56	28
Lithium	Li^+	1	7	7
Magnesium	Mg^{++}	2	24	12
Potassium	K^+	1	39	39
Sodium	Na^+	1	23	23
Acetate	$C_2H_3O_2^-$	1	59	59
Bicarbonate	HCO_3^-	1	61	61
Carbonate	CO_3^{--}	2	60	30
Chloride	Cl^-	1	35.5	35.5
Citrate	$C_6H_5O_7^{---}$	3	189	63
Gluconate	$C_6H_{11}O_7^-$	1	195	195
Lactate	$C_3H_5O_3^-$	1	89	89
Phosphate	$H_2PO_4^-$	1	97	97
	HPO_4^{--}	2	96	48
Sulfate	SO_4^{--}	2	96	48

number of anions. The total concentration of cations always equals the total concentration of anions. Any number of milliequivalents of Na^+, K^+, or any cation$^+$ always reacts with precisely the same number of milliequivalents of Cl^-, HCO_3^-, or any anion$^-$. For a given chemical compound, the milliequivalents of cation equal the milliequivalents of anion equal the milliequivalents of the chemical compound.

In preparing a solution of K^+ ions, a potassium salt is dissolved in water. In addition to the K^+ ions, the solution will also contain ions of opposite negative charge. These two components will be chemically equal in that the milliequivalents of one are equal to the milliequivalents of the other. The interesting point is that if we dissolve enough potassium chloride in water to give us 40 mEq of K^+ per liter, we also have exactly 40 mEq of Cl^-, but the solution will *not* contain the *same weight* of each ion.

A milliequivalent represents the amount, in milligrams, of a solute equal to $\frac{1}{1000}$ of its gram equivalent weight, taking into account the valence of the ions. The milliequivalent expresses the chemical activity or combining power of a substance relative to the activity of 1 mg of hydrogen. Thus, based on the atomic weight and valence of the species, 1 mEq is represented by 1 mg of hydrogen, 20 mg of calcium, 23 mg of sodium, 35.5 mg of chlorine, 39 mg of potassium, and so forth. Important values for some ions are presented in Table 10.1, and a complete listing of atomic weights is provided on the back inside cover of this text.

Converting Milliequivalents per Unit Volume to Weight per Unit Volume. To convert the concentration of electrolytes in solution expressed as milliequivalents per unit volume to weight per unit volume and vice versa, use the following.

$$mEq = \frac{mg \times valence}{atomic, molecular, or formula weight}$$

$$mg = \frac{mEq \times atomic, molecular, or formula weight}{valence}$$

Examples:

What is the concentration, in milligrams per milliliter, of a solution containing 2 mEq of potassium chloride (KCl) per milliliter?

$$\text{Molecular weight of KCl} = 74.5$$

$$\text{Equivalent weight of KCl} = 74.5$$

$$1 \text{ mEq of KCl} = \frac{1}{1000} \times 74.5 \text{ g} = 0.0745 \text{ g} = 74.5 \text{ mg}$$

$$2 \text{ mEq of KCl} = 74.5 \text{ mg} \times 2 = 149 \text{ mg/mL, } \textit{answer.}$$

Or, by using the preceding equation

$$\text{mg/mL} = \frac{2 \text{ (mEq/mL)} \times 74.5}{1}$$

$$= 149 \text{ mg/mL, } \textit{answer.}$$

What is the concentration, in grams per milliliter of a solution containing 4 mEq of calcium chloride (CaCl₂.2H₂O) per milliliter?

Recall that the equivalent weight of a binary compound may be found by dividing the formula weight by the *total valence* of the positive or negative radical.

$$\text{Formula weight of } CaCl_2.2H_2O = 147$$

$$\text{Equivalent weight of } CaCl_2.2H_2O = \frac{147}{2} = 73.5$$

$$1 \text{ mEq of } CaCl_2.2H_2O = \frac{1}{1000} \times 73.5 \text{ g} = 0.0735 \text{ g}$$

$$4 \text{ mEq of } CaCl_2.2H_2O = 0.0735 \text{ g} \times 4 = 0.294 \text{ g/mL, } \textit{answer.}$$

Or, solving by dimensional analysis:

$$\frac{1 \text{ g } CaCl_2 \cdot 2H_2O}{1000 \text{ mg } CaCl_2 \cdot 2H_2O} \times \frac{147 \text{ mg}}{1 \text{ mmole}} \times \frac{1 \text{ mmole}}{2 \text{ mEq}} \times \frac{4 \text{ mEq}}{1 \text{ mL}} = 0.294 \text{ g/mL, } \textit{answer.}$$

NOTE: The water of hydration molecules does not interfere in the calculations as long as the correct molecular weight is used.

What is the percent (w/v) concentration of a solution containing 100 mEq of ammonium chloride per liter?

$$\text{Molecular weight of } NH_4Cl \qquad = 53.5$$
$$\text{Equivalent weight of } NH_4Cl \qquad = 53.5$$
$$1 \text{ mEq of } NH_4Cl = \frac{1}{1000} \times 53.5 \qquad = 0.0535 \text{ g}$$
$$100 \text{ mEq of } NH_4Cl \qquad = 0.0535 \text{ g} \times 100 = 5.35 \text{ g/L or}$$

0.535 g per 100 mL, or 0.535%, *answer.*

Converting Milligrams Percent to Milliequivalents per Liter. To convert the concentration of electrolytes in solution expressed as milligrams percent to milliequivalents per liter, observe the following.

Examples:

A solution contains 10 mg% of K⁺ ions. Express this concentration in terms of milliequivalents per liter.

Atomic weight of K^+ = 39

Equivalent weight of K^+ = 39

1 mEq of K^+ = $\frac{1}{1000}$ × 39 g = 0.039 g = 39 mg

10 mg% of K^+ = 10 mg of K^+ per 100 mL or 100 mg of K^+ per liter

100 mg ÷ 39 = 2.56 mEq/L, *answer.*

Or, by the equation detailed previously,

$$mEq/L = \frac{100 \ (mg/L) \times 1}{39}$$

$$= 2.56 \ mEq/L, \ answer.$$

A solution contains 10 mg% of Ca^{++} ions. Express this concentration in terms of milliequivalents per liter.

Atomic weight of Ca^{++} = 40

Equivalent weight of Ca^{++} = $\frac{40}{2}$ = 20

1 mEq of Ca^{++} = $\frac{1}{1000}$ × 20 g = 0.020 g = 20 mg

10 mg% of Ca^{++} = 10 mg of Ca^{++} per 100 mL or

100 mg of Ca^{++} per liter

100 mg ÷ 20 = 5 mEq/L, *answer.*

Converting Milliequivalents per Liter to Milligrams Percent. To convert the concentration of electrolytes in solution expressed as milliequivalents per liter to milligrams percent, observe the following.

Example:

The normal magnesium (Mg^{++}) level in blood plasma is 2.5 mEq/L. Express this concentration in terms of milligrams percent.

Atomic weight of Mg^{++} = 24
Equivalent weight of Mg^{++} = $\frac{24}{2}$ = 12
1 mEq of Mg^{++} = $\frac{1}{1000}$ × 12 g = 0.012 g = 12 mg
2.5 mEq of Mg^{++} = 30 mg

30 mg/L or 3 mg per 100 mL = 3 mg%, *answer.*

Converting Weight to Milliequivalents. To convert the weight of an electrolyte to milliequivalents, observe the following.

Examples:

How many milliequivalents of potassium chloride are represented in a 15-mL dose of a 10% (w/v) potassium chloride elixir?

Molecular weight of KCl = 74.5

Equivalent weight of KCl = 74.5

1 mEq of KCl = $\frac{1}{1000}$ × 74.5 g = 0.0745 g = 74.5 mg

15-mL dose of 10% (w/v) elixir = 1.5 g or 1500 mg of KCl

$$\frac{74.5 \ (mg)}{1500 \ (mg)} = \frac{1 \ (mEq)}{x \ (mEq)}$$

$$x = 20.1 \ mEq, \ answer.$$

How many milliequivalents of magnesium sulfate are represented in 1.0 g of anhydrous magnesium sulfate ($MgSO_4$)?

$$\text{Molecular weight of } MgSO_4 = 120$$

$$\text{Equivalent weight of } MgSO_4 = 60$$

$$1 \text{ mEq of } MgSO_4 = \frac{1}{1000} \times 60 \text{ g} = 0.060 \text{ g} = 60 \text{ mg}$$

$$1.0 \text{ g of } MgSO_4 = 1000 \text{ mg}$$

$$\frac{60 \text{ (mg)}}{1000 \text{ (mg)}} = \frac{1 \text{ (mEq)}}{x \text{ (mEq)}}$$

$$x = 16.7 \text{ mEq, } \textit{answer.}$$

How many milliequivalents of Na^+ ion would be contained in a 30-mL dose of the following solution?

Disodium Hydrogen Phosphate		18 g
Sodium Biphosphate		48 g
Purified Water	ad	100 mL

Each salt is considered separately in solving the problem.

Disodium hydrogen phosphate

$$\text{Formula} = Na_2HPO_4.7H_2O$$

$$\text{Molecular weight} = 268 \text{ and the equivalent weight} = 134$$

$$\frac{18 \text{ (g)}}{x \text{ (g)}} = \frac{100 \text{ (mL)}}{30 \text{ (mL)}}$$

$$x = 5.4 \text{ g of disodium hydrogen phosphate per 30 mL}$$

$$1 \text{ mEq} = \frac{1}{1000} \times 134 \text{ g} = 0.134 \text{ g} = 134 \text{ mg}$$

$$\frac{134 \text{ (mg)}}{5400 \text{ (mg)}} = \frac{1 \text{ (mEq)}}{x \text{ (mEq)}}$$

$$x = 40.3 \text{ mEq of disodium hydrogen phosphate}$$

Because the milliequivalent value of Na^+ ion equals the milliequivalent value of disodium hydrogen phosphate, then

$$x = 40.3 \text{ mEq of } Na^+$$

Sodium biphosphate

$$\text{Formula} = NaH_2PO_4.H_2O$$

$$\text{Molecular weight} = 134 \text{ and the equivalent weight} = 134$$

$$\frac{48 \text{ (g)}}{x \text{ (g)}} = \frac{100 \text{ (mL)}}{30 \text{ (mL)}}$$

$$x = 14.4 \text{ g of sodium biphosphate per 30 mL}$$

$$1 \text{ mEq} = \frac{1}{1000} \times 134 \text{ g} = 0.134 \text{ g} = 134 \text{ mg}$$

$$\frac{134 \ (mg)}{14400 \ (mg)} = \frac{1 \ (mEq)}{x \ (mEq)}$$

$$x = 107.5 \ mEq \ of \ sodium \ biphosphate$$
$$and \ also, \quad = 107.5 \ mEq \ of \ Na^+$$

Adding the two milliequivalent values for Na^+ = 40.3 mEq + 107.5 mEq = 147.8 mEq, *answer.*

Providing a Specified Milliequivalent Level. To calculate the amount of electrolyte or its solution in a given concentration to provide a specified milliequivalent level, observe the following.

Example:

  A person is to receive 2 mEq of sodium chloride per kilogram of body weight. If the person weighs 132 lb, how many milliliters of an 0.9% sterile solution of sodium chloride should be administered?

$$Molecular \ weight \ of \ NaCl \quad = \ 58.5$$
$$Equivalent \ weight \ of \ NaCl \quad = \ 58.5$$
$$1 \ mEq \ of \ NaCl \quad = \ ^1/_{1000} \times 58.5 \ g \ = \ 0.0585 \ g$$
$$2 \ mEq \ of \ NaCl \quad = \ 0.0585 \ g \times 2 \ = \ 0.117 \ g$$

$$1 \ kg \ = \ 2.2 \ lb \quad Weight \ of \ person \ in \ kg \ = \ \frac{132 \ lb}{2.2 \ lb} \ = \ 60 \ kg$$

Because the person is to receive 2 mEq/kg, then 2 mEq or 0.117 g × 60 = 7.02 g of NaCl needed and because 0.9% sterile solution of sodium chloride contains

  9.0 g of NaCl per liter,

then

$$\frac{9.0 \ (g)}{7.02 \ (g)} = \frac{1000 \ (mL)}{x \ (mL)}$$

$$x = 780 \ mL, \ answer.$$

MILLIMOLES

As noted previously, the International System (SI) expresses electrolyte concentrations in *millimoles per liter (mmol/L)* in representing the combining power of a chemical species. For monovalent species, the numeric value of the milliequivalent and millimole are identical.

  A mole is the molecular weight of a substance in grams. A *millimole* is $^1/_{1000}$ of the molecular weight in grams.

Examples:

  How many millimoles of monobasic sodium phosphate (m.w. = 138) are present in 100 g of the substance?

$$m.w. \ = \ 138$$

$$1 \ mole \ = \ 138 \ g$$

$$\frac{1 \ (mole)}{x \ (mole)} = \frac{138 \ (g)}{100 \ (g)}$$

$$x = 0.725 \ moles \ = \ 725 \ mmol, \ answer.$$

  How many milligrams would 1 mmol of monobasic sodium phosphate weigh?

$$1 \text{ mole } = 138 \text{ g}$$
$$1 \text{ mmol } = 0.138 \text{ g} = 138 \text{ mg, } answer.$$

What is the weight, in milligrams, of 1 mmol of $HPO_4^=$?

$$\text{Atomic weight of } HPO_4^= = 95.98$$

$$1 \text{ mole of } HPO_4^= = 95.98 \text{ g}$$

$$1 \text{ mmol of } HPO_4^= = 95.98 \text{ g} \times \frac{1}{1000} = 0.09598 \text{ g}$$

$$= 95.98 \text{ mg, } answer.$$

OSMOLARITY

As indicated in Chapter 9, osmotic pressure is important to biologic processes that involve the diffusion of solutes or the transfer of fluids through semipermeable membranes. The *United States Pharmacopeia* states that knowledge of the osmolar concentrations of parenteral fluids is essential. The labels of pharmacopeial solutions that provide intravenous replenishment of fluid, nutrients, or electrolytes, and the osmotic diuretic mannitol are required to state the osmolar concentration. This information indicates to the practitioner whether the solution is hypo-osmotic, iso-osmotic, or hyper-osmotic with regard to biologic fluids and membranes.

Osmotic pressure is proportional to the *total number* of particles in solution. The unit that is used to measure osmotic concentration is the *milliosmole* (mOsmol). For dextrose, a nonelectrolyte, 1 mmol (1 formula weight in milligrams) represents 1 mOsmol. This relationship is not the same with electrolytes, however, because the total number of particles in solution depends on the degree of dissociation of the substance in question. Assuming complete dissociation, 1 mmol of NaCl represents 2 mOsmol ($Na^+ + Cl^-$) of total particles, 1 mmol of $CaCl_2$ represents 3 mOsmol ($Ca^{++} + 2Cl^-$) of total particles, and 1 mmol of sodium citrate ($Na_3C_6H_5O_7$) represents 4 mOsmol ($3Na^+ + C_6H_5O_7^-$) of total particles.

The milliosmolar value of *separate* ions of an electrolyte may be obtained by dividing the concentration, in milligrams per liter, of the ion by its atomic weight. The milliosmolar value of the *whole* electrolyte in solution is equal to the sum of the milliosmolar values of the separate ions. According to the USP, the ideal osmolar concentration may be calculated according to the equation:

$$\text{mOsmol/L} = \frac{\text{wt. of substance (g/L)}}{\text{m.w. (g)}} \times \text{number of species} \times 1000$$

In practice, as the concentration of the solute increases, physicochemical interaction among solute particles increases, and actual osmolar values decrease when compared to ideal values. Deviation from ideal conditions is usually slight in solution within the physiologic range and for more dilute solutions, but for highly concentrated solutions, the actual osmolarities may be appreciably lower than ideal values. For example, the ideal osmolarity of 0.9% Sodium Chloride Injection is:

$$\text{mOsmol/L} = \frac{9 \text{ g/L}}{58.5 \text{ g}} \times 2 \times 1000 = 308 \text{ mOsmol/L}$$

Because of bonding forces, however, *n* is slightly less than 2 for solutions of sodium chloride at this concentration, and the actual measured osmolarity of the solution is about 286 mOsmol/L.

Some pharmaceutical manufacturers label electrolyte solutions with ideal or stoichiometric osmolarities calculated by the equation just provided, whereas others list experimental or actual osmolarities. The pharmacist should appreciate this distinction.

A distinction also should be made between the terms *osmolarity* and *osmolality*. Whereas *osmolarity is the milliosmoles of solute per liter of solution, osmolality is the milliosmoles of solute per kilogram of solvent.* For dilute aqueous solutions, osmolarity and osmolality are nearly identical. For more concentrated solutions, however, the two values may be quite dissimilar. The pharmacist should pay particular attention to a product's label statement regarding molarity versus molality.

Normal serum osmolality is considered to be within the range of 275 to 295 mOsmol/kg.

Milliosmolar Values. Calculating milliosmolar values involves the following.

Examples:

A solution contains 5% of anhydrous dextrose in water for injection. How many milliosmoles per liter are represented by this concentration?

Formula weight of anhydrous dextrose   = 180
1 mmol of anhydrous dextrose (180 mg)   = 1 Osmol
5% solution contains 50 g or 50000 mg/L
50000 mg ÷ 180   = 278 mOsmol/L, *answer.*

Or, solving by dimensional analysis:

$$\frac{50,000 \text{ mg}}{1 \text{ L}} \times \frac{1 \text{ mOsmol}}{180 \text{ mg}} = 278 \text{ mOsmol/L, } answer.$$

A solution contains 156 mg of K^+ ions per 100 mL. How many milliosmoles are represented in a liter of the solution?

Atomic weight of K^+ = 39
1 mmol of K^+ (39 mg)   = 1 mOsmol
156 mg of K^+ per 100 mL   = 1560 mg of K^+ per liter
1560 mg ÷ 39   = 40 mOsmol, *answer.*

A solution contains 10 mg% of Ca^{++} ions. How many milliosmoles are represented in 1 liter of the solution?

Atomic weight of Ca^{++} = 40
1 mmol of Ca^{++} (40 mg)   = 1 mOsmol
10 mg% of Ca^{++} = 10 mg of Ca^{++} per 100 mL or
100 mg of Ca^{++} per liter
100 mg ÷ 40   = 2.5 mOsmol, *answer.*

How many milliosmoles are represented in a liter of an 0.9% sodium chloride solution?
Osmotic concentration (in terms of milliosmoles) is a function of the total number of particles present. Assuming complete dissociation, 1 mmol of sodium chloride (NaCl) represents 2 mOsmol of total particles ($Na^+ + Cl^-$).

Formula weight of NaCl = 58.5

1 mmol of NaCl (58.5 mg) = 2 mOsmol

1000 × 0.009 = 9 g or 9000 mg of NaCl per liter

$$\frac{58.5 \text{ (mg)}}{9000 \text{ (mg)}} = \frac{2 \text{ (mOsmol)}}{x \text{ (mOsmol)}}$$

x = 307.7, or 308 mOsmol, *answer.*

Practice Problems

1. What is the concentration, in milligrams per milliliter, of a solution containing 5 mEq of potassium chloride (KCl) per milliliter?

2. A solution contains 298 mg of potassium chloride (KCl) per milliliter. Express this concentration in terms of milliequivalents of potassium chloride.

3. A 10-mL ampul of potassium chloride contains 2.98 g of potassium chloride (KCl). What is the concentration of the solution in terms of milliequivalents per milliliter?

4. A person is to receive 36 mg of ammonium chloride per kilogram of body weight. If the person weighs 154 lb, how many milliliters of a sterile solution of ammonium chloride (NH_4Cl—m.w. 53.5) containing 0.4 mEq/mL should be administered?

5. A sterile solution of potassium chloride (KCl) contains 2 mEq/mL. If a 20-mL ampul of the solution is diluted to 1 liter with sterile distilled water, what is the percentage strength of the resulting solution?

6. A certain electrolyte solution contains, as one of the ingredients, the equivalent of 4.6 mEq of calcium per liter. How many grams of calcium chloride ($CaCl_2 \cdot H_2O$—m.w. 147) should be used in preparing 20 liters of the solution?

7. Sterile solutions of ammonium chloride containing 21.4 mg/mL are available commercially in 500- and 1000-mL intravenous infusion containers. Calculate the amount, in terms of milliequivalents, of ammonium chloride (NH_4Cl—m.w. 53.5) in the 500-mL container.

8. A solution contains, in each 5 mL, 0.5 g of potassium acetate ($C_2H_3KO_2$—m.w. 98), 0.5 g of potassium bicarbonate ($KHCO_3$—m.w. 100), and 0.5 g of potassium citrate ($C_6H_5K_3O_7.H_2O$—m.w. 324). How many milliequivalents of potassium (K^+) are represented in each 5 mL of the solution?

9. How many grams of sodium chloride (NaCl) should be used in preparing 20 liters of a solution containing 154 mEq/L?

10. Sterile solutions of potassium chloride (KCl) containing 5 mEq/mL are available in 20-mL containers. Calculate the amount, in grams, of potassium chloride in the container.

11. How many milliliters of a solution containing 2 mEq of potassium chloride (KCl) per milliliter should be used to obtain 2.98 g of potassium chloride?

12. A patient is to be given 1 g of sodium methicillin ($C_{17}H_{19}NaO_6S.H_2O$—m.w. 420) every 6 hours for five doses. How many milliequivalents of sodium are represented in the prescribed amount of sodium methicillin?

13. A 40-mL vial of sodium chloride solution was diluted to 1 liter with sterile distilled water. The concentration (w/v) of sodium chloride (NaCl) in the finished product was 0.585%. What was the concentration, in milliequivalents per milliliter, of the original solution?

14. How many grams of sodium bicarbonate ($NaHCO_3$—m.w. 84) should be used in preparing a liter of a solution to contain 44.6 mEq per 50 mL?

15. A solution contains 20 mg% of Ca^{++} ions. Express this concentration in terms of milliequivalents per liter.

16. Sterile sodium lactate solution is available commercially as a ⅙-molar solution of sodium lactate in water for injection. How many milliequivalents of sodium lactate ($C_3H_5NaO_3$—m.w. 112) would be provided by a liter of the solution?

17. A solution contains 322 mg of Na^+ ions per liter. How many milliosmoles are represented in the solution?

18. A certain electrolyte solution contains 0.9% of sodium chloride in 10% dextrose solution.
     (a) Express the concentration of sodium chloride (NaCl) in terms of milliequivalents per liter.
     (b) How many milliosmoles of dextrose are represented in 1 liter of the solution?

19. ℞   Potassium Chloride   10%
             Cherry Syrup q.s.   ad   480 mL
             Sig. Tablespoonful b.i.d.

     How many milliequivalents of potassium chloride are represented in each prescribed dose?

20. How many milliequivalents of potassium are in 5 million units of Penicillin V Potassium ($C_{16}H_{17}KN_2O_6S$—m.w. 388)? One milligram of Penicillin V Potassium represents 1380 Penicillin V Units.

21. The normal potassium level in the blood plasma is 17 mg%. Express this concentration in terms of milliequivalents per liter.

22. How many grams of potassium citrate ($C_6H_5K_3O_7·H_2O$—m.w. 324) should be used in preparing 500 mL of a potassium ion elixir so as to supply 15 mEq of K^+ in each 5-mL dose?

23. A potassium supplement tablet contains 2.5 g of potassium bicarbonate ($KHCO_3$—m.w. 100). How many milliequivalents of potassium (K^+) are supplied by the tablet?

24. Ringer's Injection contains 0.86% of sodium chloride, 0.03% of potassium chloride, and 0.033% of calcium chloride. How many milliequivalents of each chloride are contained in 1 liter of the injection?

25. Calculate the sodium (Na^+) content, in terms of milliequivalents, of 1 g of ampicillin sodium ($C_{16}H_{18}N_3NaO_4S$—m.w. 371).

26. A 20-mL vial of concentrated ammonium chloride solution containing 5 mEq/mL is diluted to 1 liter with sterile distilled water. Calculate: (a) the total milliequivalent value of the ammonium ion in the dilution, and (b) the percentage strength of the dilution.

27. Ringer's Solution contains 0.33 g of calcium chloride per liter.
     (a) Express the concentration in terms of milliequivalents of calcium chloride ($CaCl_2·2H_2O$—m.w. 147) per liter.
     (b) How many milliosmoles of calcium are represented in each liter of the solution?

28. How many milliosmoles of sodium are represented in 1 liter of 3% hypertonic sodium chloride solution? Assume complete dissociation.

29. A solution of sodium chloride contains 77 mEq/L. Calculate its osmolar strength in terms of milliosmoles per liter. Assume complete dissociation.

30. How many milliequivalents of potassium would be supplied daily by the usual dose (0.3 mL three times a day) of saturated potassium iodide solution? Saturated potassium iodide solution contains 100 g of potassium iodide per 100 mL.

31. Calculate the osmolar concentration, in terms of milliosmoles, represented by 1 liter of a 10% (w/v) solution of anhydrous dextrose (m.w. 180) in water.

32. An intravenous solution calls for the addition of 25 mEq of sodium bicarbonate. How many milliliters of 8.4% (w/v) sodium bicarbonate injection should be added to the formula?

33. Calcium gluconate ($C_{12}H_{22}CaO_{14}$—m.w. 430) injection 10% is available in a 10-mL ampul. How many milliequivalents of Ca^{++} does the ampul contain?

34. A flavored potassium chloride packet contains 1.5 g of potassium chloride. How many milliequivalents of potassium chloride are represented in each packet?

35. How many milliequivalents of Li^+ are provided by a daily dose of four 300-mg tablets of lithium carbonate (Li_2CO_3—m.w. 74)?

36. How many milliequivalents of ammonium (NH_4^+) ion are contained in 1 liter of 4.2% (w/v) solution of ammonium chloride?

37. A patient is to receive 10 mEq of potassium gluconate ($C_6H_{11}KO_7$—m.w. 234) four times a day for 3 days. If the dose is to be 1 teaspoonful in a cherry syrup vehicle, (a) how many grams of potassium gluconate should be used, and (b) what volume, in milliliters, should be dispensed to provide the prescribed dosage regimen?

38. A physician wishes to administer 1,200,000 units of penicillin G potassium every 4 hours. If 1 unit of penicillin G potassium ($C_{16}H_{17}KN_2O_4S$—m.w. 372) equals 0.6 μg, how many milliequivalents of K^+ will the patient receive in a 24-hour period?

39. Five milliliters of lithium citrate syrup contain the equivalent of 8 mEq of Li^+. Calculate the equivalent, in milligrams, of lithium carbonate (Li_2CO_3—m.w. 74) in each 5-mL dose of the syrup.

40. How many milligrams of magnesium sulfate ($MgSO_4$—m.w. 120) should be added to an intravenous solution to provide 5 mEq of Mg^{++} per liter?

41. The manufacturer states that a slow-release potassium chloride tablet contains 600 mg of potassium chloride in a wax matrix. How many milliequivalents of potassium chloride are supplied by a dosage of one tablet three times a day?

42. An electrolyte solution contains 222 mg of sodium acetate ($C_2H_3NaO_2$—m.w. 82) and 15 mg of magnesium chloride ($MgCl_2$—m.w. 95) in each 100 mL. Express these concentrations in milliequivalents of Na^+ and Mg^{++} per liter.

43. Ammonium chloride (NH_4Cl—m.w. 53.5) is to be used as a urinary acidifier with a dose of 150 mEq. How many 500-mg tablets should be administered?

44. A patient has a sodium deficit of 168 mEq. How many milliliters of isotonic sodium chloride solution (0.9% w/v) should be administered to replace the deficit?

45. A normal 70 kg (154 lb) adult has 80 to 100 g of sodium. It is primarily distributed in the extracellular fluid. Body retention of 1 g additional of sodium results in excess body water accumulation of approximately 310 mL. If a person retains 100

mEq of extra sodium, how many milliliters of additional water could be expected to be retained?

46. A patient receives 3 liters of an electrolyte fluid containing 234 mg of sodium chloride (NaCl—m.w. 58.5), 125 mg of potassium acetate ($C_2H_3KO_2$—m.w. 98), and 21 mg of magnesium acetate ($C_4H_6MgO_4$—m.w. 142) per 100 mL. How many milliequivalents each of Na^+, K^+, and Mg^{++} does the patient receive?

47. How many milliliters of a 2% (w/v) solution of ammonium chloride (NH_4Cl—m.w. 53.5) should be administered intravenously to a patient to provide 75 mEq?

48. Calculate the osmolarity, in milliosmoles per milliliter, of a parenteral solution containing 2 mEq/mL of potassium acetate ($KC_2H_3O_2$—m.w. 98).

49. Calculate (a) the milliequivalents per milliliter, (b) the total milliequivalents, and (c) the osmolarity of a 500-mL parenteral fluid containing 5% (w/v) of sodium bicarbonate.

50. What is the osmolarity of an 8.4% (w/v) solution of sodium bicarbonate?

51. A hospital medication order calls for the administration of 100 g of mannitol to a patient as an osmotic diuretic over a 24-hour period. Calculate (a) how many milliliters of a 15% (w/v) mannitol injection should be administered per hour, and (b) how many milliosmoles of mannitol (m.w. 182) would be represented in the prescribed dosage.

52. The usual adult dose of calcium for elevating serum calcium is 7 to 14 mEq. How many milliliters of a calcium gluceptate injection, each milliliter of which provides 18 mg of elemental calcium, would provide the recommended dosage range?

53. How many (a) millimoles, (b) milliequivalents, and (c) milliosmoles of calcium chloride ($CaCl_2 \cdot 2H_2O$—m.w. 147) are represented in 147 mL of a 10% (w/v) calcium chloride solution?

54. The oral electrolyte maintenance solution Pedialyte® has the following electrolyte content per liter: sodium, 45 mEq; potassium, 20 mEq; chloride, 35 mEq; and citrate, 30 mEq. Calculate the equivalent quantities of each in terms of milligrams.

11

Constituted Solutions, Intravenous Admixtures, and Rate of Flow Calculations

CONSTITUTION OF DRY POWDERS

Oral Solution or Oral Suspension

Some drugs, most notably antibiotics, lose their potency in a relatively short period of time when prepared in a liquid dosage form. Thus, to enhance the shelf-life of these drugs, manufacturers provide products to the pharmacy in dry powder form for *constitution* with purified water or special diluent at the time a prescription or medication order is received. Depending on the product, the dry powder may be stable for about 24 months. After constitution, the resultant solution or suspension is stable in the quantities usually dispensed, for up to 10 days at room temperature or 14 days if maintained under refrigeration.

Dry powders for constitution are packaged in self-contained bottles of sufficient size to accommodate the addition of the required volume of diluent. In addition to the quantitative amount of therapeutic agent, the powder contains such pharmaceutical ingredients as solubilizing or suspending agents, stabilizers, colorants, sweeteners, and flavorants.

On receipt of a prescription order, the pharmacist follows the label instructions for constitution,[1] adding the proper amount of purified water of other diluent to prepare the liquid form. Depending on the product's formulation, constitution results in the preparation of a clear *solution* (often called a *"syrup"*) or a *suspension*. The final volume of product is the sum of the volume of solvent or diluent added and the volume occupied by the dissolved or suspended powder mixture. These products generally are intended for infants and children, but also may be used by adults who have difficulty swallowing counterpart solid dosage form products, such as tablets and capsules.

For children and adults, constituted products for oral solution or suspension generally are formulated such that the usual dose of the drug is contained in teaspoonful amounts of product. For infants, *pediatric drops*, which also require constitution, may be used. The calculations that follow demonstrate the preparation of constituted products and how the drug concentrations may be designed to meet a particular patient's requirements.

Figure 11.1 is an example of a dry antibiotic powder for constitution and the resultant suspension following constitution.

Concentration after Constitution. Calculating the concentration of an oral liquid after constitution according to the manufacturer's directions involves the following.

Example:

   The label for a dry powder package of penicillin V potassium for oral solution directs the pharmacist to dissolve the powder in the container with sufficient purified water to make 200 mL

---

[1] Some labeling instructions use the term "reconstitute" rather than "constitute" in describing the general process. Technically, if a dry powder is prepared from its original solution by removing the solvent (as through freeze drying), and then the solution is restored by the pharmacist, the term *reconstituted* would correctly apply. Some injectable products are prepared in this fashion.

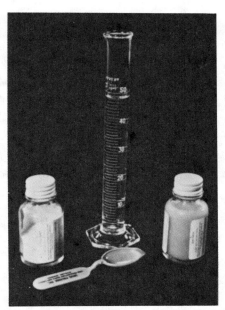

Fig. 11.1. Commercial antibiotic preparation for oral suspension following constitution with purified water. At left is the dry powder mixture; on the right is the suspension after constitution with the specified amount of purified water.

of solution. If the package contains 5 g of penicillin V potassium, how many milligrams of the antibiotic would be contained in each teaspoonful dose of the resultant solution?

5 g = 5000 mg

$$\frac{5000\ (mg)}{x\ (mg)} = \frac{200\ (mL)}{5\ (mL)}$$

$$x = 125\ mg,\ answer.$$

Or, solving be dimensional analysis:

$$\frac{5\ g}{200\ mL} \times \frac{1000\ mg}{1\ g} \times \frac{5\ mL}{1\ tsp.} = 125\ mg\ per\ teaspoonful,\ answer.$$

Volume of Dry Powder and Total Drug Content. Calculating the volume of dry powder and total drug content of a product to be constituted for oral solution or suspension involves the following.

Example:

Label instructions for an ampicillin product call for the addition of 78 mL of water to make 100 mL of constituted suspension such that each 5-mL contains 125 mg of ampicillin.

Volume of dry powder:

Because the addition of 78 mL of water results in the preparation of 100 mL of product, the volume occupied by the dry powder is:

100 mL − 78 mL = 22 mL, *answer.*

Total drug (ampicillin) present:

If in the constituted product, each 5-mL contains 125 mg of ampicillin, the total amount of ampicillin in the 100-mL product is:

$$\frac{5 \text{ mL}}{125 \text{ mg}} = \frac{100 \text{ mL}}{x}$$

$$x = 2500 \text{ mg}, \textit{answer.}$$

Modifying Label Instructions to Obtain Desired Concentration. To modify the label instructions to prepare a constituted product of a desired concentration, observe the following.

Example:

Using the product in the previous example, if a physician desires an ampicillin concentration of 100 mg/5 mL (rather than 125 mg/5 mL), how many milliliters of water should be added to the dry powder?

Because it was determined that 2500 mg of ampicillin are in the dry product, the volume of product that can be made with a concentration of 100 mg/5 mL may be calculated by:

$$\frac{2500 \text{ mg}}{x \text{ mL}} = \frac{100 \text{ mg}}{5 \text{ mL}}$$

$$x = 125 \text{ mL}, \textit{answer.}$$

Then, because it had been determined that the dry powder occupies 22 mL of volume, it is possible to determine the amount of water to add:

125 mL − 22 mL = 103 mL, *answer.*

Constitution Based on Dosage Calculation of Weight and Body Surface Area. To constitute a dry powder into an oral solution or suspension based on dosage calculation of weight or body surface area, observe the following.

Examples:

The label of a dry powder for oral suspension states that when 111 mL of water are added to the powder, 150 mL of a suspension containing 250 mg of ampicillin per 5 mL are prepared. How many milliliters of purified water should be used to prepare, in each 5-mL of product, the correct dose of ampicillin for a 60-lb child based on the dose of 8 mg/kg of body weight?

The dose of ampicillin may be determined by:

$$\frac{8 \text{ mg}}{2.2 \text{ lb}} = \frac{x \text{ mg}}{60 \text{ lb}}$$

$$x = 218 \text{ mg}$$

Then, the amount of ampicillin in the container is determined by:

$$\frac{250 \text{ mg}}{5 \text{ mL}} = \frac{x \text{ mg}}{150 \text{ mL}}$$

$$x = 7500 \text{ mg}$$

Thus, the amount of product that can be made from 7500 mg of drug such that each 5-mL contains 218 mg of drug may be found by:

$$\frac{218 \text{ mg}}{5 \text{ mL}} = \frac{7500 \text{ mg}}{x \text{ mL}}$$

$$x = 172 \text{ mL}$$

Finally, because the volume of powder occupies 39 mL (150 mL − 111 mL), the amount of water to add is determined by:

172 mL − 39 mL = 133 mL, *answer.*

The label of a dry powder for constitution into pediatric drops states that when 12 mL of purified water are added to the powder, 15 mL of a pediatric suspension containing 50 mg of amoxicillin per milliliter results. How many milliliters of water should be added to prepare the dose of amoxicillin in each 10 drops if the dropper delivers 20 drops/mL, the child has a body surface area (BSA) of 0.4 m², and the dose of the drug is based on 50 mg/m² of BSA?

The dose of amoxicillin may be determined by:

$$\frac{50 \text{ mg}}{1 \text{ m}^2 \text{ BSA}} = \frac{x \text{ mg}}{0.4 \text{ m}^2 \text{ BSA}}$$

$$x = 20 \text{ mg}$$

The volume of product to contain the 20-mg dose is determined by:

$$\frac{10 \text{ drops}}{x \text{ mL}} = \frac{20 \text{ drops}}{1 \text{ mL}}$$

$$x = 0.5 \text{ mL}$$

The amount of amoxicillin in the package is determined by:

$$\frac{50 \text{ mg}}{1 \text{ mL}} = \frac{x \text{ mg}}{15 \text{ mL}}$$

$$x = 750 \text{ mg}$$

The amount of product of the desired dose that may be prepared is determined by:

$$\frac{750 \text{ mg}}{x \text{ mL}} = \frac{20 \text{ mg}}{0.5 \text{ mL}}$$

$$x = 18.75 \text{ mL}$$

Subtracting the volume accounted for by the dry powder (15 mL − 12 mL = 3 mL), the volume of water to add is determined by:

18.75 mL − 3 mL = 15.75 mL, *answer.*

Parenteral Use

Because of instability in liquid form, some medications (particularly antibiotics) intended for injection are provided as dry powder in vials to be constituted with sterile water for injection or other designated solvent or diluent immediately before use. Generally, these medications are small-volume products intended for use by injection or as additives to large-volume parenterals.

In contrast to the dry powders intended for oral use after constitution, injectable products may contain only limited amounts of specified added ingredients to increase the stability and effectiveness of the drug (obviously, no colorants, flavorants, sweeteners, etc. are needed). So, in effect, the bulk volume of the dry contents of a vial is largely or entirely the medication.

If the quantity of the dry drug powder is small and does not contribute significantly to the final volume of the constituted solution, the volume of solvent used will approximate the final volume of solution. For example, if 1000 units of a certain antibiotic in dry form are to be dissolved, and if the powder does not account for any significant portion of the final volume, the addition of 5 mL of solvent will produce a solution containing 200 units/mL. If the dry powder, however, because of its bulk, contributes to the final volume of the constituted solution, the increase in volume produced by the drug must be considered, and this factor must then be used in calculating the amount of solvent needed to prepare a solution of a desired concentration. For example, the package directions for making injectable solutions of streptomycin sulfate specify that 4.2 mL of sterile solvent should be added to 1 g of the dry powder to produce 5.0 mL of a solution, which is to contain 200 mg/mL. The drug, in this case, accounts for 0.8 mL of the final volume. Again, in dissolving 20,000,000 units of penicillin G potassium, the addition of 32 mL of sterile solvent provides a total volume of 40 mL of a solution that contains 500,000 units/mL. The dry powder now accounts for 8 mL of the final volume.

Solvent Needed to Produce Desired Concentration When Dry Agent Does not Contribute to Final Volume. Calculating the amount of solvent needed for a given vial content of a dry powder to produce a desired concentration when the solid material does not significantly account for any portion of the constituted solution involves the following.

Examples:

Using a vial containing 200,000 units of penicillin G potassium, how many milliliters of solvent should be added to the dry powder in preparing a solution having a concentration of 25,000 units/mL?

$$\frac{25,000 \text{ (units)}}{200,000 \text{ (units)}} = \frac{1 \text{ (mL)}}{x \text{ (mL)}}$$

$$x = 8 \text{ mL, } answer.$$

Using a vial containing 200,000 units of penicillin G sodium and sodium chloride injection as the solvent, explain how you would obtain the penicillin G sodium needed in preparing the following prescription.

R̸   Penicillin G Sodium   15,000 units per mL
            Sodium Chloride Injection   ad   10 mL
            Sig. For IM Injection.

15,000 units × 10 = 150,000 units of penicillin G sodium needed

Because the dry powder represents 200,000 units of penicillin G sodium or $\frac{4}{3}$ *times* the number of units desired, $\frac{3}{4}$ of the powder will contain the required number of units.

Step 1.   Dissolve the dry powder in 4 mL of sodium chloride injection.
Step 2.   Use 3 mL of the constituted solution, *answer.*

Or, solving by dimensional analysis:

$$10 \text{ mL} \times \frac{15,000 \text{ units}}{1 \text{ mL}} \times \frac{4 \text{ mL}}{200,000 \text{ units}} = 3 \text{ mL, } answer.$$

Solvent Needed to Produce a Desired Concentration when Dry Agent Contributes to Final Volume. Calculating the amount of solvent needed for a given vial content of a dry powder to produce a desired concentration when the solid material accounts for a definite volume of the constituted solution involves the following.

Examples:

The package information enclosed with a vial containing 5,000,000 units of penicillin G potassium (buffered) specifies that when 23 mL of a sterile solvent are added to the dry powder, the resulting concentration is 200,000 units/mL. On the basis of this information, how many milliliters of sterile water for injection should be used in preparing the following solution?

℞   Penicillin G Potassium (buffered)   5,000,000 units
        Sterile Water for Injection   q.s.
        Make solution containing 500,000 units per mL
        Sig. One mL = 500,000 units of Penicillin G Potassium.

The package information states that the constituted solution prepared by dissolving 5,000,000 units of the dry powder in 23 mL of sterile solvent has a final volume of 25 mL. The dry powder, then, accounts for 2 mL of this volume.

Step 1.   The final volume of the prescription is determined as follows:

$$\frac{500,000 \text{ (units)}}{5,000,000 \text{ (units)}} = \frac{1 \text{ (mL)}}{x \text{ (mL)}}$$

$$x = 10 \text{ mL}$$

Step 2.   10 mL − 2 mL (dry powder accounts for this volume) = 8 mL, *answer.*

Streptomycin sulfate is available in 1-g vials, and the dry powder accounts for 0.8 mL of the volume of the constituted solution. Using a 1-g vial of streptomycin sulfate and sodium chloride injection as the solvent, explain how you would obtain the streptomycin sulfate needed for the following prescription.

℞   Streptomycin Sulfate   250 mg
        Sodium Chloride Injection   ad   15 mL
        Sig. For IM Injection.

Step 1.   Dissolve the dry powder in 9.2 mL of sodium chloride injection. The constituted solution will measure 10 mL and will contain 100 mg of streptomycin sulfate per milliliter.

Step 2.   Use 2.5 mL of the constituted solution, *answer.*

INTRAVENOUS ADMIXTURES

The preparation of intravenous admixtures involves the addition of one or more drugs to large-volume sterile fluids such as Sodium Chloride Injection, Dextrose Injection, Lactated Ringer's Injection, and others.[2] The additives are generally in the form of small-volume sterile solutions packaged in ampuls or vials, or sterile solids requiring constitution with a sterile solvent before transfer.

Although a wide variety of drugs and drug combinations have been used in preparing dilute infusions for intravenous therapy, some of the more common additives include electrolytes, antibiotics, vitamins, trace minerals, heparin, and, in some instances, insulin. Figure 11.2 shows the aseptic addition of an additive to a large-volume solution.

In any properly administered intravenous admixture program, all basic fluids (large-volume solutions), additives (already in solution or extemporaneously constituted), and *calculations* must be carefully checked against the medication orders. The discussion that

---

[2] By USP definition, "large-volume intravenous solution" applies to a single-dose injection intended for intravenous use packaged in containers holding more than 100 mL. The abbreviation "LVP" is commonly used to indicate "large-volume parenteral" and "SVP," "small-volume parenteral" (100 mL or less).

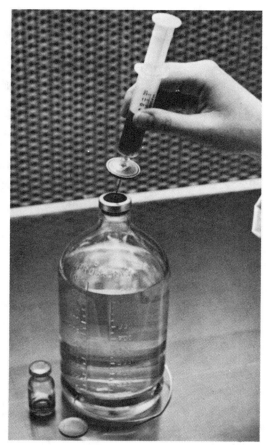

Fig. 11.2. Aseptic addition of an additive to a large-volume parenteral solution. (Courtesy of Millipore Corporation.)

follows concerns itself *solely* with some calculations that may be encountered in the extemporaneous preparation of typical intravenous admixtures.

Additive(s) Needed for Admixture with Large-Volume Fluid to Produce Infusion of Specified Content. Calculating the amount of additive(s) to be admixed with a large-volume intravenous or nutrient fluid to produce an infusion containing a required quantity of a drug or combination of drugs involves the following.

Examples:

A medication order for a patient weighing 154 lb calls for 0.25 mg of amphotericin B per kilogram of body weight to be added to 500 mL of 5% dextrose injection. If the amphotericin B is to be obtained from a constituted injection that contains 50 mg/10 mL, how many milliliters should be added to the dextrose injection?

$$1 \text{ kg} = 2.2 \text{ lb}$$

$$\frac{154 \text{ (lb)}}{2.2 \text{ (lb)}} = 70 \text{ kg}$$

$$0.25 \text{ mg} \times 70 = 17.5 \text{ mg}$$

Constituted solution contains 50 mg/10 mL

$$\frac{50 \ (mg)}{17.5 \ (mg)} = \frac{10 \ (mL)}{x \ (mL)}$$

$$x = 3.5 \ mL, \ answer.$$

Or, solving by dimensional analysis:

$$154 \ lb \times \frac{1 \ kg}{2.2 \ lb} \times \frac{0.25 \ mg}{1 \ kg} \times \frac{10 \ mL}{50 \ mg} = 3.5 \ mL, \ answer.$$

An intravenous infusion is to contain 15 mEq of potassium ion and 20 mEq of sodium ion in 500 mL of 5% dextrose injection. Using potassium chloride injection containing 6 g/30 mL and 0.9% sodium chloride injection, how many milliliters of each should be used to supply the required ions?

15 mEq of K^+ ion will be supplied by 15 mEq of KCl and 20 mEq of Na^+ ion will be supplied by 20 mEq of NaCl

$$1 \ mEq \ of \ KCl = 74.5 \ mg$$

$$15 \ mEq \ of \ KCl = 1117.5 \ mg \ or \ 1.118 \ g$$

$$\frac{6 \ (g)}{1.118 \ (g)} = \frac{30 \ (mL)}{x \ (mL)}$$

$$x = 5.59 \ or \ 5.6 \ mL, \ and$$

$$1 \ mEq \ of \ NaCl = 58.5 \ mg$$

$$20 \ mEq \ of \ NaCl = 1170 \ mg \ or \ 1.170 \ g$$

$$\frac{0.9 \ (g)}{1.17 \ (g)} = \frac{100 \ (mL)}{x \ (mL)}$$

$$x = 130 \ mL, \ answers.$$

Or, solving by dimensional analysis:

$$15 \ mEq \times \frac{74.5 \ mg}{1 \ mEq} \times \frac{1 \ g}{1000 \ mg} \times \frac{30 \ mL}{6 \ g} = 5.59 \ or \ 5.6 \ mL, \ and$$

$$20 \ mEq \times \frac{58.5 \ mg}{1 \ mEq} \times \frac{1 \ g}{1000 \ mg} \times \frac{100 \ mL}{0.9 \ g} = 130 \ mL, \ answers.$$

A medication order for a child weighing 44 lb calls for polymyxin B sulfate to be administered by the intravenous drip method in a dosage of 7500 units/kg of body weight in 500 mL of 5% dextrose injection. Using a vial containing 500,000 units of polymyxin B sulfate and sodium chloride injection as the solvent, explain how you would obtain the polymyxin B sulfate needed in preparing the infusion.

$$1 \ kg = 2.2 \ lb$$

$$\frac{44}{2.2} = 20 \ kg$$

$$7500 \ units \times 20 = 150,000 \ units$$

Step 1.   Dissolve contents of vial (500,000 units) in 10 mL of sodium chloride injection.
Step 2.   Add 3 mL of constituted solution to 500 mL of 5% dextrose injection, *answer.*

PARENTERAL NUTRITION

Parenteral nutrition or *hyperalimentation* is the feeding of a patient by the intravenous infusion of basic nutrients needed to achieve active tissue synthesis and growth. *Partial parenteral nutrition (PPN)* is support that *supplements* oral intake and provides only part of daily nutritional requirements. *Total parenteral nutrition (TPN)* provides *all* of the patient's daily nutritional requirements. Among the components generally included in parenteral nutrition fluids are dextrose, amino acids, vitamins and trace elements, and electrolytes. Other components as fat, insulin, and specific drugs may be added as prescribed.

Figure 11.3 is an example of a hospital adult parenteral nutrition form. Note that the

Fig. 11.3. Example of part of an order form for adult parenteral nutrition. (Published with the permission of Wake Medical Center, Raleigh, NC.)

prescribing physician may select the standard formulas or modifications for central or peripheral administration. Central administration lines are inserted into the superior vena cava, whereas peripheral lines are inserted into veins of the arm or hand. Because of hypertonicity, concentrated dextrose solutions may be damaging to veins. Thus, central lines are used to accommodate greater concentrations of dextrose (e.g., 25%) than peripheral lines (e.g., 10%). Special amino acid formulas are available for patients with kidney, pulmonary, and liver diseases.

In preparing solutions for parenteral nutrition, the pharmacist uses calculated quantities of small-volume parenterals (ampuls and vials) as the source(s) of most required electrolytes, and, large-volume parenterals for amino acids, dextrose, and sterile water for injection.

Caloric Requirements

The *kilocalorie* (kcal) is the unit used in metabolic studies. By definition, the kilocalorie (or large calorie) is the amount of heat required to raise the temperature of 1 kg of water from 0° to 1°C. The caloric requirements for patients vary, depending on their physical state and medical condition. The Harris-Benedict equation, which follows, is commonly used to estimate the resting metabolic energy (RME) requirements for nonprotein calories:[3]

<u>For Males:</u>

RME = 66 + (13.7 × W) + (5 × H) − (6.8 × A)

<u>For Females:</u>

RME = 655 + (9.6 × W) + (1.8 × H) − (4.7 × A)

in which W is weight in kilograms, H is height in centimeters, and A is age in years. This equation is designed to *maintain* the patient's present weight (a selected "dosing weight" for morbidly obese patients is used to keep the caloric nutrition below 3000 kcal/day). Under conditions of stress, the RME may be multiplied by factors of 1.2 to 1.4 for mild stress (as nonsurgical hospitalized patients), 1.5 to 1.75 for moderate stress (as patients with severe infection), and 1.75 to 2.0 for severe stress (as patients with severe burns). In general, 25 kcal/kg of body weight per day for an only mildly stressed hospitalized patient is considered usual. Moderately stressed patients may require 35 kcal/kg/day; postoperative patients up to 45 kcal/kg/day; and, hypercatabolic patients up to 60 kcal/kg/day.

Depending on the individual patient, calories may be provided by the administration of carbohydrate, amino acids, and lipids (fat). Fat is restricted to less than 60% of the total daily calories administered. The quantity of protein (amino acids) required is generally estimated to be about 0.75 g/kg of body weight for the average healthy adult patient who is only mildly stressed, about 0.9 g/kg for the moderately stressed patient, and about 1.25 g/kg for the severely stressed patient. On a case-by-case basis, additional amounts may be required for patients with protein loss from diarrhea, exuding skin lesions, burns, etc.

In providing parenteral nutrition, the pharmacist may first determine the total caloric requirement using the Harris-Benedict equation or some other measure. Then, the amount of protein required would be calculated based on 0.75 g/kg (or other quantity) and the caloric value of 4 kcal/g for proteins and amino acids. The remaining caloric requirement would be met by the addition of dextrose (carbohydrate) at 3.4 kcal/g (100 mL of 50%

---

[3] Gomella, L.G.: *Clinician's Pocket Reference*, 7th Ed. Norwalk, CT, Appleton & Lange, 1993.

dextrose injection provides 170 kcal), and lipid emulsions in 10% ($\cong$1 kcal/mL) or 20% ($\cong$2.0 kcal/mL) concentrations.

Component Source(s) Needed for Admixture to Provide Required Amount of Additive(s). Calculating the amount of component source(s) to be added to or admixed with a large-volume intravenous or nutrient fluid to provide the required amount of additive(s) specified in a medication order involves the following.

Examples:

The following is a formula for a desired parenteral nutrition solution. Using the source of each drug as indicated, calculate the amount of each component required in preparing the solution.

Formula	Component Source
(a) Sodium Chloride 35 mEq	Vial, 5 mEq per 2 mL
(b) Potassium Acetate 35 mEq	Vial, 10 mEq per 5 mL
(c) Magnesium Sulfate 8 mEq	Vial, 4 mEq per mL
(d) Calcium Gluconate 9.6 mEq	Vial, 4.7 mEq per 10 mL
(e) Potassium Chloride 5 mEq	Vial, 40 mEq per 20 mL
(f) Folic Acid 1.7 mg	Ampul, 5 mg per mL
(g) Multiple Vitamin Infusion 10 mL	Ampul, 10 mL

To be added to:

Amino Acids Infusion (8.5%) 500 mL
Dextrose Injection (50%) 500 mL
(a)

$$\frac{5 \text{ (mEq)}}{35 \text{ (mEq)}} = \frac{2 \text{ (mL)}}{x \text{ (mL)}}$$

$$x = 14 \text{ mL}, and$$

(b)

$$\frac{10 \text{ (mEq)}}{35 \text{ (mEq)}} = \frac{5 \text{ (mL)}}{x \text{ (mL)}}$$

$$x = 17.5 \text{ mL}, and$$

(c)

$$\frac{4 \text{ (mEq)}}{8 \text{ (mEq)}} = \frac{1 \text{ (mL)}}{x \text{ (mL)}}$$

$$x = 2 \text{ mL}, and$$

(d)

$$\frac{4.7 \text{ (mEq)}}{9.6 \text{ (mEq)}} = \frac{10 \text{ (mL)}}{x \text{ (mL)}}$$

$$x = 20.4 \text{ mL}, and$$

(e)

$$\frac{40 \text{ (mEq)}}{5 \text{ (mEq)}} = \frac{20 \text{ (mL)}}{x \text{ (mL)}}$$

$$x = 2.5 \text{ mL}, and$$

(f)

$$\frac{5 \ (mg)}{1.7 \ (mg)} = \frac{1 \ (mL)}{x \ (mL)}$$

$$x = 0.34 \ mL, \ and$$

(g)   10 mL, *answers.*

The formula for a TPN solution calls for the addition of 2.7 mEq of Ca^{++} and 20 mEq of K^+ per liter. How many milliliters of an injection containing 20 mg of calcium chloride per milliliter and how many milliliters of a 15% (w/v) potassium chloride injection should be used to provide the desired additives?

$$\begin{array}{ll} 1 \ mEq \ of \ Ca^{++} & = 20 \ mg \\ 2.7 \ mEq \ of \ Ca^{++} & = 20 \ mg \times 2.7 = 54 \ mg \end{array}$$

54 mg of Ca^{++} are furnished by 198.45 or 198 mg of calcium chloride

Because the injection contains 20 mg of calcium chloride per mL, then $198 \div 20 = 9.9 \ mL, \ and$

$$\begin{array}{ll} 1 \ mEq \ of \ K^+ & = 39 \ mg \\ 20 \ mEq \ of \ K^+ & = 39 \ mg \times 20 = 780 \ mg \end{array}$$

780 mg of K^+ are furnished by 1.49 g of potassium chloride
15% (w/v) solution contains 15 g of potassium chloride per 100 mL then

$$\frac{15 \ (g)}{1.49 \ (g)} = \frac{100 \ (mL)}{x \ (mL)}$$

$$x = 9.9 \ mL, \ answers.$$

A potassium phosphate injection contains a mixture of 224 mg of monobasic potassium phosphate (KH_2PO_4) and 236 mg of dibasic potassium phosphate (K_2HPO_4) per milliliter. If 10 mL of the injection are added to 500 mL of D5W (5% dextrose in water for injection), (a) how many milliequivalents of K^+ and (b) how many millimoles of total phosphate are represented in the prepared solution?

$$\begin{array}{ll} Formula \ weight \ of \ KH_2PO_4 & = 136 \\ 1 \ mmol \ of \ KH_2PO_4 & = 136 \ mg \end{array}$$

10 mL of injection contain 2240 mg of KH_2PO_4

and thus provide $2240 \div 136 = 16.4$ or 16 mmol of KH_2PO_4
or 16 mmol of K^+ and 16 mmol of $H_2PO_4^{=}$

$$\begin{array}{ll} Formula \ weight \ of \ K_2HPO_4 & = 174 \\ 1 \ mmol \ of \ K_2HPO_4 & = 174 \ mg \end{array}$$

10 mL of injection contain 2360 mg of K_2HPO_4
and thus provide $2360 \div 174 = 13.6$ or 14 mmol of K_2HPO_4
or 14 (mmol) $\times$ 2 (K^+) = 28 mmol of K^+, and 14 mmol of $HPO_4^{=}$
thus 10 mL of injection provide a total of :
    44 mmol of K^+ or (because the valence of K^+ is 1) 44 mEq of K^+, *and*
    30 mmol of total phosphate, *answers.*

Caloric Requirements. To calculate caloric requirements for parenteral nutrition fluids, observe the following.

Examples:

Using the Harris-Benedict equation, calculate the caloric requirement for a mildly stressed, 56-year-old hospitalized female patient weighing 121 lb and measuring 5 ft, 3 in. in height.

$$
\begin{aligned}
121 \text{ lb} &= 55 \text{ kg} \\
5'3'' &= 63 \text{ in.} = 160 \text{ cm} \\
\text{RME} &= 655 + (9.6 \times 55) + (1.8 \times 160) - (4.7 \times 56) \\
&= 655 + (528) + (288) - (263) \\
&= 1208 \text{ kcal}
\end{aligned}
$$

Using the average factor of 1.3 for a mildly stressed patient,
$$1208 \times 1.3 = 1570 \text{ kcal, } answer.$$

Calculate the daily quantity of protein required for the 55 kg patient based on 0.75 g/kg and the caloric value based on 4 kcal/g for proteins.

$$
\begin{aligned}
55 \text{ kg} \times 0.75 \text{ g/kg} &= 41.25 \text{ g protein, and} \\
41.25 \text{ g} \times 4 \text{ kcal/g} &= 165 \text{ kcal, } answers
\end{aligned}
$$

From the above two example problems, calculate the number of milliliters of 50% dextrose solution (170 kcal/dL) that may be used to provide the additional kilocalories required.

$$
\begin{aligned}
\text{Total kcal required} &= 1570 \\
\text{Kcal provided by proteins} &= 165 \\
\text{Additional kcal required} &= 1405 \ (1570 - 165)
\end{aligned}
$$

Thus,

$$
\frac{1405 \text{ kcal}}{170 \text{ kcal}} = \frac{x \text{ mL}}{100 \text{ mL}}
$$

$$
x = 826 \text{ mL, } answer
$$

RATE OF FLOW OF INTRAVENOUS FLUIDS

Small-volume injections are injected into the body site slowly using a hand-held syringe and needle. The medication is drawn into the syringe from either a single-dose *ampul* or a multiple-dose *vial*. Some syringes are packaged prefilled by the manufacturer or hospital pharmacist. Some vials contain dry powders requiring constitution with a specified liquid vehicle before use.

Large-volume parenterals for continuous intravenous administration are "hung" at the patient's bedside and allowed to drip slowly into a vein by gravity flow or through the use of electrical or battery-operated volumetric infusion pumps. Some of these pumps can be calibrated to deliver "microinfusion" volumes (e.g., 0.1 mL per hour) to as much as 2000 mL per hour, depending on the drug and the requirements of the patient. Solutions of additive drugs are placed directly into the large-volume parenteral or small-volume parenterals (minibags) containing the additive drug that may be hung "piggyback" and allowed to enter the tubing of the primary bottle of intravenous fluid and into the patient at a controlled rate. In either case, the physician specifies the rate of flow of intravenous fluids in milliliters per minute, drops per minute, amount of drug (as milligrams per hour), or, more frequently, as the approximate duration of time of administration of the total volume of the infusion. The pharmacist may be requested to make or to check the calculations involved in converting the desired total time interval into a flow rate of drops per minute.

Large-Volume Intravenous Fluid Delivery Over Specified Period. Calculating the rate of flow needed to administer a large-volume intravenous fluid during a desired time interval involves the following.

Examples:

A medication order calls for 1000 mL of D5W to be administered over an 8-hour period. Using an IV administration set that delivers 10 drops/mL, how many drops per minute should be delivered to the patient?

$$\text{Volume of fluid} = 1000 \text{ mL}$$
$$8 \text{ hours} = 480 \text{ minutes}$$

$$\frac{1000 \text{ (mL)}}{480 \text{ (min)}} = 2.1 \text{ mL per minute}$$

2.1 mL/min $\times$ 10 (drops/mL) = 21 drops per minute, *answer.*
Or, solving by dimensional analysis:

$$\frac{1000 \text{ mL}}{8 \text{ hr}} \times \frac{1 \text{ hr}}{60 \text{ min}} \times \frac{10 \text{ drops}}{1 \text{ mL}} = 20.8, \text{ or } 21 \text{ drops per minute, } answer.$$

Ten (10) milliliters of 10% calcium gluconate injection and 10 mL of multivitamin infusion are mixed with 500 mL of a 5% dextrose injection. The infusion is to be administered over 5 hours. If the dropper in the venoclysis set calibrates 15 drops/mL, at what rate, in drops per minute, should the flow be adjusted to administer the infusion over the desired time interval?

$$\text{Total volume of infusion} =$$

$$10 \text{ mL} + 10 \text{ mL} + 500 \text{ ml} = 520 \text{ mL}$$

Dropper calibrates 15 drops/mL

$$520 \times 15 \text{ drops} = 7800 \text{ drops}$$

$$\frac{7800 \text{ (drops)}}{300 \text{ (minutes)}} = 26 \text{ drops per minute, } answer.$$

Or, solving by dimensional analysis:

$$\frac{520 \text{ mL}}{5 \text{ hours}} \times \frac{1 \text{ hr}}{60 \text{ min}} \times \frac{15 \text{ drops}}{1 \text{ mL}} = 26 \text{ drops per minute, } answer.$$

An intravenous infusion contains 10 mL of a 1:5000 solution of isoproterenol hydrochloride and 500 mL of a 5% dextrose injection. At what flow rate should the infusion be administered to provide 5 μg of isoproterenol hydrochloride per minute and what time interval will be necessary for the administration of the entire infusion?

10 mL of a 1:5000 solution contain 2 mg
2 mg or 2000 μg are contained in a volume of 510 mL

$$\frac{2000 \text{ (}\mu g\text{)}}{5 \text{ (}\mu g\text{)}} = \frac{510 \text{ (mL)}}{x \text{ (mL)}}$$

$$x = 1.275 \text{ or } 1.28 \text{ mL per minute, } and$$

$$\frac{1.28 \text{ (mL)}}{510 \text{ (mL)}} = \frac{1 \text{ (minute)}}{x \text{ (minutes)}}$$

$$x = 398 \text{ minutes or approx. } 6\frac{1}{2} \text{ hours, } \textit{answers.}$$

Or, solving by dimensional analysis:

$$\frac{0.002 \text{ g}}{510 \text{ mL}} \times \frac{1,000,000 \ \mu g}{1 \text{ g}} \times \frac{1 \text{ min}}{5 \ \mu g} \times 510 \text{ mL} = 400 \text{ minutes} \approx 6\frac{1}{2} \text{ hours, } \textit{answer.}$$

Quantitative Amount of Drug in a Specified Period. Calculating the rate of flow to deliver a quantitative amount of drug in a specified period of time involves the following.

Example:

If 10 mg of a drug are added to a 500-mL large-volume parenteral fluid, what should be the rate of flow, in milliliters per hour, to deliver 1 mg of drug per hour?

$$\frac{10 \text{ (mg)}}{1 \text{ (mg)}} = \frac{500 \text{ (mL)}}{x \text{ (mL)}}$$

$$x = 50 \text{ mL per hour, } \textit{answer.}$$

In this example, if the infusion set delivers 15 drops/mL, what should be the rate of flow in drops per minute?

$$15 \text{ drops/mL} \times 50 \text{ mL/hr} = 750 \text{ drops per hour}$$

$$\frac{750 \text{ (drops)}}{x \text{ (drops)}} = \frac{60 \text{ (minutes)}}{1 \text{ (minute)}}$$

$$x = 12.5 \text{ drops/minute, } \textit{answer.}$$

Or, solving by dimensional analysis:

$$\frac{50 \text{ mL}}{1 \text{ hr}} \times \frac{1 \text{ h}}{60 \text{ min}} \times \frac{15 \text{ drops}}{1 \text{ mL}} = 12.5 \text{ drops per minute, } \textit{answer.}$$

Again, in this example, how many hours should the total infusion last?

$$\frac{50 \text{ (mL)}}{500 \text{ (mL)}} = \frac{1 \text{ (hour)}}{x \text{ (hour)}}$$

$$x = 10 \text{ hours, } \textit{answer.}$$

Using a Nomogram. A nomogram, such as is shown in Figure 11.4, may be used in determining the rate of flow of a parenteral fluid. Given the volume to be administered, the infusion time (duration), and the drops per milliliter delivered by the infusion set, the rate of flow, in drops per minute, may be determined directly.

Example:

If 1.0 liter of a parenteral fluid is to be infused over a 12-hour period using an infusion set that delivers 20 drops/mL, what should be the rate of flow in drops per minute?

First, locate the intercept of the diagonal line representing an infusion time of 12 hours with the horizontal line representing 1.0 liter of fluid. Next, follow the point of the intercept down vertically to the drop counter scale representing "20 drops/mL" to determine the answer. In the example, the horizontal line would be crossed between 20 and 30 drops per minute—closer to the 30, or approximately 28 drops per minute, *answer.*

Nomogram for number of drops per minute

The number of drops per minute required to administer a particular quantity of infusion solution in a certain time can be read off directly from this nomogram. The nomogram allows for the increase in drop size as the dropping rate increases and is based on the normal drop defined by the relationship: 20 drops distilled water at 15 °C = 1 g (± 0.05 g) when falling at the rate of 60/min. The dependence of drop size on dropping rate is allowed for by the increasing width of the scale units of the three abscissae as the dropping rate increases.

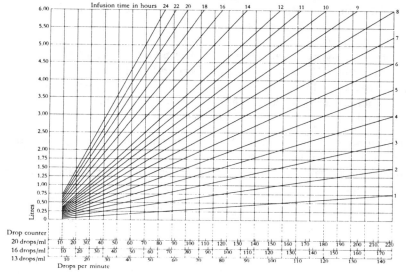

Fig. 11.4. Rate of flow versus quantity of infusion solution versus time nomogram. (From _Documenta Geigy Scientific Tables_, 7th Ed., 1970. With permission of Ciba-Geigy Limited, Basel, Switzerland.)

As a check to the proper use of the nomogram, the preceding example may be calculated as follows:

$$\text{Infusion time} = 12 \text{ hours} = 720 \text{ minutes}$$

$$\text{Infusion fluid} = 1.0 \text{ liter} = 1000 \text{ mL}$$

$$\text{Drops per milliliter} = 20$$

$$\text{Total drops in infusion liquid} = 20 \text{ drops/mL} \times 1000 \text{ mL} = 20000$$

$$\frac{20000 \text{ (drops)}}{720 \text{ (minutes)}} = 27.7 \text{ drops per minute, } \textit{answer.}$$

Or, solving by dimensional analysis:

$$\frac{20 \text{ drops}}{1 \text{ mL}} \times \frac{1000 \text{ mL}}{12 \text{ hrs}} \times \frac{1 \text{ hr}}{60 \text{ min}} = 27.7 \text{ drops per minute, } \textit{answer.}$$

Practice Problems

1. After constitution of the dry powder, each 5 mL of ampicillin for oral suspension contains 250 mg of ampicillin in package sizes to prepare 100 mL, 150 mL, or 200 mL of suspension. Which package size should be dispensed for a 20-kg child who is to take 50 mg/kg/day total, q.i.d. in equally divided and spaced doses for 10 days?

2. Manufacturer's directions call for the addition of 90 mL of water to constitute a 150-mL container of cefaclor to yield a strength of 250 mg of cefaclor per 5 mL.

If 60 mL of water were mistakenly added in constituting the product, calculate the resultant milligrams of cefaclor per 5 mL.

3. The label on a bottle of dry powder mix for constitution states that when 128 mL of water are added, 150 mL of an oral suspension, containing 250 mg of ampicillin in each 5 mL results.
    (a) How many milliliters of water should be added to the dry powder mix if a strength of 150 mg of ampicillin per 5 mL is desired?
    (b) If the dose of ampicillin is 5 mg/kg of body weight, how many milliliters of water should be added to the dry powder mix so that a child weighing 66 lb could receive the proper dose in each 5-mL of the suspension?

4. A medication order calls for 400 mg of cefazolin sodium to be administered IM to a patient every 12 hours. Vials containing 250 mg, 500 mg, and 1 g of cefazolin sodium are available. According to the manufacturer's directions, dilutions may be made as follows:

Vial Size	Solvent to Be Added	Final Volume
250 mg	2 mL	2 mL
500 mg	2 mL	2.2 mL
1 g	2.5 mL	3 mL

Explain how the prescribed amount of cefazolin sodium could be obtained.

5. Using the vial sizes in problem 4 as the source of cefazolin sodium, how many milliliters of the diluted 500-mg vial should be administered to a 40-lb child who is to receive 8 mg of cefazolin sodium per kilogram of body weight?

6. Using cefazolin sodium injection in a concentration of 125 mg/mL, complete the following table representing a *Pediatric Dosage Guide:*

Weight		Dose—25 mg/kg/day divided into 3 doses	
		Approximate single	mL of dilution
lb	kg	dose (mg/q8h)	(125 mg/mL) needed
10	4.5	37.5 or 38 mg	0.3 mL
20	_____	_____	_____
30	_____	_____	_____
40	_____	_____	_____
50	_____	_____	_____

7. A pharmacist receives a medication order for 300,000 units of penicillin G potassium to be added to 500 mL of D5W. The directions on the 1,000,000-unit package state that if 1.6 mL of solvent are added, the constituted solution will measure 2 mL. How many milliliters of the constituted solution must be withdrawn and added to the D5W?

8. A vial contains 1 g of cephadrine. Express the concentrations of the drug, in milligrams per milliliter, following constitution with sterile water for injection to the following volumes: (a) 2.2 mL, (b) 4.5 mL, and (c) 10 mL.

9. A physician orders 2 g of an antibiotic to be placed in 1000 mL of D5W. Using a constituted injection that contains 300 mg of the antibiotic per 2 mL, how many milliliters should be added to the dextrose injection in preparing the medication order?

10. A medication order for an intravenous infusion for a patient weighing 110 lb calls for 0.3 mEq of ammonium chloride per kilogram of body weight to be added to 500 mL of 5% dextrose injection. How many milliliters of a sterile solution containing 100 mEq of ammonium chloride per 20 mL should be used in preparing the infusion?

11. Acetazolamide sodium is available in 500-mg vials to be constituted to 5 mL with sterile water for injection before use. The dose of the drug for children is 5 mg/kg of body weight. How many milliliters of the injection should be administered to a child weighing 25 lb?

12. An intravenous infusion for a child weighing 60 lb is to contain 20 mg of vancomycin hydrochloride per kilogram of body weight in 200 mL of sodium chloride injection. Using a 10-mL vial containing 500 mg of vancomycin hydrochloride (dry powder), explain how you would obtain the amount needed in preparing the infusion.

13. An intravenous infusion for a patient weighing 132 lb calls for 7.5 mg of kanamycin sulfate per kilogram of body weight to be added to 250 mL of 5% dextrose injection. How many milliliters of a kanamycin sulfate injection containing 500 mg per 2 mL should be used in preparing the infusion?

14. A medication order calls for a liter of hyperalimentation solution to contain 2.125% of amino acids and 20% of dextrose. How many milliliters each of 8.5% amino acids injection, 50% dextrose injection, and sterile water for injection should be used to prepare the solution?

15. If a 50% dextrose injection provides 170 kcal in each 100 mL, how many milliliters of a 70% dextrose injection would provide the same caloric value?

16. If a 5% dextrose injection provides 17 kcal in each deciliter, how many kilocalories per 100 mL would be provided by a 70% dextrose injection?

17. Using the Harris-Benedict equation, calculate the TPN caloric requirement for a severely stressed (use average factor) 160-lb, 60-year-old male patient measuring 5 ft, 8 in. in height.

18. If amino acids have a caloric value of 4 kcal/g and the daily patient requirement is 0.75 g/kg, calculate the kilocalories administered to a patient weighing 180 lb.

19. In preparing an intravenous solution of lidocaine in D5W, a pharmacist added a concentrated solution of lidocaine (1 g per 5 mL) to 250 mL of D5W. What was the final concentration of lidocaine on a milligrams per milliliter basis?

20. An initial heparin dose of not less than 150 units/kg of body weight has been recommended for open heart surgery. How many milliliters of an injection containing 5000 heparin units/mL should be administered to a 280-lb patient?

21. A medication order for a TPN solution calls for additives as indicated in the following formula. Using the sources designated below, calculate the amount of each component required in filling the medication order.

TPN Solution Formula	Component Source
Sodium Chloride 40 mEq	10-mL vial of 30% solution
Potassium Acetate 15 mEq	20-mL vial containing 40 mEq
Vitamin B_{12} 10 μg	vial containing 1 mg in 10 mL
Insulin 8 units	vial of Insulin U-100

To be added to:
500 mL of 50% dextrose injection
500 mL of 7% protein hydrolysate injection

22. In preparing an intravenous infusion containing sodium bicarbonate, 50 mL of a 7.5% sodium bicarbonate injection were added to 500 mL of 5% dextrose injection. How many milliequivalents of sodium were represented in the total volume of the infusion?

23. A potassium phosphate solution contains 0.9 g of potassium dihydrogen phosphate and 4.7 g of potassium monohydrogen phosphate in 30 mL. If 15 mL of this solution are added to a liter of D5W, how many milliequivalents of potassium phosphate will be represented in the infusion?

24. A physician orders 20 mg of ampicillin per kilogram of body weight to be administered intravenously in 500 mL of sodium chloride injection. How many milliliters of a constituted solution containing the equivalent of 250 mg of ampicillin per milliliter should be used in filling the medication order for a 110-lb patient?

25. A solution of potassium phosphate contains a mixture of 164 mg of monobasic potassium phosphate and 158 mg of dibasic potassium phosphate per milliliter.
    (a) If a hyperalimentation fluid calls for the addition of 45 mEq of K^+, how many milliliters of the solution should be used to provide this level of potassium?
    (b) How many millimoles of total phosphate will be represented in the calculated volume of potassium phosphate solution?

26. Using the component sources as indicated, calculate the amount of each component required in preparing 1000 mL of the following parenteral nutrition solution:

Parenteral Nutrition Solution Formula	Component Source
(a) Amino Acids 2.125%	500 mL of 8.5% amino acids injection
(b) Dextrose 20%	500 mL of 50% dextrose injection
(c) Sodium Chloride 30 mEq	20-mL vial of 15% solution
(d) Calcium Gluconate 2.5 mEq	10-mL vial containing 4.6 mEq
(e) Insulin 15 units	vial of U-100 insulin
(f) Heparin 2500 units	5-mL vial containing 1000 units/mL
(g) Sterile Water for Injection to make 1000 mL	500 mL of sterile water for injection

27. How many milliliters of a constituted injection containing 1 g of drug in 4 mL should be used in filling a medication order requiring 275 mg of the drug to be added to 500 mL of D5W solution? If the solution is administered at the rate of 1.6 mL per minute, how many milligrams of the drug will the patient receive in 1 hour?

28. A physician orders a 2-g vial of cephalothin sodium to be added to 500 mL of D5W (5% dextrose in water for injection). If the administration rate is 125 mL per hour, how many milligrams of cephalothin sodium will a patient receive per minute?

29. A certain hyperalimentation fluid measures 1 liter. If the solution is to be administered over a period of 6 hours and if the administration set is calibrated at 25 drops/mL, at what rate should the set be adjusted to administer the solution during the designated time interval?

30. A physician orders 35 mg of amphotericin B and 25 units of heparin to be administered intravenously in 1000 mL of D5W over an 8-hour period to a hospitalized
patient. In filling the medication order, the available sources of the additives are a
vial containing 50 mg of amphotericin B in 10 mL and a syringe containing 10
units of heparin per milliliter.
    (a) How many milliliters of each additive should be used in filling the medication
order?
    (b) How many milliliters of the intravenous fluid per minute should the patient
receive in order to administer the fluid over the designated time interval?

31. A constituted solution containing 500,000 units of polymyxin B sulfate in 10 mL
of sterile water for injection is added to 250 mL of 5% dextrose injection. The
infusion is to be administered over 2 hours. If the dropper in the venoclysis set
calibrates 15 drops/mL, at what rate, in drops per minute, should the flow be
adjusted to administer the infusion over the designated time interval?

32. Five hundred (500) milliliters of a 2% sterile solution of ammonium chloride are
to be administered by intravenous infusion over a period of 4 hours. If the dropper
in the venoclysis set calibrates 20 drops/mL, at what rate, in drops per minute,
should the flow be adjusted to administer the infusion over the desired time interval?
Solve the problem by calculation *and* by using the nomogram in this chapter.

33. A liter of a 0.3% intravenous infusion of potassium chloride is to be administered
over 4 hours.
    (a) How many milliequivalents of potassium are represented in the infusion?
    (b) If the dropper in the venoclysis set calibrates 20 drops/mL, calculate the rate
of flow, in drops per minute, needed to administer the infusion over the desired
time interval.

34. Five hundred (500) milliliters of an intravenous solution contain 0.2% of succinylcholine chloride in sodium chloride injection. At what flow rate should the infusion
be administered to provide 2.5 mg of succinylcholine chloride per minute?

35. A physician orders 750 mg of chloramphenicol to be added to 100 mL of sodium
chloride injection and infused into a patient over 6 hours. Using a constituted
injection that contains the equivalent of 1 g of chloramphenicol per 10 mL, how
many milliliters should be added to the sterile sodium chloride solution?

36. An intravenous fluid of 1000 mL of Lactated Ringer's Injection was started in a
patient at 8 a.m. and was scheduled to run for 12 hours. At 3 p.m., 800 mL of the
fluid remained in the bottle. At what rate of flow should the remaining fluid be
regulated using an IV set that delivers 15 drops/mL to complete the administration
of the fluid in the scheduled time?

37. If a physician orders 5 units of insulin to be added to a 1-liter intravenous solution
of D5W to be administered over 8 hours, (a) how many drops per minute should
be administered using an IV set that delivers 15 drops/mL, and (b) how many units
of insulin would be administered in each 30-minute period?

38. A patient is to receive 3 μg/kg/min of nitroglycerin from a solution containing 100
mg of the drug in 500 mL of D5W. If the patient weighs 176 lb and the infusion
set delivers 60 drops/mL, (a) how many milligrams of nitroglycerin would be delivered per hour, and (b) how many drops per minute would be delivered?

39. Using the nomogram in this chapter, determine the approximate rate of infusion delivery, in drops per minute, based on 1.5 liters of fluid to be used over a period of 8 hours with an infusion set calibrated to deliver 16 drops/mL.

40. The drug alfentanil hydrochloride is administered by infusion at the rate of 2 μg/kg/min for anesthesia induction. If a total of 0.35 mg of the drug is to be administered to a 110-lb patient, how long should be the duration of the infusion?

41. The recommended maintenance dose of aminophylline for children is 1.0 mg/kg/hr by injection. If 10 mL of a 25 mg/mL solution of aminophylline is added to a 100-mL bottle of dextrose injection, what should be the rate of delivery, in milliliters per hour, for a 40-lb child?

42. A patient is to receive an infusion of a drug at the rate of 5 mg/hr for 8 hours. The drug is available in 10-mL vials containing 8 mg of drug per milliliter. If a 250-mL bottle of D5W is used as the vehicle, (a) how many milliliters of the drug solution should be added, and (b) what should be the flow rate in milliliters per minute?

43. A patient is receiving an IV drip of the following:
    Sodium Heparin 25,000 units
    Sodium Chloride Injection (0.45%) 500 mL
    (a) How many milliliter per hour must be administered to achieve a rate of 1200 units of sodium heparin per hour?
    (b) If the IV set delivers 15 drops/mL, how many drops per minute should be administered?

44. A 50-mL vial containing 1 mg/mL of the drug alteplase is added to 100 mL of D5W and administered intravenously with an infusion set that delivers 15 drop/mL. How many drops per minute should be given to administer 25 mg of the drug per hour?

45. If the loading dose of phenytoin in children is 20 mg/kg of body weight to be infused at a rate of 0.5 mg/kg/min, over how many minutes should the dose be administered to a 32-lb child?

46. If 500 mL of an intravenous solution contains 0.1 g of a drug, at what flow rate, in milliliters per minute, should the solution be administered to provide 1 mg/min of the drug?

47. If a medication order calls for a dobutamide drip, 5 μg/kg/min for a patient weighing 232 lb, what should be the drip rate, in drops per minute, if the 125 mL-infusion bag contains 250 mg of dobutamide and a microdrip chamber is used that delivers 60 drops/mL?

48. At what rate, in drops per minute, should a dose of 20 μg/kg/min of dopamine be administered to a 65-kg patient using a solution containing dopamine, 1200 μg/mL, and a drip set that delivers 60 drops/mL?

49. A pharmacist places 5 mg/mL of acyclovir sodium in 250 mL of D5W for parenteral infusion into a pediatric patient. If the infusion is to run for 1 hour and the patient is to receive 500 mg/m^2 BSA, what would be the rate of flow in milliliters per minute for a patient measuring 55 cm in height and weighing 10 kg?

50. Aminophylline is not to be administered in pediatric patients at a rate greater than 25 mg per minute to avoid excessive peak serum concentrations and possible circulatory failure. What should be the maximum infusion rate, in milliliters per minute, for a solution containing 10 mg of aminophylline in 100 mL of D5W?

12

Some Calculations Involving "Units," "μg/mg," and Other Measures of Potency

The potency of some antibiotics, endocrine products, vitamins, and biologics (e.g., vaccines) is based on their *activity*, and is expressed in terms of *units* (of activity), in *micrograms per milligram (μg/mg),* or in other standardized terms of measurement. These measures of potency meet standards approved by the Food and Drug Administration and are set forth in the *United States Pharmacopeia*. In general, they conform also to international standards (e.g., *International Unit* or *I.U.*).

Measures of degrees of activity, as units of activity, are determined by comparison against a suitable working standard, generally a USP Reference Standard. Reference standards are authentic specimens used as comparison standards in compendial tests and assays. The number of USP Units of an antibiotic, for example, is based on a comparison of activity of a sample of that antibiotic on a milligram basis to the corresponding USP Reference Standard. For instance, there are 1590 USP Units of penicillin G sodium per milligram of the USP Reference Standard of the antibiotic. Pharmaceutical products and preparations are allowed specific variances in potency; for example, the USP monograph for Sterile Penicillin G Sodium specifies a potency of not less than 1500 Penicillin G Units and not more than 1750 Penicillin G Units per milligram. The activity or potency of antibiotics is determined by their inhibitory effect on microorganisms. No relationship exists between the unit of potency of one drug and the unit of potency of another drug.

The potency of antibiotics may also be designated in terms of "μg" (micrograms) of activity. This concept originated at a time when reference standards for antibiotics were thought to consist entirely of single chemical entities and were therefore assigned potencies of "1000 μg/mg." As newer methods of antibiotic manufacture and purification were developed, however, it was determined that some highly purified antibiotics had greater than 1000 μg of activity per milligram compared to the original reference standard. Differences in potency were also found when comparing the chemical base versus the salt form. For example, ampicillin sodium has a potency equivalent to between 845 and 988 μg/mg of its parent compound ampicillin.

A comparison of units and micrograms of potency of some official drugs and their respective weight equivalents is given in Table 12.1.

Just as potencies of certain drugs are designated in units, so too, the doses of these drugs and of their preparations are measured in units. Of the drugs for which potency is expressed in units, insulin and the penicillin antibiotics are perhaps the most commonly used. In the case of insulin, several types that may vary according to the time of onset of action and the duration of action are commercially available in different strengths. These strengths are designated as U-40, U-100, and U-500, and their potencies refer to 40, 100, and 500 USP Insulin Units per milliliter of solution or suspension. Special syringes are available for measuring units of insulin, and the required dosage is then measured in milliliters, or directly in units, depending on the calibration of the syringe. Figure 12.1 shows examples of insulin syringes calibrated in Units.

Biologics are preparations produced from a living source. They include vaccines, toxoids,

Table 12.1. Drug Unitage Equivalents

Drug	Units or μg of Potency per Weight Equivalent*
Ampicillin Sodium	NLT (not less than) 845 μg and NMT (not more than) 988 μg of ampicillin per mg
Antihemophilic Factor	NLT 100 Antihemophilic Factor Units per g
Bacitracin	NLT 40 Bacitracin Units per mg
Bacitracin Zinc	NLT 40 Bacitracin Units per mg
Cephalothin Sodium	NLT 850 μg of cephalothin per mg
Chloramphenicol Palmitate	NLT 555 μg and NMT 595 μg of chloramphenicol per mg
Chymotrypsin	NLT 1000 USP Chymotrypsin Units per mg
Clindamycin Hydrochloride	NLT 800 μg of clindamycin per mg
Cod Liver Oil	NLT 255 μg (850 USP Units) of Vitamin A and NLT 2.125 μg (85 USP Units) of Vitamin D per g
Digitalis	1 USP Digitalis Unit per 100 mg
Ergocalciferol	40 USP Vitamin D Units per μg
Erythromycin	NLT 850 μg of erythromycin per mg
Erythromycin Stearate	NLT 550 μg of erythromycin per mg
Gentamycin Sulfate	NLT 590 μg of gentamycin per mg
Heparin Calcium	NLT 140 USP Heparin Units per mg
Heparin Sodium	NLT 140 USP Heparin Units per mg
Hyaluronidase	1 USP Hyaluronidase Unit per 0.25 μg of tyrosine
Insulin	NLT 26 USP Insulin Units per mg
Insulin Human	NLT 27.5 USP Insulin Human Units per mg
Kanamycin Sulfate	NLT 750 μg of kanamycin per mg
Menotropins	NLT 40 USP Follicle-stimulating Hormone Units and NLT 40 USP Luteinizing Hormone Units per mg
Neomycin Sulfate	NLT 600 μg of neomycin per mg
Nystatin	NLT 4400 USP Nystatin Units per mg
Penicillin G Benzathine	NLT 1090 and NMT 1272 Penicillin G Units per mg
Penicillin G Potassium	NLT 1440 and NMT 1680 Penicillin G Units per mg
Penicillin G Sodium	NLT 1500 and NMT 1750 Penicillin G Units per mg
Penicillin V	NLT 1525 and NMT 1780 Penicillin V Units per mg
Penicillin V Potassium	NLT 1380 and NMT 1610 Penicillin V Units per mg
Polymyxin B Sulfate	NLT 6000 Polymyxin B Units per mg
Streptomycin Sulfate	NLT 650 μg and NMT 850 μg of streptomycin per mg
Sutilains	NLT 2,500,000 USP Casein Units of proteolytic activity per g
Tobramycin	NLT 900 μg of tobramycin per mg
Trypsin	NLT 2500 USP Trypsin Units per mg
Vitamin A	1 USP Vitamin A Unit equals the biologic activity of 0.3 μg of the all-*trans* isomer of retinol

* Examples taken from the USP 23, 1995.

and immune sera, used for the development of *immunity* or resistance to disease; certain antitoxins and antivenins, used as treatment against specific antigens; and, toxins and skin antigens, used as diagnostic aids. Biologics are prepared from human serum (e.g., immune globulin), horse serum (e.g., tetanus antitoxin), chick cell culture (e.g., measles virus vaccine), and other such animate media.

The strengths of the various biologic products are expressed in a number of ways. The strength of a bacterial vaccine commonly is expressed in terms of micrograms (μg) or units of antigen per milliliter. The strength of a viral vaccine is expressed most commonly in terms of the *tissue culture infectious dose* ($TCID_{50}$), which is the quantity of virus estimated to infect 50% of inoculated cultures. Viral vaccines may also be described in terms of units, micrograms of antigen, or number or organisms per milliliter. The strength of a toxoid is generally expressed in terms of *flocculating units (Lf)*, 1 (one) Lf having the

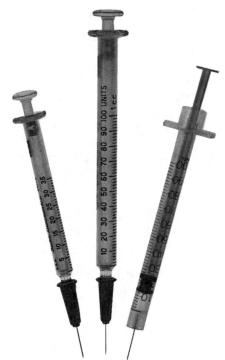

Fig. 12.1. Examples of insulin syringes calibrated in Units. (Courtesy of Becton, Dickinson and Company.)

capacity to flocculate or precipitate one unit of standard antitoxin. Units of activity are generally used to characterize the strengths of many immune sera and diagnostic antigens.

The example problems and the practice problems that follow may be solved by simple proportion or by dimensional analysis.

Amount of Drug Equivalent to Dose in Units. Calculating the amount of a drug or preparation equivalent to a dose expressed in units involves the following.

Examples:

How many milliliters of U-100 insulin should be used to obtain 40 units of insulin?

U-100 insulin contains 100 units/mL

$$\frac{100 \ (\text{units})}{40 \ (\text{units})} = \frac{1 \ (\text{mL})}{\text{x} \ (\text{mL})}$$

$$\text{x} = 0.4 \text{ mL, } answer$$

Or, solving by dimensional analysis:

$$40 \text{ units} \times \frac{1 \text{ mL}}{100 \text{ units}} = 0.4 \text{ mL, } answer.$$

A physician prescribed 100 units of insulin to be added to 500 mL of D5W in treating a patient with severe diabetic acidosis. How many milliliters of insulin injection concentrate, U-500, should be used?

U-500 insulin contains 500 units/mL

$$\frac{500 \text{ (units)}}{100 \text{ (units)}} = \frac{1 \text{ (mL)}}{x \text{ (mL)}}$$

$$x = 0.2 \text{ mL, } answer.$$

Or, solving by dimensional analysis:

$$100 \text{ units} \times \frac{1 \text{ mL}}{500 \text{ units}} = 0.2 \text{ mL, } answer.$$

How many milliliters of a heparin sodium injection containing 200,000 units in 10 mL should be used to obtain 5,000 heparin sodium units that are to be added to an intravenous dextrose solution?

$$\frac{200,000 \text{ (units)}}{5,000 \text{ (units)}} = \frac{10 \text{ (mL)}}{x \text{ (mL)}}$$

$$x = 0.25 \text{ mL, } answer.$$

Equivalency Based on "μg" Activity per Milligram. Calculating the equivalency of an antibiotic based on "μg" activity per milligram involves the following.

Example:

If neomycin sulfate has a potency of 600 μg of neomycin per milligram, how many milligrams of neomycin sulfate would be equivalent in potency to 1 mg of neomycin?

$$\frac{600 \text{ (μg of neomycin)}}{1000 \text{ (μg of neomycin)}} = \frac{1 \text{ (mg of neomycin sulfate)}}{x \text{ (mg of neomycin sulfate)}}$$

$$x = 1.67 \text{ mg, } answer.$$

Dose or Antigen Content of a Biologic Based on Potency. Calculating the dose or antigen content of a biologic based on potency involves the following.

Examples:

A biologic contains 50 Lf Units of diphtheria toxoid in each 2.5 mL of product. If a pediatric patient is to receive 10 Lf Units, how many milliliters of product should be administered?

$$\frac{50 \text{ (Lf Units)}}{10 \text{ (Lf Units)}} = \frac{2.5 \text{ (mL)}}{x \text{ (mL)}}$$

$$x = 0.5 \text{ mL, } answer.$$

Measles Virus Vaccine Live is prepared to contain 1000 $TCID_{50}$ per 0.5-mL dose. What is the $TCID_{50}$ content of a 50-mL multiple dose vial of the vaccine?

$$\frac{1000 \text{ ($TCID_{50}$)}}{x \text{ ($TCID_{50}$)}} = \frac{0.5 \text{ (mL)}}{50 \text{ (mL)}}$$

$$x = 100,000 \text{ } TCID_{50}, \text{ } answer.$$

Practice Problems

1. How many milliliters of U-40 insulin zinc suspension should be used to obtain 18 units of insulin?

2.   A patient is required to take 9 units of U-40 isophane insulin suspension and 16 units of U-100 protamine zinc insulin. What volume, in milliliters, of each type will provide the desired dosage?

3.   How many milliliters of U-100 insulin injection should be used to obtain 60 units?

4.   How many milliliters of U-40 isophane insulin suspension should be used to provide 28 units of insulin?

5.   A physician prescribes 60 mL of phenoxymethyl penicillin for oral suspension containing 4,800,000 units. How many penicillin units will be represented in each teaspoonful dose of the prepared suspension?

6.   The contents of a vial of penicillin G potassium weigh 600 mg and represent 1 million units. How many milligrams are needed to prepare 15 g of an ointment that is to contain 15,000 units of penicillin G potassium per gram?

7.   If 10 *μg* of ergocalciferol represent 400 units of vitamin D, how many 1.25 mg ergocalciferol capsules will provide a dose of 200,000 units of vitamin D?

8.   A physician prescribes 2.5 million units of penicillin G potassium daily for 1 week. If 1 unit of penicillin G potassium equals 0.6 *μg*, how many tablets, each containing 250 mg, will provide the prescribed dosage regimen?

9.   ℞   Penicillin G Potassium   5,000 units per mL
     Isotonic Sodium Chloride Solution   ad   15 mL
     Sig. Nose drops.

     Using soluble penicillin tablets, each containing 200,000 units of crystalline penicillin G potassium, explain how you would obtain the penicillin G potassium needed in compounding the prescription.

10. If 1 mg of penicillin V represents 1520 penicillin V units, how many micrograms represent 1 unit?

11. Corticotropin injection is available in a concentration of 40 units/mL. How many milliliters of the injection should be administered to provide 0.4 unit/kg for a child weighing 66 lb?

12. If 1 mg of heparin sodium is equivalent to 140 USP Heparin Units, how many micrograms of heparin sodium represent 1 unit?

13. A physician's hospital medication order calls for a patient to receive 1 unit of insulin injection subcutaneously for every 10 mg/dL of blood sugar over 175 mg/dL, with blood sugar levels and injections performed twice daily in the morning and evening. The patient's blood sugar was 200 mg/dL in the morning and 320 mg/dL in the evening. How many total units of insulin injection were administered?

14. A physician's hospital medication order calls for isophane insulin suspension to be administered to a 136-lb patient on the basis of 1 unit/kg per 24 hours. How many units of isophane insulin suspension should be administered daily?

15. A physician's hospital medication order calls for 0.5 mL of U-500 insulin injection to be placed in a 500-mL bottle of 5% dextrose injection for infusion into a patient. If the rate of infusion was set to run for 8 hours, how many units of insulin did the patient receive in the first 90 minutes of infusion?

16. Penicillin G Sodium contains 2.0 mEq of sodium per million units of penicillin. How many milligrams of sodium are contained in an I.V. drip of 20 million units per day?

17. For children, heparin sodium is administered by intermittent intravenous infusion in a range of 50 to 100 units/kg body weight every 4 hours. For a 50-lb child, calculate the range, in milliliters, of a heparin sodium injection containing 5000 units/mL to be administered daily.

18. The maintenance dose of heparin sodium in children has been recommended as 20,000 units/m^2/24 hr. Using the nomogram in Chapter 4 and a sodium heparin injection containing 1000 units/mL, calculate the daily volume to be administered to a child measuring 22 in. in height and weighing 25 lb.

19. Penicillin G potassium is available as a dry powder in a vial containing 1 million units, which when constituted with 9.6 mL of solvent, results in a 10-mL solution for injection. At a potency of 1560 units/mg, calculate the amount, in milligrams, of penicillin G potassium in each milliliter of injection.

20. Cod liver oil is available in capsules containing 0.6 mL per capsule. Using Table 12.1, calculate the amounts, in units, each of vitamins A and D in each capsule. The specific gravity of cod liver oil is 0.92.

21. Using Table 12.1, calculate the clindamycin potency equivalence, in milligrams per milliliter, of a solution containing 1 g of clindamycin hydrochloride in 10 mL of solution.

22. If a 5-mL vial of Humatrope®, a biosynthetic somatotropin of rDNA origin, contains 5 mg of somatotropin equivalent to 13 international units (IU), how many milligrams of somatotropin and how many international units would be administered in a 0.6-mL dose?

23. If a tablet contains 250 mg of erythromycin stearate, calculate the content of erythromycin, in milligrams, based on the information in Table 12.1.

24. If a suspension of chloromycetin palmitate contains the equivalent of 150 mg of chloramphenicol in each 5 mL, how many milligrams of chloramphenicol palmitate were used to prepare each 100 mL of the suspension? Use the average equivalency value from Table 12.1.

25. Pertussis vaccine contains 4 protective units per 0.5 mL. How many protective units would be contained in a 7.5-mL multiple dose vial?

26. The prophylactic dose of tetanus antitoxin is 1500 units for persons weighing less than 65 lb and 3000 to 5000 units for persons weighing more than 65 lb. The antitoxin is available in dose vials of 1,500 units, 3,000 units, 5,000 units, and 20,000 units. Which vial should a pharmacist provide for administration to a patient weighing 25 kg?

27. Each 0.01 mL of a mumps vaccine contains 400 TCID$_{50}$ of the mumps virus. If the usual dose contains 20,000 TCID$_{50}$, how many milliliters of vaccine should be administered?

28. If a biologic product contains 7.5 Lf units of diphtheria toxoid per 0.5 mL, how many flocculating units would be present in a 7.5-mL multiple dose vial?

13

Some Calculations Involving the Use of Prefabricated Dosage Forms in Compounding Procedures

As noted in Chapter 2, the extemporaneous compounding of prescriptions and medication orders is an activity for which pharmacists are uniquely qualified by virtue of their education, training, and experience. Pharmacists frequently find that bulk supplies of required drug substances are not on hand for extemporaneous compounding and that proprietary prefabricated tablets, capsules, injections, and other dosage forms provide the only convenient source of medicinal agents needed.

When using commercially prepared dosage forms as the source of medicinal agent, the pharmacist selects products that are of the most simple, economic, and convenient form. For example, uncoated tablets or capsules are preferred over coated tablets or sustained-release dosage forms. For both convenience and economy, use of the fewest dosage units is preferred; e.g., five 100-mg tablets rather than one hundred 5-mg tablets. An injection often provides a convenient source of medicinal agent when the volume of injection required is small and it is compatible with the physical characteristics of the dosage form being prepared (e.g., an oral liquid rather than dry-filled capsules).

Occasionally, when of the prescribed strength, small whole tablets, or broken *scored* (grooved) tablets, may be placed within capsule shells when capsules are prescribed. In most instances, however, tablets are crushed in a mortar and reduced to a powder. When capsules are used as the drug source, the capsule shells are opened and their powdered contents are expelled. The correct quantity of powder is then used to fill the prescription or medication order.

It is important to remember that in addition to the medicinal agent, most solid dosage forms contain additional materials, such as fillers, binders, and disintegrants. These ingredients may need to be considered in the required calculations. For example, a tablet labeled to contain 10-mg of a drug may actually weigh 200 mg because of the added ingredients. Calculations involved in the use of injections generally are simplified because injections are labeled according to quantity of drug per unit volume, e.g., milligrams per milliliter (mg/mL).

In addition to the use of tablets for compounding, some tablets are used as the measured source of a drug substance in the preparation of solutions. Official monographs describe *Tablets for Solution* (e.g., Halazone Tablets for Solution), *Tablets for Oral Solution* (e.g., Penicillin G Potassium Tablets for Oral Solution), and *Tablets for Topical Solution* (e.g., Cocaine Hydrochloride Tablets for Topical Solution), which are intended to be added to a given volume of water to produce a solution of a desired concentration.

Obtaining a Specified Quantity of a Drug Substance. To obtain a desired quantity of a drug substance using prefabricated dosage forms, observe the following.

Examples:

Only capsules, each containing 25 mg of indomethacin, are available. How many capsules should be used to obtain the amount of indomethacin needed in preparing the following prescription?

> ℞   Indomethacin   2 mg/mL
>   Cherry Syrup   ad   150 mL
>   Sig. 5 mL b.i.d.

Because 2 mg/mL of indomethacin are prescribed, 300 mg are needed in preparing the prescription. Given that each capsule contains 25 mg of indomethacin, then, 300 (mg) ÷ 25 (mg) = 12 capsules are needed, *answer.*

The drug loseride is available as 50-mg tablets. Before preparing the following prescription, a pharmacist determined that each tablet weighed 120 mg. Explain how to obtain the proper quantity of loseride.

> ℞   Loseride   15 mg
>   Lactose, qs ad   300 mg
>   Prepare 24 such capsules.
>   Sig. One cap. 2× a day.

15 (mg) × 24 = 360 mg of loseride needed
Crush 8 tablets, which contain:

400 mg (8 × 50 mg) of loseride and
960 mg (8 × 120 mg) of total powder

$$\frac{400 \text{ (mg loseride)}}{360 \text{ (mg loseride)}} = \frac{960 \text{ (mg total)}}{x \text{ (mg total)}}$$

$$x = 864 \text{ mg quantity of powder to use, } answer.$$

How many milliliters of an injection containing 40 mg of triamcinolone per milliliter may be used in preparing the following prescription?

> ℞   Triamcinolone   0.05%
>   Ointment Base ad   120 g
>   Sig. Apply to affected area.

120 (g) × 0.0005 = 0.06 g = 60 mg triamcinolone needed

$$\frac{40 \text{ (mg)}}{60 \text{ (mg)}} = \frac{1 \text{ (mL)}}{x \text{ (mL)}}$$

$$x = 1.5 \text{ mL, } answer.$$

The only source of sodium chloride is in the form of tablets, each containing 1 g. Explain how you would obtain the amount of sodium chloride needed for the following prescription.

> ℞   Ephedrine Sulfate   0.5
>   Isotonic Sodium Chloride Solution (0.9%)   50.0
>   Sig. For the nose.

50 (g) × 0.009 = 0.450 g of sodium chloride needed

Because one tablet contains 1 g of sodium chloride or $^{20}/_9$ *times* the amount desired, $^9/_{20}$ of the tablet will contain the required quantity, or 0.450 g. The required amount of sodium chloride may be obtained as follows:

Step 1.   Dissolve *one* tablet in enough purified water to make 20 mL of dilution.

Step 2.   Take 9 mL of the dilution, *answer.*

The only source of potassium permanganate is in the form of tablets for topical solution, each containing 0.3 g. Explain how you would obtain the amount of potassium permanganate needed for the following prescription.

> ℞   Potassium Permanganate Solution   250 mL
>   1 : 5000
>   Sig. Use as directed.

$$1 : 5000 = 0.02\%$$

250 (g) × 0.0002 = 0.050 g or 50 mg of potassium permanganate needed

Because one tablet for topical solution contains 300 mg of potassium permanganate or 6 *times* the amount needed, ⅙ of the tablet will contain the required amount or 50 mg. The required quantity of potassium permanganate may be obtained as follows:

Step 1.   Dissolve *one* tablet for topical solution in enough purified water to make 60 mL of dilution.

Step 2.   Take 10 mL of the dilution, *answer.*

Practice Problems

1. ℞   Potassium Permanganate Solution   500 mL
            1 : 10,000
         Sig. Use as directed.

    Using tablets, each containing 0.3 g of potassium permanganate, explain how you would obtain the amount of potassium permanganate needed for the prescription.

2. ℞   Triamcinolone   0.05%
         Ointment Base   ad   120 g
         Sig. Apply.

    A pharmacist has no triamcinolone powder but does have (a) triamcinolone cream 0.5% and (b) triamcinolone tablets, 4 mg. What quantity of each could be used in preparing the prescription?

3. How many milliliters of a 0.9% solution of sodium chloride can be made from 10 tablets for solution each containing 2.25 g of sodium chloride?

4. ℞   Phenacaine Hydrochloride Solution 1%   7.5 mL
         Scopolamine Hydrobromide Solution 0.2%   7.5 mL
         Sig. For the eye.

    How many tablets, each containing 600 μg of scopolamine hydrobromide, should be used in preparing the prescription?

5. ℞   Hexachlorophene
         Hydrocortisone   aa   0.25%
         Coal Tar Solution   30.0 mL
         Hydrophilic Ointment   ad   120.0 g
         Sig. Apply.

    How many tablets, each containing 20 mg of hydrocortisone, should be used in preparing the prescription?

6. How many milliliters of an injection containing 40 mg of a drug per milliliter would provide the amount of the drug needed to prepare 120 mL of a 0.2% suspension?

7. ℞   Allopurinol   65 mg/5 mL
        Cologel   40 mL
        Syrup   ad   150 mL
        M. ft. susp.
        Sig. As directed.

    How many scored 100-mg allopurinol tablets may be used in preparing the prescription?

8. How many tablets for solution, each containing 4 mg of halazone, should be added to 1 gallon of purified water to provide a concentration of 1:250,000 (w/v)?

9. How many tablets for topical solution, each containing 300 mg of potassium permanganate, should be added to 1 gallon of purified water to provide a concentration of 0.012% (w/v)?

10. A prescription for 240 mL of a cough mixture calls for 2 mg of hydrocodone bitartrate per teaspoonful. How many tablets, each containing 5 mg of hydrocodone bitartrate, should be used in preparing the cough mixture?

11. ℞   Dantrolene   5 mg/mL
        Citric Acid   150 mg
        Purified Water   10 mL
        Syrup   ad   125 mL
        M. ft. susp.
        Sig. As directed.

    If the only source of dantrolene is 100-mg capsules, each containing 200 mg of drug-diluent powder mix, (a) how many capsules must be opened, and (b) how many milligrams of the powder mix should be used in preparing the prescription?

12. ℞   Cocaine Hydrochloride   1 g
        Isotonic Sodium Chloride Solution   100 mL
        Sig. For the nose.

    The only source of sodium chloride is in the form of 2.25-g tablets. Explain how you would obtain the amount of sodium chloride needed for the prescription. Isotonic sodium chloride solution contains 0.9% of sodium chloride.

13. How many Dantrium® Capsules, each containing 25 mg of dantrolene, are needed to prepare 100 mL of a pediatric suspension containing 5 mg of dantrolene per milliliter?

14. The only source of sodium chloride is in the form of tablets, each containing 2.25 g. How many tablets should be used in preparing 1 liter of a stock solution of such strength that 20 mL diluted 100 mL with purified water will yield a 0.9% (w/v) solution?

15. How many tablets, each containing 25 mg of spironolactone, are needed to prepare 200 mL of a pediatric suspension to contain 5 mg of spironolactone per milliliter?

16. A physician prescribes 30 capsules, each containing 300 mg of ibuprofen, for a patient. The pharmacist has on hand 400-mg and 600-mg ibuprofen tablets. How

many each of these tablets could be used to obtain the amount of ibuprofen needed in preparing the prescription?

17. ℞   Indomethacin Powder   1%
           Carbopol 941 Powder   2%
           Purified Water   10%
           Alcohol   ad   90 mL
           Sig. Use as directed.

How many 75-mg capsules of indomethacin should be used in preparing the prescription?

18. ℞   Minoxidil   0.3%
           Vehicle/N   ad   50   mL
           Sig. Apply to affected areas of the scalp b.i.d.

Tablets, containing 2.5 mg and 10 mg of minoxidil, are available. Explain how you would obtain the amount of minoxidil needed in preparing the prescription, using the available sources of the drug.

19. ℞   Nystatin   100,000 units/g
           Chloramphenicol   250 mg
           Unibase
           Petrolatum   aa   ad   30 g
           Sig. Apply to hands twice daily.

How many tablets, each containing 500,000 units of nystatin, could be used to obtain the nystatin needed in compounding the prescription?

20. ℞   Aminophylline   500 mg
           Sodium Pentobarbital   75 mg
           Carbowax Base   ad   2 g
           Ft. suppos. no. 12
           Sig. Insert one at night.

How many capsules, each containing 100 mg of sodium pentobarbital, should be used to provide the sodium pentobarbital needed in preparing the prescription?

21. ℞   Codeine Sulfate   0.06 g/f℥
           Benylin Expectorant   ad   120   mL
           Sig. Teaspoonful q.i.d.

Tablets, each containing 15 mg of codeine sulfate, are available. How many tablets should be used to provide the codeine sulfate needed in preparing the prescription?

22. ℞   Carafate®   400 mg/5 mL
           Cherry Syrup   40 mL
           Sorbitol Solution   40 mL
           Flavor   q.s.
           Purified Water   ad   125 mL
           Sig. 5 mL t.i.d.

How many 1-g Carafate® tablets should be used in preparing the prescription?

14

Some Calculations Associated with Drug Availability and Pharmacokinetics

The availability to the biologic system of a drug substance formulated into a pharmaceutical product is integral to the goals of dosage form design and paramount to the effectiveness of the medication.

Before a drug substance can be absorbed by the biologic system, it must be released from its dosage form (e.g., tablet) or drug delivery system (e.g., transdermal patch) and dissolved in the physiologic fluids. Several factors play a role in a drug's biologic availability, including the physical and chemical characteristics of the drug itself, such as its particle size and solubility, and the features of the dosage form or delivery system, such as the nature of the formulative ingredients and the method of manufacture. The area of study that deals with the properties of drug substances and dosage forms that influence the release of the drug for biologic activity is termed *biopharmaceutics*. The term *bioavailability* refers to the *relative amount* of drug from an administered dosage form that enters the systemic circulation.

Pharmacokinetics is the study and characterization of the time course of the absorption, distribution, metabolism, and excretion (ADME) of drugs. *Drug absorption* is the process of uptake of the compound from the site of administration into the systemic circulation. *Drug distribution* refers to the transfer of the drug from the blood to extravascular fluids and tissues. *Drug metabolism* is the enzymatic or biochemical transformation of the drug substance to (usually less toxic) metabolic products, which may be eliminated more readily from the body. *Drug excretion* is the final elimination of the drug substance or its metabolites from the body such as through the kidney (urine), intestines (feces), skin (sweat), saliva, and/or milk.

The relationship between the processes of absorption, distribution, metabolism, and excretion influences the therapeutic and toxicologic effects of drugs. The application of pharmacokinetic principles in the treatment of individual patients in optimizing drug therapy is referred to as *clinical pharmacokinetics*.

DRUG AVAILABILITY FROM DOSAGE FORMS AND DELIVERY SYSTEMS

The availability of a drug from a dosage form or delivery system is determined by measuring its dissolution characteristics *in vitro* (outside the biologic system) and/or its absorption patterns *in vivo* (within the biologic system). Generally, data are collected that provide information on both *rate* and *extent* of drug dissolution and/or absorption. The data collected may be plotted on graph paper to depict concentration versus time curves for the drug's dissolution and/or absorption.

Plotting and Interpreting Drug Dissolution Data. Drug dissolution data are obtained in vitro for tablets or capsules using the USP Dissolution Test, which defines the apparatus and methods to be used.[1] The data obtained may be presented in tabular form and depicted graphically, as in the following example.

Example:

The following dissolution data were obtained from a 250-mg capsule of ampicillin. Plot the data on graph paper and determine the approximate percentage of ampicillin dissolved following 15, 30, and 45 minutes of the study.

Time Period (minutes)	Ampicillin Dissolved (mg)
5	12
10	30
20	75
40	120
60	150

Plotting the data:

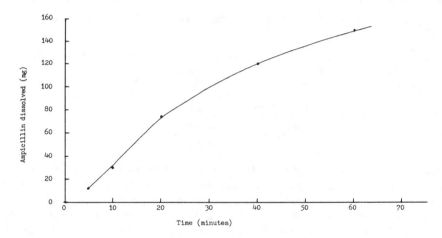

Determining the intercepts at 15, 30, and 45 minutes:

At 15 minutes, approximately 50 mg or 20% of the ampicillin,
At 30 minutes, approximately 100 mg or 40% of the ampicillin,
At 45 minutes, approximately 125 mg or 50% of the ampicillin, *answers.*

Amount of Drug Bioavailable from a Dosage Form. If drug dissolution or drug absorption studies demonstrate consistently that only a portion of a drug substance in a dosage form is "available" for biologic absorption, the drug's bioavailability factor (F), which represents the decimal percent of a drug substance available, may be used to calculate bioavailability.

Example:

If the bioavailability factor (F) for a drug substance in a dosage form is 0.60, how many milligrams of drug would be available for absorption from a 100-mg tablet of the drug?

---

[1] *United States Pharmacopeia XXII,*, United States Pharmacopeial Convention, Inc., Washington, D.C., 1990, pp. 1578-1579.

The bioavailability factor (F) indicates that only 60% of the drug present in the dosage form is available for absorption. Thus:

100 mg $\times$ 0.60 = 60 mg, *answer.*

"Bioequivalent" Amounts of "Bioinequivalent" Dosage Forms. The bioavailability of a given drug substance may vary when in different dosage forms or in the same dosage form but from a different manufacturer. Thus, it may be desired to calculate the equivalent doses for two *bioinequivalent* products.

Example:

If the bioavailability (F) of digoxin in a 0.25-mg tablet is 0.60 compared to the bioavailability (F) of 0.75 in a digoxin elixir (0.05 mg/mL), calculate the dose of the elixir equivalent to the tablet.

First, calculate the amount of "bioavailable" digoxin in the tablet:

0.25 mg $\times$ 0.60 = 0.15 mg, bioavailable amount of digoxin in the tablet

Next, calculate the amount of "bioavailable" digoxin per milliliter of the elixir:

0.05 mg $\times$ 0.75 = 0.0375 mg, bioavailable amount of digoxin per milliliter of the elixir

Finally, determine the quantity of elixir that will provide 0.15 mg of bioavailable digoxin:

By proportion:

$$\frac{0.0375 \ (\text{mg})}{0.15 \ (\text{mg})} = \frac{1 \ (\text{mL})}{\text{x} \ (\text{mL})}$$

$$\text{x} = 4 \ \text{mL, } answer.$$

Plotting and Interpreting a Blood Drug Concentration-Time Curve. Following the administration of a medication, if blood samples are drawn from the patient at specific time intervals and analyzed for drug content, the resulting data may be plotted on ordinary graph paper to prepare a blood drug concentration-time curve. The vertical axis of this type of plot characteristically presents the concentration of drug present in the blood (or serum or plasma) and the horizontal axis presents the times the samples were obtained after administration of the drug. When the drug is first administered (time zero), the blood concentration of the drug should also be zero. As an orally administered drug passes into the stomach and/or intestine, it is released from the dosage form, fully or partially dissolves, and is absorbed. As the sampling and analysis continue, the blood samples reveal increasing concentrations of drug, until the maximum (peak) concentration (C_{max}) is reached. Then, the blood level of the drug decreases progressively and, if no additional dose is given, eventually falls back to zero.

For conventional dosage forms, such as tablets and capsules, the C_{max} will usually occur at only a single time point, referred to as T_{max}. The amount of drug is usually expressed in terms of its concentration in relation to a specific volume of blood, serum, or plasma. For example, the concentration may be expressed as g/100 mL, μg/mL, mg/dL, or mg% (mg/100 mL). The quantity of a dose administered and its bioavailability, dissolution, and absorption characteristics influence the blood level concentration for a drug substance. The rate or speed of drug absorption determines the T_{max}, the time of greatest blood drug concentration after administration, the faster the rate of absorption, the sooner the T_{max}.

In a blood drug concentration-time curve, the area-under-the-curve (AUC) is considered representative of the *total* amount of drug absorbed into systemic circulation. The area under the curve may be measured mathematically, using a technique known as the trapezoidal rule. The procedure may be found in other texts and references.[2]

Example:

From the following data, plot a serum concentration-time curve and determine (a) the peak height concentration (C_{max}) and (b) the time of the peak height concentration (T_{max}).

Time Period (hours)	Serum Drug Concentration ($\mu g/mL$)
0.5	1.0
1.0	2.0
2.0	4.0
3.0	3.8
4.0	2.9
6.0	1.9
8.0	1.0
10.0	0.3
12.0	0.2

Plotting the data and interpretation of the curve:

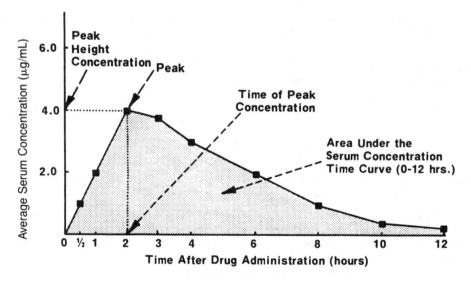

Determining the intercept for C_{max} and T_{max}:

$$C_{max} = 4.0\ \mu g/mL$$
$$T_{max} = 2\ \text{hours, } answers.$$

[2] Gibaldi, M.: *Biopharmaceutics and Clinical Pharmacokinetics*, 4th Ed. Philadelphia, Lea & Febiger, 1991, p. 377.

SOME INTRODUCTORY CONCEPTS AND CALCULATIONS INVOLVED IN PHARMACOKINETICS

As defined previously, pharmacokinetics is the study and characterization of the time course of absorption, distribution, metabolism, and excretion of drugs. Many of the calculations involved in pharmacokinetics are complex and the subject of advanced textbooks devoted to this important field. The intention in the following discussion is to define and describe some of the more introductory concepts and calculations.

Plasma Concentration of Unbound versus Bound Drugs. Once absorbed into the circulation, a portion of the total drug plasma concentration (C_T) is bound to plasma proteins (usually albumin) and a portion remains unbound or free. It is the unbound drug (C_U) that is available for further transport to its site of action in the body. The fraction of unbound drug compared to bound drug (C_B) is primarily a function of the affinity of the drug molecules for binding to the plasma proteins and the concentration of the latter (some patients may have a reduced or elevated serum albumin concentration). Some drug molecules may be over 90% bound to plasma proteins, whereas others may be bound only slightly. Any change in the degree of binding of a given drug substance can alter its distribution and elimination, and thus its clinical effects.

The fraction of unbound drug in the plasma compared to the total plasma drug concentration, bound and unbound, is termed *alpha* (or α).

Thus,

$$\alpha = \frac{C_U}{C_U + C_B} = \frac{C_U}{C_T}$$

If one knows the value of α for a drug and the total plasma concentration (C_T), the concentration of free drug in the plasma may be determined by a rearranged equation:

$$C_U = \alpha \times (C_T)$$

Example:

If the alpha (α) value for the drug digoxin is 0.70, what would be the concentration of free drug in the plasma if the total plasma concentration of the drug were determined to be 0.7 ng/mL?

$$\begin{aligned} C_U \quad &= (0.70) \times (0.7 \text{ ng/mL}) \\ &= 0.49 \text{ ng/mL, } \textit{answer.} \end{aligned}$$

Apparent Volume of Distribution of a Drug Substance. The apparent volume of distribution for a drug is not a "real" volume, but rather a hypothetic volume of body fluid that would be required to dissolve the total amount of drug at the same concentration as that found in the blood. The volume of distribution is an indicator of the extent of a drug's distribution throughout the body fluids and tissues. The information is useful in understanding how the body processes and distributes a given drug substance. After a dose of a drug is administered intravenously, a change in the concentration of the drug in the blood means a corresponding change in the drug's concentration in another body fluid or tissue. This sequence allows an understanding of the pattern of the drug's distribution.

It may be useful in understanding the concept of volume of distribution to imagine a 100-mg amount of a drug substance dissolved in an undetermined volume of water. If the analysis of a sample of the resultant solution revealed a drug concentration of 20 mg per liter, it can be seen that the total volume of water in which the drug was dissolved equaled 5 liters.

$$\frac{20 \ (mg)}{100 \ (mg)} = \frac{1 \ (liter)}{x \ (liters)}$$

$$x = 5 \ liters$$

Different drugs administered in the same amount will show different volumes of distribution because of different distribution characteristics. For example, drugs that remain in the blood after intravenous administration because of drug binding to plasma proteins or to blood cells show high blood concentrations and low volumes of distribution. Conversely, drugs that exit the circulation rapidly and diffuse into other body fluids and tissues show low blood concentrations and high volumes of distribution.

If the volume of distribution in an adult is 5 liters, the drug is considered confined to the circulatory system, as it would be immediately after a rapid intravenous injection (IV bolus). If the volume of distribution is between 10 and 20 liters, or between 15 and 27% of the body weight, it is assumed that the drug has been distributed into the extracellular fluids; if it is between 25 and 30 liters, or between 35 and 42% of body weight, it is assumed that the drug has been distributed into the intracellular fluid; if it is about 40 liters, or 60% of the body weight, the assumption is that the drug has been distributed in the whole body fluid.[3] If the apparent volume of distribution actually exceeds the body weight, it is assumed that the drug is being stored in body fat, bound to body tissues, or is distributed in peripheral compartments.

The equation for determining the volume of distribution (Vd) is:

$$Vd = \frac{D}{C_P}$$

in which D is the total amount of drug in the body, and C_p is the drug's plasma concentration. The apparent volume of distribution may be expressed as a simple volume or as a percentage of body weight.

Example:

A patient received a single intravenous dose of 300 mg of a drug substance that produced an immediate blood concentration of 8.2 μg of drug per milliliter. Calculate the apparent volume of distribution.

$$Vd = \frac{D}{C_P}$$

$$= \frac{300 \ mg}{8.2 \ \mu g/mL} = \frac{300 \ mg}{8.2 \ mg/L}$$

$$= 36.6 \ L, \ answer.$$

Total Amount of Drug Given Volume of Distribution and Plasma Concentration. Calculating the total amount of drug in a body, given the volume of distribution and the plasma drug concentration, involves the following.

Example:

Four hours following the intravenous administration of a drug, a patient weighing 70 kg was found to have a drug blood level concentration of 10 μg/mL. Assuming the apparent volume of

---

[3] Ritschel, W.A.: *Handbook of Basic Pharmacokinetics*, 2nd Ed. Hamilton, IL, Drug Intelligence Publications, Inc., 1982, p. 219.

distribution is 10% of body weight, calculate the total amount of drug present in body fluids 4 hours after the drug was administered.

$$Vd = \frac{D}{C_P} \qquad D = (Vd) \times (C_p)$$

$$Vd = 10\% \text{ of } 70 \text{ kg} = 7 \text{ kg} = 7 \text{ L}$$

$$C_P = 10 \ \mu g/mL = 10 \text{ mg/L}$$

$$7 \text{ L} = \frac{D}{10 \text{ mg/L}}$$

$$D = (7 \text{ L}) \times (10 \text{ mg/L})$$

$$= 70 \text{ mg, } \textit{answer}$$

Elimination Half-Life and Elimination Rate Constant. The elimination phase of a drug from the body is reflected by a decline in the drug's plasma concentration. The *elimination half-life* ($t^{1/2}$) is the time it takes for the plasma drug concentration (as well as the amount of drug in the body) to fall by one half. For example, if it takes 3 hours for the plasma concentration of a drug to fall from 6 to 3 mg/L, its half-life would be 3 hours. It would take the same period of time (3 hours) for the concentration to fall from 3 to 1.5 mg/L, or from 1.5 to 0.75 mg/L. Many drug substances follow first-order kinetics in their elimination from the body, meaning that the rate of drug elimination per unit of time is proportional to the amount present at that time. As demonstrated previously, the elimination half-life is independent of the amount of drug in the body, and the amount of drug eliminated is less in each succeeding half-life. After five elimination half-lives, it may be expected that virtually all of a drug (97%) originally present will have been eliminated. The student might wish to examine this point, starting with a 100-mg dose of a drug (after first half-life, 50 mg, etc.).

Blood level data from a drug may be plotted against time on regular graph paper to obtain an exponential curve, or it may be plotted on semilogarithmic graph paper to obtain a straight line. From the latter, the elimination half-life may be determined, as shown in the example that follows in this section.

The elimination rate constant (K_e) characterizes the elimination process and may simply be regarded as the *fractional rate of drug removal per unit time, expressed as a decimal fraction* (e.g., 0.01 min^{-1}, meaning 1% per minute). The elimination rate constant for a first-order process may be calculated using the equation:

$$K_e = \frac{0.693}{t_{1/2}}$$

The derivation of this equation is described for the exponential decay of radioisotopes (see Chapter 15).

Examples:

A patient received 12 mg of a drug intravenously and blood samples were drawn and analyzed at specific time intervals, resulting in the following data. Plot the data on semilogarithmic graph paper and determine the elimination half-life of the drug.

Plasma Drug Level Concentration (μg/100 mL)	Time (hours)
26.5	1
17.5	2
11.5	3
7.6	4
5.0	5
3.3	6

Plotting the data:

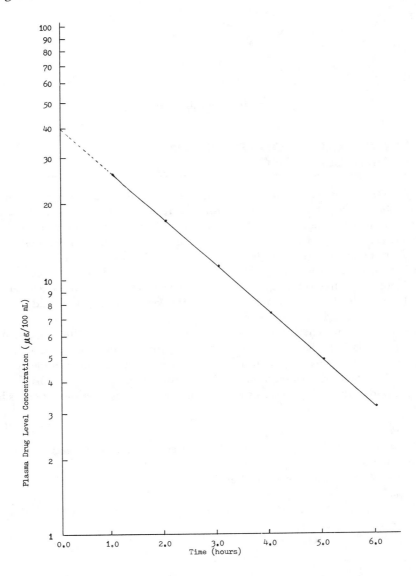

From the plotted data, the straight line may by extrapolated to time zero to determine the initial plasma drug concentration, which is found to be 40 μg/100 mL. The time it takes to reduce that level to one-half, or 20 μg/100 mL, is the elimination half-life. The 20 μg/100 mL concentration intersects the straight line at 1.7 hours.

Therefore, the elimination half-life is 1.7 hours, *answer.*

Note: The same answer may be obtained by selecting any plasma drug concentration (for example, 10 μg/100 mL), determining the time of that plasma level from the intercept, repeating the process for one-half of that drug level (5 μg/100 mL), and determining the elapsed time by subtraction to obtain the elimination half-life.

Example:

Calculate the elimination rate constant for a drug that has an elimination half-life of 50 minutes.

$$K_e = \frac{0.693}{t_{1/2}}$$

$$= \frac{0.693}{50 \text{ min}}$$

$$= 0.0139 \text{ min}^{-1}, \text{ } answer.$$

DOSAGE CALCULATIONS BASED ON CREATININE CLEARANCE

Dose of a Drug. The two major mechanisms by which drugs are eliminated from the body are through hepatic (liver) metabolism and renal (kidney) excretion. When renal excretion is the major route, a loss of kidney function will dramatically affect the rate at which the drug is cleared from the body. Polar drugs are eliminated predominantly by renal excretion and are generally affected by decreased kidney function.

With many drugs, it is important to reach and maintain a specific drug concentration in the blood to realize the proper therapeutic effect. The initial blood concentration attained from a specific dose depends, in part, on the weight of the patient and the volume of body fluids in which the drug is distributed.

The ideal body weight (IBW) provides an excellent estimation of the distribution volume, particularly for some polar drugs that are not well distributed in adipose (fat) tissue. These calculations have been used clinically with the aminoglycoside antibiotics and with digoxin to determine doses and to predict blood levels. The IBW may be calculated readily through the use of the following formulas based on the patients's height and sex.

For males:
IBW = 50 kg + 2.3 kg for each inch of patient's height over 5 feet
or, in pounds
110 lb + 5 lb for each inch over 5 feet
For females:
IBW = 45.5 kg + 2.3 kg for each inch of patient height over 5 feet
or, in pounds
100 lb + 5 lb for each inch over 5 feet

Examples:

Calculate the ideal body weight for a male patient weighing 164 lb and measuring 5 ft, 8 in. in height.

IBW = 110 lb + (8 × 5 lb)
110 lb + 40 lb = 150 lb, answer.

Calculate the ideal body weight for a female patient weighing 60 kg and measuring 160 cm in height.

160 cm = 63 inches = 5 ft, 3 in.
IBW = 45.5 kg + (3 × 2.3 kg)
45.5 kg + 6.9 kg = 52.4, *answer.*

NOTE: In instances in which the IBW is determined to be greater than the actual body weight, the latter is used in dosage calculations.

The kidneys receive about 20% of the cardiac output (blood flow) and filter approximately 125 mL per minute of plasma. As kidney function is lost, the quantity of plasma filtered per minute decreases, with an accompanying decrease in drug clearance. The filtration rate of the kidney can be estimated by a number of methods. One of the most useful, however, is the estimation of the creatinine clearance rate (CrCl) through the use of the following empiric formulas based on the patient's age, weight, and serum creatinine value.[4] The creatinine clearance rate represents the volume of blood plasma that is cleared of creatinine by kidney filtration per minute. It is expressed in milliliters per minute.

By the Jelliffe Equation:[5]
For males:
Creatinine Clearance Rate
(CrCl)

$$= \frac{98 - 0.8 \times (\text{patient's age in years} - 20)}{\text{Serum Creatinine (as mg/dL)}}$$

For females:
Creatinine Clearance Rate
(CrCl)

$$= 0.9 \times \text{CrCl determined using formula for males}$$

By the Cockcroft and Gault Equation:[6]
For males:

$$\text{CrCl} = \frac{(140 - \text{patient's age in years}) \times \text{body weight in kg}}{72 \times \text{Serum Creatinine in mg/dL}}$$

For females:

$$\text{CrCl} = 0.85 \times \text{CrCl determined using formula for males}$$

Example:

Determine the creatinine clearance rate for an 80-year-old male patient weighing 70 kg and having a serum creatinine of 2 mg/dL. Use both the Jelliffe and Cockcroft-Gault equations.

---

[4] Creatinine, which is a break-down product of muscle metabolism, is generally produced at a constant rate and in quantities that depend on the muscle mass of the patient. Because creatinine is eliminated from the body essentially through renal filtration, reduced kidney performance results in a reduced creatinine clearance rate. The normal adult value of serum creatinine is 0.7 to 1.5 mg/dL.

[5] Jelliffe, R.W.: Estimation of creatinine clearance when urine cannot be collected. Lancet, *1*:975, 1971; Jelliffe, R.W.: Creatinine clearance, bedside estimate. Ann. Intern. Med., 79:604, 1973.

[6] Cockcroft, D.W. and Gault, M.H.: Prediction of creatinine clearance from serum creatinine. Nephron, *16*:31, 1976.

By the Jelliffe Equation:

$$CrCl = \frac{98 - 0.8 \times (80 - 20)}{2 \ (mg/dL)}$$

$$= \frac{98 - (0.8 \times 60)}{2 \ (mg/dL)} = \frac{98 - 48}{2 \ (mg/dL)} = \frac{50}{2 \ (mg/dL)}$$

$$= 25 \ mL/min, \ answer.$$

By the Cockcroft and Gault Equation:

$$CrCl = \frac{(140 - 80) \times 70}{72 \times 2 \ (mg/dL)}$$

$$= \frac{60 \times 70}{144}$$

$$= \frac{4200}{144}$$

$$= 29.2 \ mL/min, \ answer.$$

Adjusting Creatinine Clearance for Body Surface Area. It is sometimes desirable to adjust the calculated creatinine clearance for body surface area to account for this possible variable in determining drug dosage. This adjustment is accomplished through the use of a nomogram of body surface area (BSA) as described previously (see Chapter 4) and the following formula:

$$\frac{BSA}{1.73} \times CrCl = Adjusted \ CrCl$$

Example:

If a patient weighing 120 lb and measuring 60 in. in height has a calculated creatinine clearance of 40 mL per minute, adjust the CrCl based on body surface area.

Using the nomogram in Chapter 4, the patient's BSA is determined to be 1.50 m². Thus,

$$\frac{1.50 \ m^2}{1.73 \ m^2} \times 40 \ mL/min = 34.7 \ mL/min, \ adjusted \ CrCl, \ answer.$$

Normal creatinine clearance rate may be considered 100 mL per minute. Thus, in the preceding example, the patient would exhibit 25 to 35% of normal creatinine clearance.

The creatinine clearance rate method for determining drug dose is used primarily in aminoglycoside therapy in which reduced renal function is a factor. The primary drugs involved are gentamicin, tobramycin, amikacin, and kanamycin.

Once the creatinine clearance rate and the ideal body weight have been calculated, the *loading dose* (initial dose) required to reach a certain drug concentration in the patient and the *maintenance dose* needed to maintain the specified concentration can be calculated.

The loading dose is based solely on the ideal body weight of the patient (except in obese patients), whereas the maintenance dose is based on the ideal body weight *and* the renal clearance rate of the drug.

To calculate the **loading dose** *(LD), perform the following:*

LD = ideal body weight (IBW) in kg or lb × drug dose per kg or lb

To calculate the **maintenance dose** (MD), *perform the following:*

For the "normal" patient:

$$MD = IBW \; (kg) \times dose \; per \; kg \; per \; dosing \; interval$$

For the "renally impaired" patient:

$$MD = \frac{CrCl \; (patient)}{CrCl \; (normal)} \times dose \; for \; "normal" \; patient$$

Example:

Determine the loading and maintenance doses of gentamicin for a 76-year-old male patient weighing 190 lb with a height of 6 feet and having a serum creatinine of 2.4 mg/dL. The physician desires a loading dose of 1.5 mg/kg of ideal body weight and a maintenance dose of 1.0 mg/kg of ideal body weight to be administered every 8 hours after the initial dose.

$$
\begin{aligned}
IBW &= 110 \; lb + (5 \; lb \times 12) \\
&= 110 \; lb + 60 \; lb \\
&= 170 \; lb \; or \; 77.3 \; kg
\end{aligned}
$$

$$
\begin{aligned}
CrCl &= \frac{98 - 0.8 \times (76 - 20)}{2.4 \; (mg/dL)} \\[2mm]
&= \frac{98 - 44.8}{2.4 \; (mg/dL)} = \frac{53.2}{2.4 \; (mg/dL)} = 22.2 \; mL \; per \; minute
\end{aligned}
$$

$$LD = 77.3 \; kg \times 1.5 \; mg/kg = 116 \; mg, \; answer.$$

MD for "normal" patient:

$$
\begin{aligned}
&= 77.3 \; kg \times 1.0 \; mg/kg \; every \; 8 \; hours \\
&= 77.3 \; mg \; every \; 8 \; hours
\end{aligned}
$$

MD for "renally impaired" patient:

$$= \frac{22.2 \; mL \; per \; minute}{100 \; mL \; per \; minute} \times 77.3 \; mg$$

$$= 17.2 \; mg \; every \; 8 \; hours, \; answer.$$

Use of Creatinine Clearance Dosage Tables

For certain drugs, tables of dosage guidelines may be presented in the labeling/literature to adjust for impaired renal function. For example, the usual dose of the anti-infective drug cefmetazole sodium is 2 g every 6 to 12 hours, with dosage adjusted based on the location and severity of the infection and the patient's renal function. For adult patients with impaired renal function, guidelines for dosage based on creatinine clearance with adjustment for body surface area are given in Table 14.1.:[7]

Table 14.1. Creatinine Clearance Dosage Guidelines

Renal Function	Creatine Clearance (mL/min/1.73m²)	Dose (grams)	Frequency
Mild impairment	90–50	1–2	Q 12h
Moderate impairment	49–30	1–2	Q 16h
Severe impairment	29–10	1–2	Q 24h
Essentially no function	<10	1–2	Q 48h

---

[7] Zefazone (cefmetazole sodium) product literature, 1991. The Upjohn Company, Kalamazoo, MI 49001.

Example:

Using the table of dosage guidelines for cefmetazole sodium and adjusting for body surface area (BSA), determine the dose and daily dose schedule for a patient weighing 70 kg, measuring 70 in. in height, and having a creatinine clearance (CrCl) of 48 mL per minute.

Using the nomogram in Chapter 4, the patient is determined to have a BSA of 1.87 m^2. Applying the formula for the adjustment of CrCl based on BSA, the patient's CrCl is then determined:

$$\frac{1.87 \text{ m}^2}{1.73 \text{ m}^2} \times 48 \text{ mL/min} = 51.9 \text{ or } 52 \text{ mL/min}$$

By use of the dosage table, the adjusted CrCl indicates a dosage of:

1 to 2 g every 12 hours, *answer.*

Practice Problems

1. If the bioavailability factor (F) for a 100-mg tablet of a drug is 0.70 compared to the bioavailability factor of 1.0 for an injection of the same drug, how many milliliters of the injection containing 40 mg/mL would be considered bioequivalent to the tablet?

2. If 5 mL of an elixir containing 2 mg/mL of a drug is bioequivalent to a 15-mg tablet having a bioavailability factor of 0.60, what is the bioavailability factor of the elixir?

3. If at equilibrium, two thirds of the amount of a drug substance in the blood is bound to protein, what would be the alpha (α) value of the drug?

4. The alpha (α) value for a drug in the blood is 0.90, equating to 0.55 ng/mL. What is the concentration of total drug in the blood?

5. A patient received an intravenous dose of 10 mg of a drug. A blood sample was drawn and it contained 40 μg/100 mL. Calculate the apparent volume of distribution for the drug.

6. The volume of distribution for a drug was found to be 10 liters with a blood level concentration of 2 μg/mL. Calculate the total amount of drug present in the patient.

7. Calculate the elimination rate constant for a drug having an elimination half-life of 1.7 hours.

8. Plot the following data on semilogarithmic graph paper and determine (a) the elimination half-life of the drug and (b) the elimination rate constant.

Plasma Drug Concentration (μg/100 mL)	Time (hours)
8.5	0.5
6.8	1.0
5.4	1.5
4.0	2.0
3.2	2.5
2.5	3.0

9. What percentage of an originally administered intravenous dose of a drug remains in the body following three half-lives?

10. If the half-life of a drug is 4 hours, approximately what percent of the drug administered would remain in the body 15 hours after administration?

11. Determine the loading and maintenance doses of tobramycin for a 72-year-old female patient weighing 187 lb and measuring 5 ft, 3 in. in height with a serum creatinine of 2.8 mg/dL. The loading dose desired is 1.0 mg/kg of ideal body weight and 1.66 mg/kg every 8 hours as the maintenance dose.

12. Determine the loading and maintenance doses of amikacin for a 42-year-old female patient weighing 210 lb and measuring 5 ft in height with a serum creatinine of 1.8 mg/dL. The physician requests a loading dose of 7.5 mg/kg of ideal body weight and a maintenance dose of 5 mg/kg of ideal body weight to be administered continually at intervals of 8 hours.

13. If 100 mg of a drug are administered intravenously and the resultant drug plasma concentration is determined to be 2.5 μg/mL, calculate the apparent volume of distribution.

14. If a dose of 1 g of a drug is administered intravenously to a patient and the drug plasma concentration is determined to be 65 μg/mL, calculate the apparent volume of distribution.

15. If 500 mg of a drug are administered orally and 300 mg are absorbed into the circulation, calculate the bioavailability factor (F).

16. Calculate the creatinine clearance rate for a 20-year-old male patient weighing 70 kg with a serum creatinine of 1 mg/dL. If a patient is 5 ft, 8 in. tall, adjust the creatinine clearance based on body surface area.

17. The volume of distribution for chlordiazepoxide has been determined to be 34 liters. Calculate the expected drug plasma concentration of the drug, in micrograms per deciliter, immediately after an intravenous dose of 5 mg.

18. Using the creatinine clearance dosing table in this chapter and the nomogram for body surface area in Chapter 4, what would be the dose and dosage schedule of cefmetazole sodium for a patient weighing 50 kg, measuring 66 in. in height, and having a creatinine clearance (unadjusted for BSA) of 31 mL per minute?

19. In normal subjects, blood makes up about 7% of the body weight.
    (a) Calculate the approximate blood volume, in liters, for a man weighing 70 kg.
    (b) If the drug Zantac® reached peak blood levels of about 500 ng/mL 2 to 3 hours after an oral dose, calculate the total amount of the drug, in milligrams, in the blood of the patient described in (a) when peak blood levels are achieved.

15

Some Calculations Involving Radioactive Pharmaceuticals

RADIOISOTOPES

The atoms of a given element are not necessarily alike. In fact, certain elements actually consist of several different components, called *isotopes*, that are chemically identical but physically may differ slightly in mass. Isotopes, then, may be defined as atoms that have the same nuclear charge, and hence the same atomic number, but masses that differ. The mass number physically characterizes a particular isotope.

Isotopes may be classified as stable and unstable. Stable isotopes never change unless affected by some outside force; unstable isotopes are distinguishable by radioactive transformations and hence are said to be radioactive. The radioactive isotopes of the elements are called *radioisotopes* or *radionuclides*. They may be divided into two types: naturally occurring and artificially produced radionuclides.

The use of naturally occurring radioisotopes in medicine dates back some 75 years when radium was first introduced in radiologic practice. It was not until after 1946, however, that artificially produced radioisotopes were readily available to hospitals and to the medical profession. Since that time, radionuclides have become important tools in medical research, and selected radioisotopes have been recognized as extremely valuable diagnostic and therapeutic agents. Monographs for a number of radioactive pharmaceuticals are now official in the *United States Pharmacopeia*. Examples of some radioactive pharmaceuticals are listed in Table 15.1.

These and many other radioactive pharmaceutical products are commercially available to properly trained and licensed personnel. Pharmacists, especially those engaged in hospital practice, who have a knowledgeable background in nuclear pharmacy may be required to make certain modifications and dilutions of the products that usually are available from pharmaceutical manufacturers. They may also be required to make certain corrections for radioactive decay in making dosage calculations.

RADIOACTIVITY

The breakdown of an unstable isotope is characterized by radioactivity. In the process of radioactivity, an unstable isotope undergoes changes until a stable state is reached, and in the transformation, it emits energy in the form of radiation. This radiation may consist of *alpha particles, beta particles,* and *gamma rays.* The stable state is reached as a result of *radioactive decay,* which is characteristic of all types of radioactivity. Individual radioisotopes differ in the rate of radioactive decay, but in each case, a definite time is required for half of the original atoms to decay. This time is called the *half-life* of the radioisotope. Each radioisotope, then, has a distinct half-life. The half-lives of some commonly used radioisotopes are given in Table 15.2.

The rate of decay is always a constant fraction of the total number of undecomposed atoms present. Mathematically, the rate of disintegration may be expressed as follows:

$$-\frac{dN}{dt} = \lambda N \qquad (1)$$

**Table 15.1. Examples of Some Radioactive
Pharmaceuticals**

Ammonia N 13 Injection
Chromic Phosphate P 32 Suspension
Cyanocobalamin Co 57 Capsules
Cyanocobalamin Co 57 Oral Solution
Fludeoxyglucose F 18 Injection
Fluorodopa F 18 Injection
Gallium Citrate Ga 67 Injection
Indium In 111 Pentetate Injection
Iodinated I 131 Albumin Aggregated Injection
Iodinated I 125 Albumin Injection
Iodinated I 131 Albumin Injection
Iodohippurate Sodium I 123 Injection
Iodohippurate Sodium I 131 Injection
Iothalamate Sodium I 125 Injection
Rose Bengal Sodium I 131 Injection
Rubidium Chloride Rb 82 Injection
Sodium Chromate Cr 51 Injection
Sodium Fluoride F 18 Injection
Sodium Iodide I 123 Capsules
Sodium Iodide I 123 Solution
Sodium Iodide I 131 Capsules
Sodium Iodide I 131 Solution
Sodium Pertechnetate Tc 99m Injection
Sodium Phosphate P 32 Solution
Technetium Tc 99m Albumin Aggregated Injection
Technetium Tc 99m Albumin Injection
Technetium Tc 99m Disofenin Injection
Technetium Tc 99m Etidronate Injection
Technetium Tc 99m Gluceptate Injection
Technetium Tc 99m Medronate Injection
Technetium Tc 99m Oxidronate Injection
Technetium Tc 99m Pentetate Injection
Technetium Tc 99m (pyro- and trimeta-) Phosphates Injection
Technetium Tc 99m Pyrophosphate Injection
Technetium Tc 99m Succimer Injection
Technetium Tc 99m Sulfur Colloid Injection
Thallous Chloride Tl 201 Injection
Water O 15 Injection
Xenon Xe 133 Injection

in which N is the number of undecomposed atoms at time t, and λ is the decay constant or the fraction disintegrating per unit of time.

The constant may be expressed in any unit of time, i.e., reciprocal seconds, minutes, hours, etc. The numeric value of the decay constant will be 24 times as great when expressed in days, for example, as when expressed in hours. This equation may be integrated to give the expression of the *exponential decay law,* which may be written,

$$N = N_0 e^{-\lambda t} \qquad (2)$$

in which N is the number of atoms remaining at elapsed time t, N_0 is the number of atoms originally present (when t = 0), λ is the decay constant for the unit of time in terms of which the interval t is expressed, and e is the base of the natural logarithm 2.71828 (see Appendix J).

Because the rate of decay may also be characterized by the half-life ($T_{1/2}$), the value of N in equation 2 at the end of a half period is $\frac{1}{2}N_0$. The equation then becomes,

Table 15.2. Half-Lives of Some Radioisotopes

Radioisotope	Half-life
^{198}Au	2.70 days
^{14}C	5,700 years
^{45}Ca	180 days
^{57}Co	270 days
^{60}Co	5.27 years
^{51}Cr	27.8 days
^{59}Fe	45.1 days
^{67}Ga	78.3 hours
^{203}Hg	46.6 days
^{123}I	13.2 hours
^{125}I	60 days
^{131}I	8.08 days
^{111}In	2.83 days
^{42}K	12.4 hours
^{81m}Kr	13.1 seconds
^{99}Mo	2.6 years
^{22}Na	2.6 years
^{24}Na	15.0 hours
^{32}P	14.3 days
^{35}S	87.2 days
^{75}Se	120 days
^{85}Sr	64 days
^{99m}Tc	6.0 hours
^{201}Tl	73.1 hours
^{133}Xe	5.24 days
^{169}Yb	32.0 days

$$\tfrac{1}{2}N_0 = N_0^{-\lambda T_{1/2}} \tag{3}$$

Solving equation 3 by natural logarithms results in the following expression:

$$\ln \tfrac{1}{2} = -\lambda T_{1/2}$$

$$\text{or} \quad \lambda T_{1/2} = \ln 2$$

$$\text{then} \quad \lambda T_{1/2} = 2.303 \log 2$$

$$\text{and} \quad T_{1/2} = \frac{0.693}{\lambda} \tag{4}$$

The half-life ($T_{1/2}$), then, is related to the disintegration constant λ by equation 4. Hence, if one value is known, the other can be readily calculated.

UNITS OF RADIOACTIVITY

The quantity of activity of a radioisotope is expressed in absolute units (total number of atoms disintegrating per unit time). The basic unit is the *curie* (Ci), which is defined as that quantity of a radioisotope in which 3.7×10^{10} (37 billion) atoms disintegrate per second. The *millicurie* (mCi) is one thousandth of a curie and the *microcurie* (μCi) is one millionth of a curie. The *nanocurie* (nCi), also known as the *millimicrocurie*, is one billionth of a curie (10^{-9} Ci).

The International System (SI) (see Chapter 3) unit for radioactivity is the *becquerel* (Bq),

Table 15.3. Conversion Equivalents

$$1 \ Ci = 3.7 \times 10^{10} \ Bq = 3.7 \times 10^4 \ MBq = 37 \times 10^3 \ MBq$$

$$1 \ mCi = 37 \ MBq$$
$$1 \ \mu Ci = 0.037 \ MBq$$

$$1 \ Bq = 2.7 \times 10^{-11} \ Ci$$
$$1 \ MBq = 10^6 \ Bq = 2.7 \times 10^{-5} \ Ci$$
$$= 2.7 \ 10^{-2} \ mCi = 0.027 \ mCi$$
$$= 27 \ \mu Ci$$

which is defined as 1 disintegration per second. Because the becquerel is so small, it is more convenient to use multiples of the unit, such as the *megabecquerel* (MBq), which is equal to 10^6 disintegrations per second, and the *gigabecquerel* (GBq), which is equal to 10^9 disintegrations per second.

The *United States Pharmacopeia* has adopted the becquerel unit to eventually replace the long-familiar curie as a matter of international agreement. For the present, both units are used to label radioactivity, and the doses of many radiopharmaceuticals are expressed in megabecquerels as well as in millicuries and/or microcuries.

Table 15.3 provides equivalents for conversion from the curie unit (and its subunits) to the becquerel unit (and its multiples), and vice versa.

Millicuries and Microcuries to Megabecquerels. Converting radioactivity units from millicuries and microcuries to megabecquerels involves the following.

Example:

A thallous chloride Tl 201 injection has a labeled activity of 550 microcuries (μCi). Express this activity in terms of megabecquerels.

$$550 \ \mu Ci = 0.55 \ mCi$$
$$1 \ mCi = 37 \ MBq$$
$$\frac{1 \ (mCi)}{0.55 \ (mCi)} = \frac{37 \ (MBq)}{x \ (MBq)}$$
$$x = 20.35 \ MBq, \ answer.$$

Megabecquerels to Millicuries and Microcuries. Converting radioactivity units from megabecquerels to millicuries and microcuries involves the following.

Example:

Sodium chromate Cr 51 injection is administered in a dose of 3.7 MBq for the determination of blood volume. Express this dose in terms of microcuries.

$$1 \ MBq = 0.027 \ mCi$$

$$\frac{1 \ (MBq)}{3.7 \ (MBq)} = \frac{0.027 \ (mCi)}{x \ (mCi)}$$

$$x = 0.1 \ mCi$$

$$= 100 \ \mu Ci, \ answer.$$

Other units that may be encountered in practice, but are not used in the calculations that follow, include the roentgen and the rad. The *roentgen* is the international unit of x rays or gamma radiation. It is the quantity of x rays or gamma radiation that produces, under standard conditions of temperature and pressure, ions carrying 1 electrostatic unit of electrical charge of either sign. The *rad* (acronym for radiation absorbed dose) is a unit of measurement of the absorbed dose of ionizing radiation. It corresponds to an energy transfer of 100 ergs/g of any absorbing material (including tissues).

Half-Life Determination When Disintegration Constant is Known. Calculating the half-life of a radioisotope when its disintegration constant is given involves the following.

Example:

 The disintegration constant of a radioisotope is 0.02496 day^{-1}. Calculate the half-life of the radioisotope.

$$T_{1/2} = \frac{0.693}{\lambda}$$

$$\text{Substituting, } T_{1/2} = \frac{0.693}{0.02496 \text{ day}^{-1}}$$

$$T_{1/2} = 27.76 \text{ or } 27.8 \text{ days, } answer.$$

Disintegration Constant Determination When Half-Life is Known. Calculating the disintegration constant of a radioisotope when its half-life is given involves the following.

Example:

 The half-life of ^{198}Au is 2.70 days. Calculate its disintegration constant.

$$T_{1/2} = \frac{0.693}{\lambda}$$

$$\text{Substituting, } 2.70 \text{ days} = \frac{0.693}{\lambda}$$

$$\lambda = \frac{0.693}{2.70 \text{ days}} = 0.2567 \text{ day}^{-1}, answer.$$

Disintegration Constant and Half-Life Determinations When Initial and Time t Activities are Known. Calculating the disintegration constant and the half-life of a radioisotope when its initial activity and its activity at time *t* are given involves the following.

Example:

 The original quantity of a radioisotope is given as 500 μCi (18.5 MBq)/mL. If the quantity remaining after 16 days is 125 μCi (4.625 MBq)/mL, calculate (a) the disintegration constant and (b) the half-life of the radioisotope.

(a) Equation 2, written in logarithmic form, becomes

$$\ln \frac{N}{N_0} = -\lambda t$$

or

$$\lambda = \frac{2.303}{t} \log \frac{N_0}{N}$$

Substituting,

$$\lambda = \frac{2.303}{16} \log \frac{500}{125} \text{ or, } \frac{2.303}{16} \log \frac{18.5 \text{ (MBq)}}{4.625 \text{ (MBq)}}$$

$$\lambda = \frac{2.303}{16} (0.6021)$$

$$\lambda = 0.08666 \text{ day}^{-1,} answer.$$

(b) Equation 4 may now be used to calculate the half-life.

$$T_{1/2} = \frac{0.693}{\lambda}$$

$$\text{Substituting, } T_{1/2} = \frac{0.693}{0.08666 \text{ day}^{-1}} = 8.0 \text{ days, } \textit{answer.}$$

Remaining Activity at Any Time t. Calculating the activity of a radioisotope remaining at any time *t* after the original assay involves the following.

Examples:

A sample of ^{131}I has an initial activity of 30 μCi (1.11 MBq). Its half-life is 8.08 days. Calculate its activity, in microcuries (megabecquerels), at the end of exactly 20 days.

$$\text{By substituting } \lambda = \frac{0.693}{T_{1/2}} \text{ and } e^{-0.693} = \frac{1}{2}$$

In equation 2, the activity of a radioactive sample decreases with time according to the following expression:

$$N = N_0 \left(2^{-t/T_{1/2}} \right) = N_0 \left(\frac{1}{2^{t/T_{1/2}}} \right)$$

$$\text{Since} \qquad t/T\frac{1}{2} = \frac{20}{8.08} = 2.475$$

$$\text{then} \qquad N = 30 \left(\frac{1}{2^{2.475}} \right)$$

$$\text{Solving by logarithms log } N = \log 30 - \log 2 \ (2.475)$$
$$= 1.4771 - 0.7450$$
$$\log N = 0.7321$$
$$N = 5.39 \text{ or } 5.4 \text{ μCi, } \textit{answer.}$$

Or, using megabecquerel units:

$$N = 1.11 \left(\frac{1}{2^{2.475}} \right)$$

$$\text{Solving by logarithms log } N = \log 1.11 - \log 2 \ (2.475)$$
$$= 0.0453 - 0.7450$$
$$\log N = -0.6997$$
$$N = 0.1997 \text{ or } 0.2 \text{ MBq, } \textit{answer.}$$

A vial of Sodium Phosphate P 32 Solution has a labeled activity of 500 μCi (18.5 MBq)/ mL. How many milliliters of this solution should be administered exactly 10 days after the original assay to provide an activity of 250 Ci (9.25 MBq)? The half-life of ^{32}P is 14.3 days.
The activity exactly 10 days after the original assay is given by

$$N = N_0 \left(\frac{1}{2^{t/T_{1/2}}} \right)$$

$$\text{Since} \qquad t/T_{1/2} = \frac{10}{14.3} = 0.6993$$

$$\text{then} \qquad N = 500 \left(\frac{1}{2^{0.6993}} \right)$$

$$\log N = \log 500 - \log 2 \ (0.6993)$$
$$= 2.6990 - 0.2105$$
$$\log N = 2.4885$$
$$N = 308 \ \mu\text{Ci/mL, activity after radioactive decay}$$

$$\frac{308 \ (\mu\text{Ci})}{250 \ (\mu\text{Ci})} = \frac{1 \ (\text{mL})}{\text{x} \ (\text{mL})}$$
$$\text{x} = 0.81 \ \text{mL, } \textit{answer.}$$

Or, using megabecquerel units:

$$N = 18.5 \left(\frac{1}{2^{0.6993}} \right)$$

$$\log N = \log 18.5 - \log 2 \ (0.6993)$$

$$= 1.2672 - 0.2105$$

$$\log N = 1.0567$$

$$= 11.39 \ \text{MBq/mL, activity after radioactive decay}$$

$$\frac{11.39 \ (\text{MBq})}{9.25 \ (\text{MBq})} = \frac{1 \ (\text{mL})}{\text{x} \ (\text{mL})}$$

$$\text{x} = 0.81 \ \text{mL, } \textit{answer.}$$

Practice Problems

1. Cyanocobalamin Co 57 capsules are administered in doses of 0.5 to 1.0 μCi in a test for pernicious anemia. Express this dosage range in terms of becquerel units.

2. If 1 mCi of radioactivity is equivalent to 37 MBq in activity, how many becquerels of radioactivity would be the equivalent of 1 Ci?

3. A gallium citrate Ga 67 injection has a labeled activity of 366 MBq. Express this activity in terms of millicuries.

4. If 1.85 MBq of radioactivity is equivalent to 50 μCi, how many millicuries would be represented in 7.4 MBq?

5. If 50 μCi of radioactivity is equivalent to 1.85 MBq of activity, how many megabecquerels of radioactivity would be the equivalent of 10 mCi?

6. Express an administered dose of 5 mCi sodium phosphate P 32 solution in terms of megabecquerels.

7. Calculate the half-life of a radioisotope that has a disintegration constant of 0.00456 day^{-1}.

8. Calculate the half-life of ^{203}Hg, which has a disintegration constant of 0.0149 day^{-1}.

9. Calculate the disintegration constant of ^{64}Cu, which has a half-life of 12.8 hours.

10. Calculate the disintegration constant of ^{35}S, which has a half-life of 87.2 days.

11. The original quantity of a radioisotope is given as 100 mCi (3700 MBq). If the quantity remaining after 6 days is 75 mCi (2775 MBq), calculate the disintegration constant and the half-life of the radioisotope.

12. A series of measurements on a sample of a radioisotope gave the following data:

Days	Counts per Minute
0	5600
4	2000

Calculate the disintegration constant and the half-life of the radioisotope.

13. The original activity of a radioisotope is given as 10 mCi (370 MBq) per 10 mL. If the quantity remaining after exactly 15 days is 850 μCi (31.45 MBq)/mL, calculate the disintegration constant and the half-life of the radioisotope.

14. If the half-life of a radioisotope is 12 hours, what will be the activity after 4 days of a sample that has an original activity of 1 Ci (37000 MBq)? Express the activity in terms of microcuries (megabecquerels).

15. Sodium iodide I 131 capsules have a labeled potency of 100 μCi (3.7 MBq). What will be their activity exactly 3 days after the stated assay date? The half-life of ^{131}I is 8.08 days.

16. A sodium chromate Cr 51 injection has a labeled activity of 50 mCi (1850 MBq) at 5:00 p.m. on April 19. Calculate its activity at 5:00 p.m. on May 1. The half-life of ^{51}Cr is 27.8 days.

17. Iodinated I 125 Albumin Injection contains 0.5 mCi (18.5 MBq) of radioactivity per milliliter. How many milliliters of the solution should be administered exactly 30 days after the original assay to provide an activity of 60 μCi (2.22 MBq)? The half-life of ^{125}I is 60 days.

18. An Ytterbium Yb 169 Pentetate Injection has a labeled radioactivity of 5 mCi (185 MBq)/mL. How many milliliters of the injection should be administered 10 days after the original assay to provide an activity of 100 μCi (3.7 MBq)/kg of body weight for a person weighing 110 lb? The half-life of ^{169}Yb is 32.0 days.

19. A sodium pertechnetate Tc 99m injection has a labeled activity of 15 mCi (555 MBq)/mL. If the injection is administered 10 hours after the time of calibration, (a) what will be its activity, and (b) how many milliliters of the injection will be required to provide a dose of 15 mCi (555 MBq)? The half-life of ^{99m}Tc is 6.0 hours.

20. A sodium phosphate P 32 solution contains 1 mCi (37 MBq)/mL at the time of calibration. How many milliliters of the solution will provide an activity of 500 μCi (18.5 MBq) 1 week after the original assay? The half-life of ^{32}P is 14.3 days.

Appendices

The Common Systems and Intersystem Conversion

In addition to the metric system, the avoirdupois and apothecaries' systems of measurement are used in the United States; and, in spite of the predominant use of the official metric system in pharmacy and medicine, some physicians continue to use the apothecaries' systems of measuring volume and weight in their prescriptions. The pharmacist, therefore, must have a practical knowledge of the so-called *common systems of measure*.

APOTHECARIES' FLUID MEASURE

$$
\begin{aligned}
60 \text{ minims } (\mathfrak{m}) &= 1 \text{ fluidrachm or fluidram (f3 or 3)}^1 \\
8 \text{ fluidrachms } (480 \text{ minims}) &= 1 \text{ fluidounce (f}\bar{\mathfrak{z}} \text{ or } \bar{\mathfrak{z}})^1 \\
16 \text{ fluidounces } &= 1 \text{ pint (pt or 0)} \\
2 \text{ pints } (32 \text{ fluidounces}) &= 1 \text{ quart (qt)} \\
4 \text{ quarts } (8 \text{ pints}) &= 1 \text{ gallon (gal or C)}
\end{aligned}
$$

This table may also be written:

gal	qt	pt	f$\bar{\mathfrak{z}}$	f3	$\mathfrak{m}$
1	4	8	128	1024	61440
	1	2	32	256	15360
		1	16	128	7680
			1	8	480
				1	60

APOTHECARIES' MEASURE OF WEIGHT

$$
\begin{aligned}
20 \text{ grains } (gr) &= 1 \text{ scruple } (\Theta) \\
3 \text{ scruples } (60 \text{ grains}) &= 1 \text{ drachm or dram (3)} \\
8 \text{ drachms } (480 \text{ grains}) &= 1 \text{ ounce } (\bar{\mathfrak{z}}) \\
12 \text{ ounces } (5760 \text{ grains}) &= 1 \text{ pound } (\text{℔})
\end{aligned}
$$

This table may also be written:

℔	$\bar{\mathfrak{z}}$	3	Θ	gr
1	12	96	288	5760
	1	8	24	480
		1	3	60
			1	20

A typical set of Apothecaries' Weights consists of the following units:

$$\bar{\mathfrak{z}}\text{ii} \quad \bar{\mathfrak{z}}\text{i} \quad \bar{\mathfrak{z}}\text{ss} \quad 3\text{ii} \quad 3\text{i} \quad 3\text{ss} \quad \Theta\text{ii} \quad \Theta\text{i} \quad \Theta\text{ss}$$

5-grain, 4-grain, 3-grain, 2-grain, 1-grain, ½-grain

---

[1] When it is clear that a liquid is to be measured, physicians commonly omit the *f* in this symbol.

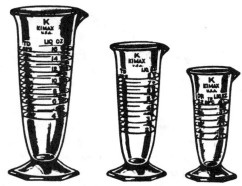

Fig. AA.1. Apothecaries' Graduates. (Courtesy of Kimble Glassware Co.)

AVOIRDUPOIS MEASURE OF WEIGHT

437½ or 437.5 grain (gr) = 1 ounce (oz)
16 ounces (7000 grains) = 1 pound (lb)

This table may also be written:

lb	*oz*	*gr*
1	16	7000
	1	437.5

Only one denomination has a value common to the apothecaries' and avoirdupois systems of measuring weight, namely, the *grain*. The other denominations bearing the same name have different values.

Bulk or stock packages of powdered drugs and chemicals (and occasionally some liquids when they are sold by weight) are customarily provided to the pharmacist in avoirdupois units of weight by manufacturers and wholesalers. The pharmacist likewise sells bulk packages of nonprescription drug and chemical items by the avoirdupois system. When compounding prescriptions, however, the pharmacist uses the apothecaries' and metric systems to weigh and measure ingredients.

In contrast with the invariable use of *simple* quantities in the metric system, measurements in the common systems are recorded whenever possible in *compound quantities*, i.e., quantities expressed in two or more denominations. So, 20 f℥ may be used during the process of calculating, but as a final result, it should be recorded as 1 pt 4 f℥. The process of reducing a quantity to a compound quantity beginning with the highest possible denomination is called *simplification*. Decimal fractions may be used in calculation, but the subdivision of a minim or a grain in a final result is recorded as a *common fraction*.

When prescriptions are written in the common system, the numbers are written in Roman numerals and *follow* the abbreviations or symbols for the denominations.

Examples:

℞	Codeine Sulfate		gr iv
	Ammonium Chloride		ℨ iss
	Cherry Syrup	ad	f℥ iv
	Sig. ℨi as directed.		

FUNDAMENTAL COMPUTATIONS

Compound Quantity to a Simple Quantity. Before a compound quantity can be used in a calculation, it must usually be expressed in terms of a single denomination. To do so, reduce each of the denominations in the compound quantity to the required denomination and add the results.

Examples:

Reduce ℥ss ʒii ℈i to grains.

$$℥ss = ½ \times 480 \text{ gr} = 240 \text{ gr}$$
$$ʒii = 2 \times 60 \text{ gr} = 120 \text{ gr}$$
$$℈i = 1 \times 20 \text{ gr} = \underline{20 \text{ gr}}$$
$$380 \text{ gr, } answer.$$

Reduce f℥iv fʒiiss to fluidrachms.

$$f℥iv = 4 \times 8 \text{ fʒ} = 32 \quad \text{fʒ}$$
$$fʒiiss = \underline{2½ \text{ fʒ}}$$
$$34½ \text{ fʒ, } answer.$$

Simple Quantities to Weighable or Measurable Denominations. Before being weighed, a given quantity should be expressed in denominations equal to the actual weights on hand. Before a volume is measured, a given quantity should be expressed in denominations represented by the calibrations on the graduate.

Examples:

Change 165 grains to weighable apothecaries' units.

By selecting larger weight units to account for as many of the required grains as possible, beginning with the largest, we find that we may use the following weights:

$$ʒii, ℈ss, ℈ss, 5 \text{ gr, } answer.$$

$$\textit{Check: } ʒii = 120 \text{ gr}$$
$$℈ss = 30 \text{ gr}$$
$$℈ss = 10 \text{ gr}$$
$$5 \text{ gr} = \underline{5 \text{ gr}}$$
$$165 \text{ gr, } total.$$

In enlarging a formula, we are to measure 90 fʒ of a liquid. Using two graduates, if necessary, in what denominations may we measure this quantity?

$$11 \text{ f℥ and } 2 \text{ fʒ, } answer.$$

$$\textit{Check: } 11 \text{ f℥} = 88 \text{ fʒ}$$
$$2 \text{ fʒ} = \underline{2 \text{ fʒ}}$$
$$90 \text{ fʒ, } total.$$

Addition or Subtraction. To add or subtract quantities in the common systems, reduce to a common denomination, add or subtract, and reduce the result (unless it is to be used in further calculations) to a compound quantity.

Examples:

A formula contains ℈ii of ingredient A, ʒi of ingredient B, ℥iv of ingredient C, and gr viiss of ingredient D. Calculate the total weight of the ingredients.

$$Эii = 2 \times 20 \text{ gr} = 40 \text{gr}$$
$$Зi = 1 \times 60 \text{ gr} = 60 \text{gr}$$
$$Зiv = 4 \times 60 \text{ gr} = 240 \text{gr}$$
$$\text{gr viiss} = 7\frac{1}{2} \text{ gr}$$
$$347\frac{1}{2} \text{ gr} = 5 \, З \, 2 \, Э \, 7\frac{1}{2} \text{ gr, } \textit{answer.}$$

A pharmacist had 1 gallon of alcohol. At different times, he dispensed fЗiv, Oii, fЗviii, and fЗiv. What volume of alcohol was left?

$$f\text{З}iv = 4 f\text{З}$$
$$Oii = 2 \times 16 \, f\text{З} = 32 f\text{З}$$
$$f\text{З}viii = 8 f\text{З}$$
$$f\text{З}iv = \frac{1}{2} f\text{З}$$
$$44\frac{1}{2} \, f\text{З}, \textit{ total dispensed.}$$

$$1 \text{ gal} = 128 f\text{З}$$
$$- 44\frac{1}{2} \, f\text{З}$$
$$83\frac{1}{2} \, f\text{З} = 5 \text{ pt } 3 \, f\text{З} \, 4 \, f\text{з, } \textit{answer.}$$

Multiplication and Division. A *simple* quantity may be multiplied or divided by any *pure* number, such as *12 × 10 oz = 120 oz or 7 lb 8 oz.*

If, however, *both* terms in division are derived from denominate numbers (as when we express one quantity as a fraction of another), they must be reduced to a *common* denomination before division.

A *compound* quantity is most easily multiplied or divided, and with least chance of careless error, if it is first reduced to a *simple* quantity: *2 × 8 fЗ 6 fз = 2 × 70 fз = 140 fз or 17 fЗ 4 fз.*

The *result* of multiplication should be (1) left as it is, if it is to be used in further calculations, (2) simplified, or (3) reduced to weighable or measurable denominations.

Examples:

A prescription for 24 powders calls for gr ¼ of ingredient A, Эss of ingredient B, and gr v of ingredient C in each powder. How much of each ingredient should be used in compounding the prescription?

$$24 \times \text{gr } \frac{1}{4} = 6 \text{ gr of ingredient A,}$$
$$24 \times \frac{1}{2}Э = 12 \, Э, \text{ or } 4 \, З \text{ of ingredient B,}$$
$$24 \times \text{gr v} = 120 \text{ gr, or } 2 \, З \text{ of ingredient C, } \textit{answers.}$$

A formula for 24 capsules contains Эss of one ingredient, Зi of another, and Зiiss of a third. How many grains of each ingredient will be contained in each capsule?

$$Эss = 10 \text{ gr, and } ^{10}\!/_{24} \text{ gr} = {}^{5}\!/_{12} \text{ gr,}$$
$$Зi = 60 \text{ gr, and } ^{60}\!/_{24} \text{ gr} = 2\frac{1}{2} \text{ gr,}$$
$$Зiiss = 150 \text{ gr, and } ^{150}\!/_{24} \text{ gr} = 6\frac{1}{4} \text{ gr, } \textit{answers.}$$

How many 15-minim doses can be obtained from a mixture containing fЗiii of one ingredient and fзii of another?

$$f\text{З}iii = 3 \times 480 \, \text{m} = 1440 \, \text{m}$$
$$f\text{з}ii = 2 \times 60 \, \text{m} = \underline{ 120\text{m}}$$
$$1560 \, \text{m, } \textit{total.}$$
$$^{1560}\!/_{15} \text{ doses} = 104 \text{ doses, } \textit{answer.}$$

RELATIONSHIP OF AVOIRDUPOIS AND APOTHECARIES' WEIGHTS

As noted previously, the *grain* is the same in both the avoirdupois and apothecaries' systems of weight, but other denominations with the same names are not equal.

To convert from either system to the other, first reduce the given quantity to grains in the one system, and then reduce to any desired denomination in the other system.

The custom of buying chemicals by avoirdupois weight and compounding prescriptions by apothecaries' weight leads to problems, many of which can be most conveniently solved by proportion.

Examples:

Convert ℥ii ʒii to avoirdupois weight.

$$℥ii = 2 \times 480 \text{ gr} = 960 \text{ gr}$$
$$ʒii = 2 \times 60 \text{ gr} = 120 \text{ gr}$$

Total: 1080 gr

$$1 \text{ oz} = 437.5 \text{ gr}$$

$$\frac{1080}{437.5} \text{ oz} = 2 \text{ oz, } 205 \text{ gr, } answer.$$

How many grains of a chemical are left in a 1-oz (avoir.) bottle after ʒvii are dispensed from it?

$$1 \text{ oz} = 1 \times 437.5 \text{ gr} = 437.5 \text{ gr}$$
$$ʒvii = 7 \times 60 \text{ gr} = 420.0 \text{ gr}$$

Difference: 17.5 gr, *answer.*

If a drug costs $8.75 per oz (avoir.), what is the cost of 2 ʒ?

$$1 \text{ oz} = 437.5 \text{ gr, and } 2 ʒ = 120 \text{ gr}$$

$$\frac{437.5 \text{ (gr)}}{120 \text{ (gr)}} = \frac{8.75 \text{ (\$)}}{x \text{ (\$)}}$$

$$x = \$2.40, \ answer.$$

Practice Problems

1. Reduce each of the following quantities to grains:
    (a) ʒii ℈iss.
    (b) ℥ii ʒiss.
    (c) ℥i ʒss ℈i.
    (d) ʒi ℈i gr x.

2. Reduce Oi f℥ii to fluidrachms.

3. Reduce each of the following quantities to weighable apothecaries' denominations:
    (a) 158 gr
    (b) 175 gr
    (c) 210 gr
    (d) 75 gr
    (e) 96 gr

4. ℞   Phenobarbital   gr ¼
         Aspirin   gr iv
         Lactose   ad   gr vi
         D.T.D. cap. #48
         Sig. cap. i t.i.d.

What combination of individual apothecaries' weights from a standard set could a pharmacist use to weigh the amount of lactose required to fill prescription?

5. A pharmacist had 1 gallon of phenobarbital elixir. At different times, he dispensed Oi, f℥vi, fℨiv, Oss, f℥iss, and f℥xii. What volume, in fluidounces, of the elixir was left?

6. How many f℥ii-bottles of cough syrup can be obtained from 5 gallons of the cough syrup?

7. Children's chewable aspirin tablets contain 1¼ grains of aspirin in each tablet. How many tablets can be prepared from 1 avoirdupois pound of aspirin?

8. How many grains of a chemical are left in a 1-oz (avoir.) bottle after enough of it has been used to make 2000 tablets each containing $\frac{1}{200}$ gr of the chemical?

9. If a chemical costs \$10.75 per oz (avoir.), what is the cost of ℨiii?

10. How many $\frac{1}{400}$-gr tablets of nitroglycerin can a manufacturer prepare from a quantity of a trituration of nitroglycerin that contains $\frac{1}{8}$ oz of the drug?

11. A chewing gum laxative contains 1½ gr of phenolphthalein in each chewable tablet. How many tablets can be prepared from 6 avoirdupois ounces of phenolphthalein?

12. In checking a narcotic file, a pharmacist found that the following quantities of codeine sulfate had been used from a bottle originally containing 1 oz (avoir.):
    ℞1—gr v
    ℞2— Əi
    ℞3—ℨss
    ℞4—Əss
    ℞5—gr iiss
How many grains of codeine sulfate were left in the bottle?

13. A formula for a cough syrup is as follows:

Phenylpropanolamine	640 grains
Dextromethorphan HBr	512 grains
Alcohol	2 fluidounces
Cherry Syrup, to make	5 gallons

  (a) What compound apothecaries' quantities of phenylpropanolamine and dextromethorphan HBr should be weighed in preparing the formula?

  (b) What fraction of a grain of phenylpropanolamine would be contained in each fluidram of the finished product?

14. ℞   Codeine sulfate   gr iii
         Aspirin   ℨiss
         Phenacetin   ℨi
         Caffeine   Əi
         M. ft. caps. no. xxiv
         Sig. One capsule p.r.n. pain.

How many grains of each ingredient would be contained in each capsule?

15. ℞   Colchicine Tablets   gr $\frac{1}{100}$
           Disp. no. xii
           Sig. Two tablets q. 2 h. as directed.

How many such tablets can be made from a 1-oz (avoir.) package of colchicine?

16. ℞   Aminophylline   ℥ss
           Ephedrine Hydrochloride   gr vi
           Amobarbital   gr v
           M. ft. cap. no. xv
           Sig. One capsule t.i.d. p.r.n. asthma.

    (*a*) How many grains of aminophylline would be contained in each capsule?
    (*b*) What fraction of a grain of ephedrine hydrochloride would be contained in each capsule?

INTERSYSTEM CONVERSION

In pharmacy and medicine, the metric system currently predominates in use over the common systems. Most prescriptions and medication orders are written in the metric system and labeling on most prefabricated pharmaceutical products have drug strengths and dosages described in metric units. Manufacturing formulas are similarly expressed almost exclusively in metric units, replacing to a great extent use of the common systems of measurement.

On occasion, however, it may be necessary to translate a weight or measurement from units of one system to units of another system. This translation is called *conversion*.

The measurement of a denomination of one system in terms of another system is properly called a *conversion factor*. Any one conversion factor is sufficient to serve as a bridge between two systems. In practice, however, it is convenient to have a choice of several. We may use the equation *1 g = 15.432 gr,* for example, in converting a number of grams to grains, but in converting grains to grams, a more useful equation is *1 gr = 0.065 g or 65 mg.* Again, it is convenient to have one equation for converting a large denomination directly to a large denomination, and another for converting a small denomination to a small denomination.

A common question is how accurate our conversions should be. When a high degree of precision is required, *exact conversion equivalents* rounded to three significant figures should be used. In most pharmacy practice applications, however, the equivalents listed in Table AA.1 are sufficient, with two- or three-figure accuracy desired. *These equivalents should be memorized.*

Note that such equivalents may be used in two ways. For example, to convert a number of fluidounces to milliliters, *multiply* by 29.57; to convert a number of milliliters to fluidounces, *divide* by 29.57.

Some individuals prefer to set up a ratio of a known equivalent and solve conversion problems by proportion. For example, in determining the number of milliliters in 8

Table AA.1. Table of Practical Conversion Equivalents

Conversion Equivalents of Length

1 m	=	39.37	in
1 in	=	2.54	cm

Conversion Equivalents of Volume

1 mL	=	16.23	ℳ
1 ℳ	=	0.06	mL
1 f℥	=	3.69	mL
1 f℥	=	29.57	mL
1 pt	=	473	mL
1 gal (U.S.)	=	3785	mL

Conversion Equivalents of Weight

1 g	=	15.432	gr
1 kg	=	2.20	lb (avoir.)
1 gr	=	0.065	g or 65 mg
1 oz (avoir.)	=	28.35	g
1 ℥	=	31.1	g
1 lb (avoir.)	=	454	g
1 lb (apoth.)	=	373.2	g

Other Equivalents

1 oz (avoir.)	=	437.5	gr
1 ℥	=	480	gr
1 gal (U.S.)^2	=	128	f℥
1 f℥ (water)	=	455	gr

fluidounces, an equivalent relating *milliliters to fluidounces is selected* (1 f℥ = 29.57 mL) and the problem is solved by proportion as follows:

$$\frac{1 \ (f℥)}{8 \ (f℥)} = \frac{29.57 \ (mL)}{x \ (mL)}$$

$$x = 236.56 \ mL, \ \textit{answer.}$$

In using the ratio and proportion method, the equivalent that contains both the units named in the problem is the best one to use. Sometimes, more than one equivalent may be appropriate. For instance, in converting grams to grains, or vice versa, the gram-to-grain relationship is found in the following basic equivalents, 1 g = 15.432 gr and 1 gr = 0.065 g, as well as in *derived equivalents,* such as 31.1 g = 480 gr and 28.35 g = 437.5 gr. It is best to use the basic equivalents when converting from one system to another and to select the equivalent that provides the answer most readily.

In response to the question: *Must we round off results so as to contain no more significant figures than are contained in the conversion factor?*, the answer is *yes.* If we desire greater accuracy, we should use a more accurate conversion factor. But to the question: *If a formula includes the one-figure quantity 5 g, and we convert it to grains, must we round off the result to 1 significant figure?*, the answer is decidedly *no.* We should interpret the quantity given in a formula as expressing the precision we are expected to achieve in compounding—usually not less than three-figure accuracy. Hence, 5 g in a formula or prescription should be interpreted as meaning *5.00 g* or greater precision.

---

[2] The "U.S." gallon is specified because the British Imperial gallon and other counterpart measures differ substantially, as follows: British Imperial gallon, 4545 mL; pint, 568.25 mL; f℥, 28.412 mL; f℥, 3.55 mL; and, ℳ, 0.059 mL. Note, however, that the metric system of weights and measures is used in both the *United States Pharmacopeia* and the *British Pharmacopoeia.*

> For prescriptions and all other problems stated in the apothecaries' or avoirdupois systems of measurement, it is recommended that all such quantities be converted to equivalent metric quantities before solving in the usual manner described in this text.

CONVERSION OF LINEAR QUANTITIES

Metric Lengths to Common Equivalents. We may reduce any given metric length to meters and then multiply this quantity by *39.37* (the number of inches equivalent to each meter) to get inches. If the metric quantity is small, it may be more convenient to reduce it to centimeters and then divide by *2.54* to get inches.

Example:

The fiber length of a sample of purified cotton is 6.35 mm. Express the length in inches.

$$6.35 \text{ mm} = 0.635 \text{ cm}$$

Solving by proportion:

$$\frac{1 \text{ (in.)}}{x \text{ (in.)}} = \frac{2.54 \text{ (cm)}}{0.635 \text{ (cm)}}$$

$$x = 0.250 \text{ in., or } \frac{1}{4} \text{ in., } \textit{answer.}$$

Or, solving by dimensional analysis:

$$6.35 \text{ mm} \times \frac{1 \text{ cm}}{10 \text{ mm}} \times \frac{1 \text{ in}}{2.54 \text{ cm}} = 0.250 \text{ in, } \textit{answer.}$$

Common Lengths to Metric Equivalents. If given a length of a yard or more, reduce it to inches and divide by *39.37* to get meters. If given a shorter length, reduce it to inches and multiply by *2.54* to get centimeters.

Example:

A medicinal plaster measures $4\frac{1}{2}$ in. by $6\frac{1}{2}$ in. What are its dimensions in centimeters?
Assuming three-figure precision in the measurement,

$$4\frac{1}{2} \text{ or } 4.50 \times 2.54 \text{ cm} \quad = 11.4 \text{ cm wide,}$$
$$6\frac{1}{2} \text{ or } 6.50 \times 2.54 \text{ cm} \quad = 16.5 \text{ cm long, } \textit{answers.}$$

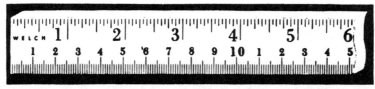

Fig. AA.2. Portion of meter stick showing relation between centimeters and inches. (Courtesy of W. M. Welch Scientific Co.)

CONVERSION OF LIQUID QUANTITIES

Metric Volumes to Apothecaries' Fluid Equivalents. For small volumes, multiply the number of milliliters by *16.23* to get minims and then reduce the result to measurable units if necessary.

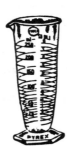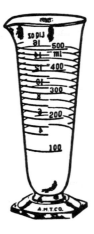

Fig. AA.3. Dual-scale conical graduates, calibrated in metric and apothecaries' units of volume. (Courtesy of Corning Glass Works and Arthur H. Thomas Co.)

For larger volumes, reduce the given volume to milliliters and divide by *29.57* to get fluidounces or by *473* to get pints.

Examples:

Convert 0.4 mL to minims.
To achieve two-figure precision,

$$0.40 \times 16.23 \, \text{m} = 6.492 \text{ or } 6.5 \, \text{m}, \textit{answer.}$$

Or, solving by dimensional analysis:

$$0.4 \text{ mL} \times \frac{16.23 \, \text{m}}{1 \text{ mL}} = 6.492 \text{ or } 6.5 \, \text{m}, \textit{answer.}$$

Convert 2.5 L to fluidounces.

$$2.5 \text{ L} = 2500 \text{ mL}$$

Solving by proportion:

$$\frac{1 \, (\text{f}\text{з})}{\text{x} \, (\text{f}\text{з})} = \frac{29.57 \, (\text{mL})}{2500 \, (\text{mL})}$$

$$\text{x} = 84.5 \, \text{f}\text{з}, \textit{answer.}$$

Or, solving by dimensional analysis:

$$2.5 \text{ L} \times \frac{1000 \text{ mL}}{1 \text{ L}} \times \frac{1 \, f\text{з}}{29.57} = 84.5 \, f\text{з}, \textit{answer.}$$

Apothecaries' Fluid Volume to Metric Equivalents. For small volumes, reduce to minims and divide by *16.23* to get milliliters.

For larger volumes, reduce to fluidounces and multiply by *29.57* to get milliliters.

Examples:

Convert fзiiss to milliliters.

$$\text{fзiiss} = 2\frac{1}{2} \times 60 \, \text{m} = 150 \, \text{m}$$

Solving by proportion:

$$\frac{1 \ (mL)}{x \ (mL)} = \frac{16.23 \ (\mathrm{m})}{150 \ (\mathrm{m})}$$

$$x = 9.24 \ mL, \ answer.$$

Or, solving by dimensional analysis:

$$2.5 \ f\mathfrak{Z} \times \frac{60 \ \mathrm{m}}{1 \ f\mathfrak{Z}} \times \frac{1 \ mL}{16.23 \ \mathrm{m}} = 9.24 \ mL, \ answer.$$

Convert Oiiss to milliliters.

$$\text{Oiiss} = 2\tfrac{1}{2} \times 16 \ f\mathfrak{Z} = 40 \ f\mathfrak{Z}$$

$$40 \times 29.57 \ mL = 1182.8 \ or \ 1180 \ mL, \ answer.$$

Or, solving by dimensional analysis:

$$2.5 \ pt \times \frac{16 f\mathfrak{Z}}{1 \ pt} \times \frac{29.57 \ mL}{1 \ f\mathfrak{Z}} = 1182.8 \ or \ 1180 \ mL, \ answer.$$

CONVERSION OF WEIGHTS

Metric Weights to Common Weights. Reduce a given quantity to grams and multiply by *15.432* or divide by *0.065* (whichever gives the answer more readily) to get grains, and reduce the quantity to any desired denomination.

For a larger quantity, divide the number of grams by *31.1* to get apothecaries' ounces, or by *28.35* to get avoirdupois ounces.

For a still larger quantity, divide the number of grams by *454* to get avoirdupois pounds.

Examples:

Convert 12.5 g to grains.

$$12.5 \times 15.432 \ gr = 192.9 \ or \ 193 \ gr, \ answer.$$

Alternate solution (about 0.5% less accurate):

$$\frac{12.5}{0.065} \ gr = 192.3 \ or \ 192 \ gr, \ answer.$$

Convert 5 mg to grains.

Solving by proportion:

$$\frac{1 \ (gr)}{x \ (gr)} = \frac{65 \ (mg)}{5 \ (mg)}$$

$$x = \tfrac{5}{65} \ gr = \tfrac{1}{13} \ gr, \ answer.$$

Convert 15 kg to avoirdupois pounds.

Solving by proportion:

$$\frac{1 \ (kg)}{15 \ (kg)} = \frac{2.2 \ (lb)}{x \ (lb)}$$

$$x = 33.0 \ lb, \ answer.$$

Common Weights to Metric Equivalents. Reduce a given small quantity to grains and multiply by 65 to get milligrams, or reduce the quantity to grains and multiply by *0.065* or divide by *15.432* (whichever gives the answer more readily) to get grams. Reduce the result to any required denomination.

For larger quantities, reduce to apothecaries' ounces and multiply by *31.1*, or to avoirdupois ounces and multiply by *28.35* to get grams.

For still larger quantities, reduce to apothecaries' pounds and multiply by *454* to get grams, and then reduce, if required, to kilograms. Alternatively, and more directly, reduce the given quantity to avoirdupois pounds and divide by *2.2* to get kilograms.

Examples:

Convert 6.2 gr to milligrams.

$$6.2 \times 65 \text{ mg} = 403 \text{ or } 400 \text{ mg, } answer.$$

Or, solving by dimensional analysis:

$$6.2 \text{ gr} \times \frac{1 \text{ g}}{15.432 \text{ gr}} \times \frac{1000 \text{ mg}}{1 \text{ g}} = 401.8 \text{ or } 400 \text{ mg, } answer.$$

How many grams are represented by 850 grains?

Solving by proportion:

$$\frac{1 \text{ (gr)}}{850 \text{ (gr)}} = \frac{0.065 \text{ (g)}}{x \text{ (g)}}$$

$$x = 55.25 \text{ or } 55 \text{ g, } answer.$$

Convert 176 avoirdupois pounds to kilograms.

$$\frac{176}{2.2} \text{ kg} = 80.0 \text{ kg, } answer.$$

Practice Problems

1. A brand of nitroglycerin transdermal patch measures 2.5 inches in diameter. Express this dimension in centimeters.

2. A mercury barometer reads 760 mm. Express this pressure in inches.

3. Convert 2 gal and 30 f℥ to liters.

4. If a mixture of powders weighing 30 g is divided into 100 dosage units, how many grains will each dosage unit weigh?

5. The inhalant dose of amyl nitrite is 0.18 mL. Express the dose in minims.

6. Ergonovine maleate ampuls each contain $\frac{1}{300}$ gr of drug. How many micrograms of ergonovine maleate are in each ampul?

7. Adhesive tape made from film has a tensile strength, determined warpwise, of not less than 3 kg per 2.54 cm of width. Convert these quantities to common system equivalents.

8. Urethral suppositories are traditionally prepared to the following lengths: 50 mm for females and 125 mm for males. Convert these dimensions to inches.

9. The average diameter of the oil globules in an emulsion is 2.5 μm. What is the average size in inches?

10. A pharmacist received a prescription calling for 30 capsules, each to contain $\frac{1}{200}$ gr of nitroglycerin. How many 0.4-mg nitroglycerin tablets would supply the amount required?

11. If a physician prescribed 4 grams of aspirin to be taken by a patient daily, about how many 5-grain tablets should the patient take each day?

12. A certain elixir contains 0.325 g of potassium thiocyanate per teaspoonful (5 mL). At \$15.35/lb, what is the cost of the potassium thiocyanate required to make 1 gallon of the elixir?

13. ℞   Codeine Sulfate   30 mg
        Acetaminophen   325 mg
        M. ft. cap. D.T.D. no. 24
        Sig. One capsule t.i.d. for pain.

    How many grains each of codeine sulfate and acetaminophen should be used in compounding the prescription?

14. If a child accidentally swallowed 2 fluidounces of Feosol® Elixir, containing $\frac{2}{3}$ gr of ferrous sulfate per 5 mL, how many milligrams of ferrous sulfate did the child ingest?

15. Sustained release tablets of nitroglycerin contain the following amounts of drug: $\frac{1}{25}$ gr, $\frac{1}{10}$ gr, and $\frac{1}{50}$ gr. Express these quantities as milligrams.

16. A physician advises an adult patient to take a children's tablet (81 mg of aspirin per tablet) daily as a precaution against a heart attack. Instead, the patient decides to cut 5-gr aspirin tablets into dosage units. How many doses could be obtained from each 5-gr tablet?

17. A hematinic tablet contains 525 mg of ferrous sulfate, which is equivalent to 105 mg of elemental iron. How many grains each of ferrous sulfate and elemental iron would a patient receive from one tablet?

18. The usual dose of colchicine for an acute gout attack is $\frac{1}{120}$ gr every hour for 8 doses. How many milligrams of colchicine are represented in the usual dose?

19. Nitrostat® Sublingual Tablets are available as $\frac{1}{200}$-gr tablets. What is the approximate equivalent in milligrams?

20. The clearance between the rotor and stator of a colloid mill is set so that particles having a diameter of approximately 0.0005 inch will be produced. What is the size, in micrometers, of the dispersed particles?

21. If f℥i of a cough syrup contains 10 gr of sodium citrate, how many milligrams are contained in 5 mL?

22. A formula for a cough syrup contains $\frac{1}{8}$ gr of codeine phosphate per teaspoonful (5 mL). How many grams of codeine phosphate should be used in preparing 1 pint of the cough syrup?

23. Premarin® Tablets are available in strengths of 0.3 mg, 0.625 mg, 0.9 mg, 1.25

mg, and 2.5 mg. If a physician wrote "Premarin® Tablets, $\frac{1}{50}$ gr," which of the available strengths should be dispensed?

24. A physician instructs an adult patient to take 165-mg aspirin tablets. How many grains of aspirin are present per tablet?

25. If 1000 mL of an intravenous fluid contain 2 g of an added antibiotic, how many grains of the antibiotic were administered to a patient who received 1 pint of the fluid?

26. If 15 mL of a potassium chloride solution contain 1.5 g of potassium chloride, equivalent to 20 mEq each of potassium and chloride, how many grams of potassium chloride and how many milliequivalents of both potassium and chloride would be present in a 60-minim dose of the solution?

27. A drug substance has been shown to be embryotoxic in rats at doses of 50 mg/kg/day. Express the dose on the basis of micrograms per pound per day.

28. Peak body stores of digoxin should be maintained at 8 to 12 μg/kg of body weight for optimum effect. Express these values in nanograms per pound.

29. Tetracycline has been shown to form a calcium complex in bone-forming tissue in infants given oral tetracycline in doses of 0.011 g/lb of body weight every 6 hours. Express the dose in terms of milligrams per kilogram of body weight.

B Some Pharmacoeconomic Calculations

The term *pharmacoeconomics* encompasses the economic aspects of drugs, from the costs associated with drug discovery and development to the costs of drug therapy analyzed against therapeutic outcomes. It includes many additional considerations, including drug product acquisition costs at the retail, institutional, and consumer levels; inventory, financial, and human resource management; cost/benefit relationships of drug therapy decisions, non-drug treatment alternatives, and health outcomes; factors associated with drug product selection and drug formulary decisions; impact of proper drug utilization on incidence of hospitalization and length of stay; economic and health consequences of patient noncompliance, drug misuse, and adverse drug reactions; demographics of medication use by patients of various age groups, gender, and socioeconomic status; as well as other factors.

Pharmacoeconomics is the subject of much current research with a broad array of information available in the primary literature and through various references and textbooks dedicated to this topic. The purpose of Appendix B is necessarily limited to some introductory calculations associated with drug and drug product selection, drug acquisition costs, and dispensing fees.

COST CONSIDERATIONS OF DRUG AND DRUG PRODUCT SELECTION

Drug therapy and other means of treatment (e.g., surgery) are intended to serve the health care interests of the patient while being cost effective. In prescribing drug therapy, clinical as well as economic factors are important considerations in the selection of the drug substance and drug product. For example, if an expensive drug reduces morbidity and hospitalization time, it is considered both therapeutically advantageous and cost effective. If, however, a less expensive drug would provide therapeutic benefit comparable to the more expensive drug, the less costly drug is likely to be selected for use.

In general, new drug entities and/or novel dosage forms that are protected by patents and are available from only a single source are more expensive than older, off-patent drugs available from multiple manufacturers or distributors. *Multisource pharmaceuticals* are generally lower priced because, unlike the innovator product, they do not bear the original research costs incurred in developing and bringing the new drug to market. Multisource pharmaceuticals generally are available to the pharmacist both as brand name and generic products and at a range of prices. For economic reasons, the prescribing physician, patient, health care institution, state or federally sponsored program, or other third party payer may request or reimburse only for the dispensing of a generic product, when available.

It is common practice for drug use decision-makers, such as hospital drug formulary committees, to establish a list of drugs approved for use and funding that balances therapeutic outcome and cost-containment goals. Drug and drug product selection choices may be presented to prescribers on a cost-per-day or cost-per-course of treatment basis.

Cost Differential Between Drugs. Computing the cost differential between two or more drug products involves the following.

Example:

An antihypertensive drug is available from various manufacturers at prices per 100 tablets ranging from $6.25 to $25.50, with a mean price of $10.75. If a patient presents a prescription for a 6-month supply of the drug calling for two tablets to be taken daily, calculate the differentials in the cost of the drug to the pharmacy between the highest, mean, and lowest cost products.

6 month supply   = approximately 180 days
2 tablets a day × 180 days   = 360 tablets

lowest price:

$$\$6.25/100 \text{ tablets} = \$0.0625/\text{tablet} \times 360 \text{ tablets} = \$22.50$$

Mean price:

$$\$10.75/100 \text{ tablets} = \$0.1075/\text{tablet} \times 360 \text{ tablets} = \$38.70$$

Highest price:

$$\$25.50/100 \text{ tablets} = \$0.255/\text{tablet} \times 360 \text{ tablets} = \$91.80$$

Differentials:
Highest price to lowest price:

$$\$91.80 - \$22.50 = \$69.30, \textit{answer.}$$

Highest price to mean price:

$$\$91.80 - \$38.70 = \$53.10, \textit{answer.}$$

Mean price to lowest price:

$$\$38.70 - \$22.50 = \$16.20, \textit{answer.}$$

Depending on which product is dispensed, these differentials would be reflected in the prescription price charged to the patient.

Relative Cost of Alternative Regimens. Computing the relative cost of drug-regimen alternatives involves the following.

Examples:

An antianginal drug is available in a three-times-a-day tablet at $42.50/100 tablets; in a twice-a-day tablet at $64.00/100 tablets; and in a once-a-day tablet at $80.20/100 tablets. Which form would be most economical to a compliant patient?

Cost for each type:

Three-times-a-day, $0.425/tablet × 3   = $1.28/day
Twice-a-day, $0.64/tablet × 2   = $1.28/day
Once-a-day, $0.802/tablet × 1   = $0.80/day
The once-a-day tablet is most economical, *answer.*

Using a hospital drug formulary, a physician narrows her choice of cephalosporin antimicrobial agents to three: one administered every 8 hours and costing the hospital $5.50 per dose, another administered every 6 hours and costing $4.74 per dose, and the third administered every 24 hours and costing $24.40 per dose. Discounting personnel time, which drug is most economical? (Note that personnel time in preparing and administering drug therapy and any associated costs, such as intravenous administration sets, must be considered when evaluating the *total cost* of drug therapy.)

First drug: $5.50/dose $\times$ 3   = $16.50/day
Second drug: $4.74/dose $\times$ 4   = $18.96/day
Third drug: $24.40/dose, $\times$ 1   = $24.40/day
The first drug is most economical, *answer*.

DISCOUNTS

Pharmacists purchase prescription and nonprescription drugs and other merchandise from wholesalers, distributors, and manufacturers. A pharmacy's actual acquisition cost (AAC) for a given product is the *trade price*, or the basic list price to the pharmacy, less all discounts that are applied.

Discounts provided by suppliers may be based on quantity buying and/or payment of invoices within a specified time period. In addition, for nonprescription products, discounts may be available for certain seasonal or other promotional products, bonuses in terms of free merchandise, and advertising and display allowances. These discounts provide the pharmacy with a means of increasing the gross profit on selected merchandise.

Net Cost Given List Price and Allowable Discount. Computing the net cost of merchandise, given the list price and allowable discount, involves the following.

Example:

The list price of an antihistamine elixir is $6.50 per pint, less 40%. What is the net cost per pint of the elixir?

List Price		Discount		Net Cost
100%	−	40%	=	60%
$6.50	×	0.60	=	$3.90, *answer*.

Several discounts may be allowed on promotional deals. For example, the list price on some merchandise may be subject to a trade discount of 33.5%, plus a quantity discount of 12% and a cash discount of 2% for prompt payment of the invoice. This chain of deductions, sometimes referred to as a *series discount*, may be converted to a single discount equivalent. In such cases, the discounts in the series cannot be figured by adding them; rather, the first discount is deducted from the list price and each successive discount is taken on the balance remaining after deduction of the preceding discount. The order in which the discounts in a series discount are taken is immaterial.

Net Cost Given List Price and a Series of Discounts. Computing this net cost involves the following.

Example:

The list price of 12 bottles (100 count) of analgesic tablets is $36.00, less a trade discount of $33\frac{1}{3}$%. If purchased in quantities of 12 dozens, an additional discount of 10% is allowed by the manufacturer, plus a 2% cash discount for payment of the invoice within 10 days of billing. Calculate the net cost of 144 bottles (100 count) of the analgesic tablets when purchased under the terms of the offer.

List price of 12 (100 count)   = $36.00
List price of 144 (100 count)   = $432.00

100% − $33\frac{1}{3}$%   = $66\frac{2}{3}$%   100% − 10% = 90%   100% − 2% = 98%
$432.00 × $66\frac{2}{3}$%   = $288.00, cost after $33\frac{1}{3}$% is deducted
$288.00 × 90%   = $259.20, cost after 10% is deducted
$259.20 × 98%   = $254.02, net cost, *answer*.

Single Discount Equivalent to a Series of Discounts. To compute a single discount equivalent to a series of discounts, subtract each discount in the series from 100% and multiply the net percentages. The product thus obtained is subtracted from 100% to give the single discount equivalent to the series of discounts.

Example:

A promotional deal provides a trade discount of 33.5%, an off invoice allowance of 12%, and a display allowance of 5%. Calculate the single discount equivalent to these deductions.

$$100\% - 33.5\% \quad = 66.5\% \quad 100\% - 12\% = 88\% \quad 100\% - 5\% = 95\%$$

$$0.665 \times 0.88 \times 0.95 \quad = 0.556 \text{ or } 55.6\% = \% \text{ to be paid}$$
$$\text{Discount} \quad = 100\% - 55.6\% = 44.4\%, \textit{answer.}$$

MARKUP

The term *markup*, sometimes used interchangeably with the term *margin of profit (gross profit)*, refers to the difference between the cost of merchandise and its selling price. For example, if a pharmacist buys an article for $1.50 and sells it for $2.50, the markup (or gross profit) as a dollars-and-cents item is $1.00.

Markup percent (percent of gross profit) refers to the markup (gross profit) divided by the selling price. The expression of the percent of markup may be somewhat ambiguous because it may be based on either the cost or the selling price of merchandise. In modern retail practice, this percentage is invariably based on selling price, and when reference is made to markup percent (or percent of gross profit), it means the percentage that the markup is of the selling price. If, however, a pharmacist chooses, for convenience, to base percent markup on the cost of merchandise, he or she may do so providing not overlooked is the fact that the markup on cost must yield the desired percent of gross profit on the selling price.

Calculating the selling price of merchandise to yield a given percent of gross profit on the cost involves the following.

Example:

The cost of 100 antacid tablets is $2.10. What should be the selling price per 100 tablets to yield a 66⅔% gross profit on the cost?

$$\text{Cost} \times \% \text{ of gross profit} \quad = \text{Gross profit}$$
$$\$2.10 \times 66\tfrac{2}{3}\% \quad = \$1.40$$
$$\text{Cost} + \text{Gross profit} \quad = \text{Selling price}$$
$$\$2.10 + \$1.40 \quad = \$3.50, \textit{answer.}$$

Calculating the selling price of merchandise to yield a given percent of gross profit on the selling price involves the following.

Example:

The cost of 100 antacid tablets is $2.10. What should be the selling price per 100 tablets to yield a 40% gross profit on the selling price?

$$\text{Selling price} \quad = 100\%$$
$$\text{Selling price} - \text{Gross profit} \quad = \text{Cost}$$
$$100\% - 40\% \quad = 60\%$$

$$\frac{60 \ (\%)}{100 \ (\%)} = \frac{(\$) \ 2.10}{(\$) \ x}$$

$$x = \$3.50, \ answer.$$

Calculating the cost of merchandise given the selling price and percent of gross profit on the cost involves the following.

Example:

A bottle of headache tablets is sold for $2.25, thereby yielding a gross profit of 60% on the cost. What was the cost of the bottle of tablets?

$$
\begin{aligned}
\text{Cost} + \text{Gross Profit} &= \text{Selling Price} \\
x + 0.6x &= \$2.25 \\
1.6x &= \$2.25 \\
x &= \$1.40, \ answer.
\end{aligned}
$$

Calculating the percent markup on the cost that will yield a desired percent of gross profit on the selling price involves the following.

Example:

What should the percent markup on the cost of an item be to yield a 40% gross profit on the selling price?

$$
\begin{aligned}
\text{Selling price} &= 100\% \\
\text{Selling price} - \text{Gross profit} &= \text{Cost} \\
100\% - 40\% &= 60\%
\end{aligned}
$$

$$\frac{\text{Cost as \% of selling price}}{\text{Selling price as \%}} = \frac{\text{Gross profit as \% of selling price}}{x \ (\%)}$$

$$x = \% \ \text{gross profit on the cost}$$

$$\frac{60 \ (\%)}{100 \ (\%)} = \frac{40 \ (\%)}{x \ (\%)}$$

$$x = 66\tfrac{2}{3}\%, \ answer.$$

PRESCRIPTION PRICING

Each pharmacy should have a uniform and consistently applied system of prescription pricing that ensures a fair return on investment and costs and enables the pharmacy to provide the needed services to the community.

Although many methods of prescription pricing have been used over the years, the following are the most common:[1]

1. *Percent Markup*. In this common method, the desired percent markup is taken of the cost of the ingredients and *added to* the cost of the ingredients to obtain the prescription price. The percent markup applied may be varied depending on the cost of the ingredients,

---

[1] Adapted from Ansel, H.C.: The prescription. In *Remington's Pharmaceutical Sciences*, 18th Ed. Easton, PA, Mack Publishing Co., 1990, pp. 1828-1844.

with a lower percent markup generally used for prescription items of higher cost and a higher percent markup applied for prescription items of lower cost.

Cost of ingredients + (cost of ingredients × % markup) = prescription price

Example:

If the cost of the quantity of a drug product to be dispensed is $4.00 and the pharmacist applies an 80% markup on cost, what would be the prescription price?

$4.00 + ($4.00 × 80%) = $4.00 + $3.20 = $7.20, answer.

2. *Percent Markup Plus a Minimum Professional Fee.* In this method, both a percent markup and a minimum professional fee are added to the cost of the ingredients. The percent markup in this method is usually lower than that used in the method just described. The minimum fee is established to recover the combined cost of the container, label, overhead, and professional services.

Cost of ingredients + (cost of ingredients × % markup) + minimum professional fee = prescription price

Example:

If the cost of the quantity of a drug product to be dispensed is $4.00 and the pharmacist applies a 40% markup on cost plus a professional fee of $2.25, what would be the prescription price?

$4.00 + ($4.00 × 40%) + $2.25 = $4.00 + $1.60 + $2.25 = $7.85, answer.

3. *Professional Fee.* This method involves the addition of a specified professional fee to the cost of the ingredients used in filling a prescription. The professional fee includes all the dispensing costs and professional remuneration. A *true* professional fee is independent of the cost of the ingredients and thus does not vary from one prescription to another. Some pharmacists, however, use a *variable* or *sliding* professional fee method whereby the amount of the fee varies on the basis of the cost of the ingredients. By this method, the greater the cost of prescription ingredients, the greater the fee, the rationale being that the cost of inventory maintenance must be recovered in this manner.

A pharmacy may determine its professional fee by (1) averaging the amount previously charged, above the cost of ingredients, for prescriptions dispensed over a specified period of time, or (2) using a more exacting cost analysis method in which all costs attributed to the prescription department are divided by the prescription volume in determining the actual cost of filling a prescription, with the profit and desired fee then determined. Pharmacies that charge a professional fee commonly make adjustments for prescriptions requiring compounding to compensate for the extra time, materials, and equipment used.

Cost of ingredients + professional fee = prescription price

Example:

If the cost of the quantity of a drug product to be dispensed is $4.00 and the pharmacist applies a professional fee of $4.25, what would be the prescription price?

$4.00 + $4.25 = $8.25, answer.

Many governmental agencies, such as state human services departments, and many insurance companies have adopted the professional fee method for the reimbursement of pharmacists in filling prescriptions covered under their programs. Such third-party payers establish the professional fee to be used with pharmacists interested in participating in the programs. In addition, because the actual acquisition cost of a given drug product may vary substantially between pharmacies, depending on the discounts received, most third-party payer use the "average wholesale price (AWP)" less an established percentage as the cost basis for the drug in reimbursement programs. The AWP is obtained from commercial listings. The reimbursed amount is calculated from a predetermined formula, e.g., "AWP less 10% plus $4.50 professional fee." Many third-party programs have a "copayment" provision, which requires the patient to pay a portion of the charge for each prescription filled.

Examples:

If a third-party payer reimburses a pharmacy "AWP less 15%" plus a professional fee of $4.75, what would be the total reimbursement on a prescription calling for 24 capsules having an AWP of $25.00 per 100 capsules?

$$\begin{align}
\text{AWP for 24 capsules} &= \$6.00, \text{ less } 15\% = \$5.10 \\
\$5.10 + \$4.75 &= \$9.85, \textit{answer.}
\end{align}$$

If a pharmacy provider contract calls for a copayment of $2.00 to be paid directly to the pharmacy for each prescription the patient has filled, how much would the third party reimburse the pharmacy in the preceding example?

$9.85 − $2.00 = $7.85, *answer.*

A patient's individual or group health insurance coverage often provides reimbursement benefits only after a patient reaches a self-paid level (the stated "deductible" amount) of his or her health care expenses, after which the coverage may pay fully or partially for certain covered expenses.

Example:

A patient's health insurance covers 80% of prescription drug costs after a $200.00 deductible is reached. If after making payments of $184.00 toward the deductible amount, a patient pays a pharmacy $86.00 for a prescription, how much can he expect to be reimbursed by his insurance carrier?

$$\begin{align}
\$200.00 - \$184.00 &= \$16.00, \text{ remaining toward the deductible amount} \\
\$86.00 - \$16.00 &= \$70.00, \text{ covered expense} \\
\$70.00 \times 80\% &= \$56.00 \text{ reimbursement, } \textit{answer.}
\end{align}$$

Practice Problems

1. The drug hydralazine may be administered intravenously when needed to control hypertension at 20-mg doses in D5W every 12 hours for 48 hours, after which the patient is converted to oral dosage, 10-mg tablets four times per day for 2 days, then 25-mg tablets four times per day for the next 5 days. If the 20-mg i.v. ampul costs $6.00; 10-mg tablets, $18.00/100 tablets; 25-mg tablets, $26.00/100 tablets; and D5W, $10.00 per bottle, calculate the *average daily* costs of intravenous versus oral therapy.

2. A physician has a choice of prescribing the following ACE inhibitor drugs to treat hypertension, with the pharmacist's cost of each, per 100 tablets, given in parentheses: benazepril, 10 mg ($63.00); captopril, 25 mg ($59.00); enalapril, 5 mg ($84.00); and fosinopril, 10 mg ($70.00). Each drug is once-a-day dosing except for captopril tablets, which are taken twice a day. Calculate the 30-day medication cost for each drug.

3. The cost to a hospital of the drug vecuronium is $16.97 per 10-mg vial. If the drug is administered by intermittent injection at 0.15 mg/kg/hr for 24 hours, calculate the daily cost of the drug used for a 70-kg patient.

4. If the drug in the preceding problem may be administered to the same patient by continuous infusion (rather than by intermittent injection) with a 0.1 mg/kg loading dose and subsequent doses of 0.05 mg/kg for the next 23 hours, calculate the daily cost of the drug by this route of administration.

5. The intravenous dosing schedules and costs of the following cephalosporin antimicrobial agents are: cefazolin, 1 g every 8 hours ($3.00); cefoxitin, 1 g every 6 hours ($6.24); and ceftriaxone, 1 g every 24 hours ($31.39). Compare the daily cost of each drug.

6. The drug diltiazem is available as follows: 60-mg tablets taken q.i.d. ($63.00/100 tablets); 120-mg sustained release capsules taken b.i.d. ($110.00/100 capsules); and 240-mg sustained release capsules taken once daily ($162.00/100 capsules). Compare the cost per month of each dosage form.

7. Calculate the single discount equivalent to each of the following series of deductions:
   (a) A trade discount of 40%, a quantity discount of 5% and a cash discount of 2%.
   (b) A trade discount of 33⅓%, a 10% off invoice allowance, and a 6% display allowance.
   (c) A trade discount of 30%, a display allowance of 5%, and a cash discount of 2%.

8. If an ointment is listed at $5.40/lb, less 33⅓%, what is the net cost of 10 lb?

9. A pain relief lotion is listed at $52.35 per dozen 6-oz bottles, less a discount of 33.5%. The manufacturer offers 2 bottles free with the purchase of 10 on a promotional deal. What is the net cost per bottle when the lotion is purchased on the deal?

10. A cough syrup is listed at $54.00 per gallon, less 40%. What is the net cost of 1 pint of the cough syrup?

11. A pharmacist receives a bill of goods amounting to $1,200.00, less a 5% discount for quantity buying and a 2% cash discount for paying the invoice within 10 days. What is the net amount of the bill?

12. If a cough syrup is listed at $54.00 per dozen 4-oz bottles, less a discount of 33.4%, and the manufacturer provides 1 unit free with 11 on an order for 1 gross, what is the net cost per bottle of the cough syrup?

13. A decongestant spray lists at $42.24 per dozen units, less a discount of 33⅓%, plus an additional promotional discount of 10%. Calculate the net cost per unit.

14. The list price of an antacid tablet is $168.75 per 5000, less 40%. What is the net cost of 100 tablets?

15. Calculate the difference in the net cost of a bill of goods amounting to $2500 if the bill is discounted at 45%, and if it is discounted at 33% and 12%.

16. ℞   Glycerin   120.0
        Boric Acid Solution

Witch Hazel	aa ad	500.0

Sig. Apply to affected areas.

Witch hazel is listed at $12.00 per gallon, less 34.5%. What is the net cost of the amount needed in filling the prescription?

17. ℞   Belladonna Tincture   30.0
       Phenobarbital Elixir   ad   240.0
       Sig. 5 mL in water a.c.

Belladonna tincture costs $12.40 per pint, and the phenobarbital elixir was bought on a special deal at $31.50 per gallon, less 15%. Calculate the net cost of the ingredients in the prescription.

18. Zinc oxide ointment in 1-oz tubes is purchased at $10.80 per 12 tubes. At what price per tube must it be sold to yield a gross profit of $66\frac{2}{3}\%$ on the cost?

19. A jar of cleansing cream is sold for $7.50, thereby yielding a gross profit of 60% on the cost. What did it cost?

20. A bottle of mouth wash costs $2.40. At what price must it be sold to yield a gross profit of 40% on the selling price?

21. If a surgical lubricating jelly is listed at $21.75 per dozen tubes, with discounts of 15% and 5% when purchased in gross lots, what is the net cost per tube?

22. A topical antibacterial ointment is listed at $3.70 per tube, less 35%, and the manufacturer allows 6 tubes free with the purchase of 66 tubes.
    (a) What is the net cost per tube?
    (b) At what price per tube must the ointment be sold to yield a gross profit of 45% on the selling price?

23. Twelve (12) bottles of 100 analgesic tablets cost $18.96 when bought on a promotional deal. If the tablets sell for $2.69 per 100, what percent of gross profit is realized on the selling price?

24. If chloroform (specific gravity 1.475) costs $6.00/lb, at what price per pint must it be sold to yield a gross profit of 50% on the selling price?

25. A pharmacist buys 20,000 tablets for $400.00 with discounts of 16% and 2%. At what price per 100 must the tablets be sold to yield a gross profit of 40% on the selling price?

26. A pharmacist buys glycerin (specific gravity 1.25) for $4.25/lb. At what price must 8 fluidounces be sold to realize a gross profit of 50% on the selling price?

27. A pharmacist sells a bottle of tablets for $3.75, thereby realizing a gross profit of 60% on the cost. Calculate the cost of the tablets.

28. An oil is purchased for $7.00 per liter. If a pint is sold for $8.00, what percent of gross profit on the selling price is realized?

29. Calculate the difference between a single discount of 40% and successive discounts of 33.5% and 6.5%.

30. A pharmacist finds that a gross profit of 40% on the selling price is realized if a medicine is sold for $7.50 per bottle. What percentage of gross profit does this represent if based on the cost of the medicine?

31. A pharmacist sells a jar of a cosmetic cream for $9.75, thereby realizing a profit of 60% on the selling price. Calculate the cost of the cosmetic cream.

32. A pharmacist bought 5 gallons of an elixir for $150.00, which was 20% off the list price. Four (4) gallons of the elixir were sold at 10% off the list and the balance at 10% above list. What was the percent of gross profit, the basis of the calculation to be the selling price?

33. A pharmacist purchased 1 dozen bottles of an ophthalmic solution listed at $75.00 per dozen. A discount of 35% was allowed on the purchase plus a 2% discount for paying the bill before the tenth day of the month. At what price per unit must the solution be sold to yield a gross profit of 50% on the selling price?

34. At what price must a pharmacist mark an item that costs $2.60 so that the selling price can be reduced 25% for a special sale and still yield a gross profit of 35% on the cost price?

35. A prescription item costs a pharmacist $8.40. Using a markup of 50% on the cost, what would be the price of the dispensed prescription?

36. A prescription item costs a pharmacist $12.20. Using a markup of 25% on the cost plus a professional fee of $4.75, calculate the prescription price.

37. A pharmacist decided to determine a professional fee by calculating the average markup on a series of previously filled prescriptions. A sample of 100 prescriptions had a total cost to the pharmacist of $850 and a total prescription price of $1,310. Calculate the average professional fee that could be used in prescription pricing.

38. A recent annual survey of pharmacies revealed the following:
    Number of Rxs filled: 45,097
    Number of refill Rxs: 18,595
    Number of third party Rxs: 20,912
    Rx dollar volume: $1,039,005
    Total (store) dollar volume: $5,102,809
    Using these data, calculate (a) the average prescription price, (b) the percentage of new prescriptions filled, (c) the percentage of third-party prescriptions, and (d) the percentage of store volume attributed to the prescriptions.

C Graphical Methods

The accurate and effective presentation and interpretation of data are important components of pharmacy and the biomedical sciences. Data obtained from laboratory research, through clinical investigations, and as a result of studies of drug utilization, health care statistics, demographics, and economics are prominently presented in the scientific and professional literature. These data provide the basis for further research and for professional judgment. Therefore, it is important for students in all health professions to become familiar with the various techniques of data presentation and interpretation.

In pharmacy, as in other sciences, the study of the influence of one variable on another is common. Curves, and the equations they represent, give a clear picture of tabulated data and the relationship between variables. Pharmacists are often called on to plot experimental data, interpret graphical material and equations, and manipulate the relationship between curves and their equations.

For simple first-degree equations, in which the variable contains no exponent greater than 1, a straight line will result when the two variables are plotted on rectangular graph paper (rectangular coordinates). Such pharmaceutical phenomena as the influence of temperature on solubility, decomposition of drug suspensions, influence of drug dose on pharmacologic response, and standard assay curves usually give straight line relationships when plotted on rectangular graph paper.

Exponential or logarithmic relationships are common in pharmaceutical studies. Drug degradation in solution, chemical equilibria, and vapor pressure changes are some examples of exponential phenomena. If a logarithmic or exponential relationship occurs between the two variables, a straight line usually can be obtained by plotting the logarithm of one variable against the other variable or plotting the data on semilogarithmic graph paper.

LINEAR RELATIONSHIPS ON RECTANGULAR GRAPH PAPER

Several straight lines and their corresponding equations on rectangular graph paper are presented in Figure AC.1. The plotting of data on rectangular coordinates should be familiar to all students. The horizontal axis is called the X axis, and the magnitude of the independent variable is plotted along this horizontal scale. The other variable, the dependent variable, is measured along the vertical or Y axis. A point on any of the curves in Figure AC.1 is defined by two coordinates. The x value, or abscissa, is the distance from the Y axis, and the y value, or ordinate, is the distance from the X axis. By convention, the x value is designated first and the y value second. For example, the point 1, 3 when substituted into the equation $y = -2x + 5$ gives $3 = -2 + 5$ and, as expected, satisfies the equation. The point 0, 4.5 satisfies the equation $y = 4.5$, whereas the point 2.5, 0 satisfies the equation $x = 2.5$ because both of these curves run parallel to the X or Y axis, respectively.

The fundamental algebraic equation that describes first-degree or straight line equations is:

$$y = mx + b$$

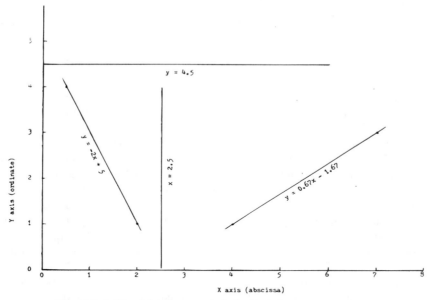

Fig. AC.1. Straight lines and their first-degree equations.

in which m and b are constants. The constant m is the slope of the line. It is a ratio of a change in y with a corresponding change in x and is expressed as $m = \Delta y/\Delta x$. The constant b is the y intercept when $x = 0$ and can usually be determined by extrapolating the straight line to the Y axis.

The most convenient equation for determining the equation for the straight line that passes through two given points is the two-point form of the straight line equation,

$$y - y_1 = \frac{y_2 - y_1}{x_2 - x_1}(x - x_1)$$

The results of measuring the ultraviolet absorbance (UV) of various concentrations of drug A and drug B in solutions are shown in Table AC.1.

Table AC.1. Data for Ultraviolet Absorbance of Various Concentrations of Drug

x Drug Concentration ($\mu g/mL$)	y Absorbance Drug A	y Absorbance Drug B
1.0	0.10	0.195
2.0	0.20	0.33
3.0	0.30	0.465
4.0	0.40	0.60
5.0	0.50	—

The data of Table AC.1 are plotted in Figure AC.2, and the results are two straight lines with positive slopes. By selecting two widely separated points $(1, 0.1)$ and $(5, 0.5)$ on the drug A curve and substituting the values into the two-point equation as follows,

$$y - 0.1 = \frac{0.5 - 0.1}{5 - 1}(x - 1)$$

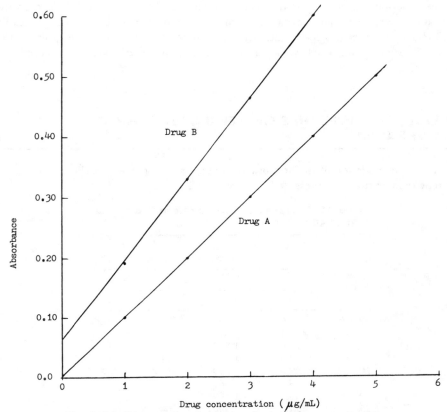

Fig. AC.2. Plot of absorbance against drug concentration.

the equation for the straight line becomes

$$y - 0.1 = \frac{0.4}{4.0} (x - 1)$$
$$y - 0.1 = 0.1 (x - 1)$$
$$y - 0.1 = 0.1x - 0.1$$
$$y = 0.1x$$

Because the line passes through the origin, the constant b in the straight line equation is 0.

The equation of the line for drug B is obtained the same way, using the points (1, 0.195) and (4, 0.60) and substituting into the two-point equation to give:

$$y - 0.195 = \frac{0.6 - 0.195}{4 - 1} (x - 1)$$

$$y - 0.195 = \frac{0.405}{3} (x - 1)$$

$$y - 0.195 = 0.135x - 0.135$$

$$y = 0.135x + 0.06$$

This equation can now be used to calculate one variable given a value for the other. For example, what is the concentration of drug B in solution when the absorbance reading is 0.30? Substituting into the equation gives $0.30 = 0.135x + 0.06$ and solving for x gives 1.78 μg/mL. The same value can also be determined directly from the curve in Figure AC.2.

LINEAR RELATIONSHIPS ON SEMILOGARITHMIC GRAPH PAPER

Data for the degradation of an antibiotic in aqueous solution over a period of time at two different temperatures are presented in Table AC.2.

Table AC.2. Decrease of Antibiotic in Solution at 30° and 40°C

| Time (Days) x | Concentration (mg/mL) (y) and Logarithm of Concentration (Log y) | | | |
| | at 30°C | | at 40°C | |
	y	Log y	y	Log y
0	80.0	1.903	80	1.903
2	72.1	1.858	63	1.799
3	69.0	1.839	56.2	1.750
5	62.0	1.792	44.8	1.651
10	49.0	1.690	25.2	1.401
15	38.5	1.586	14.2	1.152
20	30.5	1.480	—	—
25	24.0	1.380	—	—

Three different ways of plotting these data are shown in Figures AC.3 to AC.5. In Figure AC.3, the experimental measurements are plotted directly on rectangular graph paper to give curvilinear lines typical of exponential phenomena. In Figure AC.4, the logarithms of the concentrations are plotted against time on rectangular coordinate paper and the resulting curves are straight lines. In Figure AC.5, the concentration values are plotted on semilogarithmic paper and the curves are straight lines equivalent to those in Figure AC.4. Figure AC.5 is convenient for reading the concentration values directly from the graph, whereas Figure AC.4 is more convenient for obtaining the straight line equation of each curve.

The straight line equation that describes the degradation of antibiotic in solution at 40°C is determined by using the two-point equation:

$$\log y - \log y_1 = \frac{\log y_2 - \log y_1}{x_2 - x_1}(x - x_1)$$

$$\log y - 1.903 = \frac{1.152 - 1.903}{15 - 0}(x - 0)$$

$$\log y - 1.903 = 0.05x$$

$$\log y = -0.05x + 1.903$$

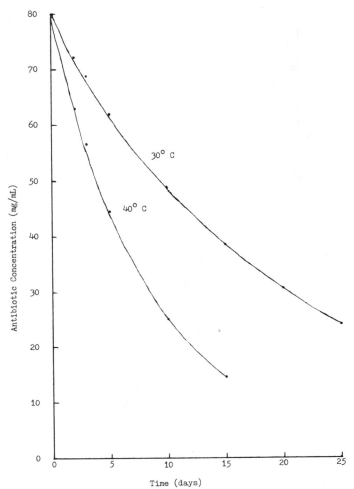

Fig. AC.3. Concentration values plotted on rectangular graph paper.
Figs. AC.3 to AC.5. Three different ways of plotting the concentration of antibiotic (y)
as a function of time (x).

OTHER METHODS OF DATA PRESENTATION:
TABLES AND CHARTS

As demonstrated in the preceding discussion, plots of data are commonly used to describe the relationships between two or more variables. Absolute data often are best presented by *tables,* which indicate the precise values. Others methods of data treatment, such as *histograms, bar charts, and circular* or *pie charts,* effectively illustrate trends represented by the data.[1,2]

   Tables are a common and useful means of presenting established data, such as the Table of Atomic Weights (back inside cover), as well as experimental research results,

---

[1] Simmonds, D., ed.: *Charts and Graphs.* Lancaster, England, MTP Press Limited, 1980.
[2] Bolton, S.: Data graphics. In *Pharmaceutical Statistics: Practical and Clinical Applications,* New York, Marcel Dekker, Inc., 1984, pp. 32–49.

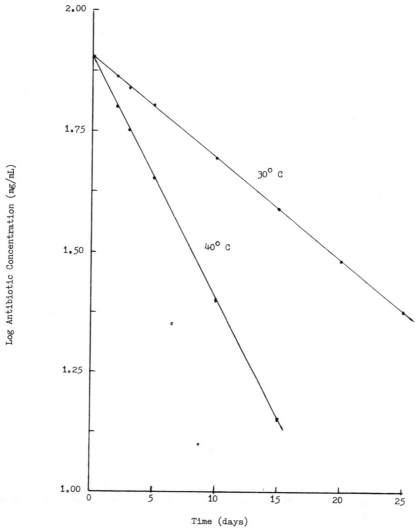

Fig. AC.4. Logarithms of concentration values plotted against time on rectangular coordinate paper.

exemplified by Table AC.3. When properly constructed with clear column headings, tables provide a quick and accurate means of finding the data item desired through right angle vertical and horizontal location.

Example:

Using Table AC.3, determine the C_{max} for subject 1 and the T_{max} for subject 7.

    Following the horizontal for subject 1 to the "C_{max}" column, the figure is 2.1 ng/mL, *answer.*

    Following the horizontal for subject 7 to the "T_{max}" column, the value is 6.0 hours, *answer.*

    Bar graphs are familiar to most persons because they are used widely in professional

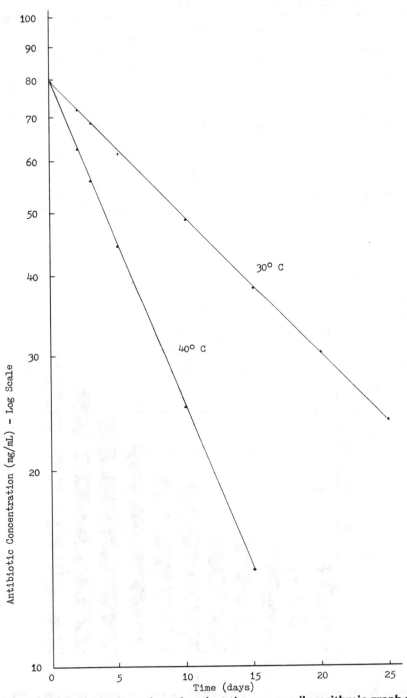

Fig. AC.5. Concentration values plotted against time on semilogarithmic graph paper.

Table AC.3. Noncompartmental Pharmacokinetic Parameters After Rectal Administration of Droperiodal to Healthy Volunteers

Subject	C_{max} (ng/ml)	T_{max} (hr)	MAT (hr)	F (%)	K_a (hr^{-1})	AUC_{inf} (ng-hr/ml)
1	2.1	6.0	4.61	65	0.217	42
2	2.0	8.0	3.94	51	0.254	40
3	1.8	10.0	5.84	55	0.171	38
4	2.3	6.0	1.39	38	0.719	31
5	2.3	4.0	2.23	49	0.448	42
6	2.2	10.0	4.53	41	0.221	33
7	1.8	6.0	3.64	38	0.275	32
8	2.7	8.8	4.77	65	0.210	49
Mean	2.1	7.3	3.87	50	0.314	38
SD	0.3	2.3	1.44	11	0.184	6

From Gupta, S.K.: Pharmacokinetics of Droperiodal in Healthy Volunteers Following Intravenous Infusion and Rectal Administration from an Osmotic Drug Delivery Module. Pharm. Res., 9:694, 1992, with permission.)

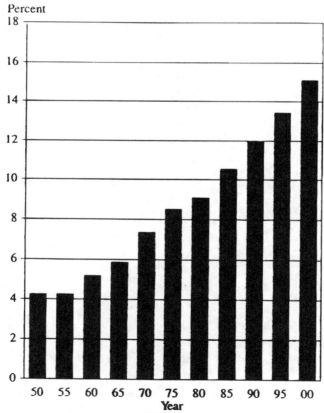

Fig. AC.6. Health expenditures as a percent of the gross national product (GNP). (From Schondelmeyer, S. W.: Trends with third parties and managed health care: A pharmacy perspective, in *The Changing Health Care Environment: Its Impact on Pharmacy and the Pharmaceutical Industry*. Proceedings of the Midwest Conference, November 11-14, 1987. Indianapolis, IN, Eli Lilly and Company, 1988, p. 17.)

and lay publications. Bar graphs contain a series of horizontal rectangles with the length of each bar reflecting the quantity of the (usually *different*) item it represents. Each bar may be subdivided to identify additional comparisons within the group represented.

In contrast to bar graphs, *column graphs* generally are used to compare the *same* item with bars arranged vertically. By joint-pairing columns (adjoining columns side-by-side) in the same grouping, two or more items may be compared.

A *histogram* is a type of graph that defines a frequency distribution.[3] In a histogram, the horizontal scale represents the characteristic or class intervals (as years) being measured and the vertical scale indicates the corresponding frequency of occurrence (usually in percent) (Fig. AC.6). Histograms are useful in displaying groups of data for the ease of their visual interpretation. In preparing histograms, the rectangles may be of equal or unequal widths, defining the magnitude of the class. When the rectangles are of equal width, the heights of the rectangles are proportional to the frequency; i.e., twice the height, twice the frequency. If the rectangles are not of equal width, the heights must be accommodated accordingly (i.e., twice the width, half the height), and it is more difficult to visually interpret the histogram.

Example:

Using Figure AC.6, it may be stated that health expenditures as a percent of the gross national product have doubled approximately every _____ (fill in blank) years.

Comparing the bars at 4% and 8%, and those at 6% and 12%, it appears that the percent has doubled approximately every 25 years, *answer.*

Circular charts or pie charts are prepared by subdividing a circle into sections by radial lines to indicate the portion of the whole represented by related items. Pie charts are common in the lay press and in scientific and professional literature and should be familiar to most students.

Practice Problems

1. In Figure AC.1, what is the y intercept for the equation $y = -2x + 5$? For $y = 0.67x - 1.67$?

2. On regular coordinate graph paper, plot the curves for the following equations.
    (a) $y = -4.0 \times 10^{-2}x + 1.5$
    (b) $y = 500x + 3$
    (c) $3y = 9x + 21$

3. A drug suspension containing 250 mg of drug per 5 mL was placed in a 50°C storage oven. Samples were removed periodically and assayed for drug content. The following results were obtained.

Time (Days)	5	10	20	30	40	50
Drug Concentration (mg/5 mL)	232	213	175	133	102	65

    (a) Plot the data on rectangular coordinate paper.
    (b) Calculate the straight line equation.
    (c) What is the concentration after 15 days?

---

[3] Simmonds, D., ed. *Charts and Graphs.* Lancaster, England, MTP Press Limited, 1980.

(d) The rate of decomposition K is equal to the slope of the curve. What is this rate of decomposition?

4. From Figure AC.4, calculate the straight line equation for the degradation of antibiotic solution at 30°C. How much antibiotic would be left in solution after 30 days?

5. An area of a wound was determined every 4 days by drawing the outline of the wound on a sterile sheet of transparent plastic. After applying an antibiotic cream on the initial day (0), the following results were obtained:

Time (Days)	0	4	8	12	16	20
Area (cm^2)	60	46.5	36	28	21.5	16.7

(a) Plot the data on regular coordinate graph paper.
(b) Plot the data on semilogarithmic graph paper.
(c) Plot the log area versus time on regular coordinate graph paper.
(d) Calculate the straight line equation.
(e) How much time would elapse before the wound reduced to 50% of the original size? To 5 cm^2?
(f) If the rate constant of this equation is defined as $k = 2.3\ m$, calculate k.

D Basic Statistical Concepts

Statistics may be defined as the science of the collection, classification, and interpretation of facts on the basis of relative number or occurrence as a ground for induction. Accordingly, all statistical studies begin with the gathering of reliable data. This information, or "raw data," whether it deals with measurements in business or science, is subsequently tabulated and analyzed for significance and validity by means of a number of mathematical and graphical procedures.

In this brief presentation, some elementary concepts that form the basis for these procedures are discussed in order to acquaint the student with the fundamentals of the "statistical approach."

THE ARRAY

When numeric facts are collected, they are initially recorded in haphazard fashion. Before the data can be analyzed effectively, however, a logical arrangement of it must be made. In other words, the "raw data" must be tabulated. One such simple arrangement is called the *array*. It consists of listing the items in a set of values or variables in order of magnitude, from smallest to largest or largest to smallest. Thus, the array rearranges the values but does not summarize them. The data are organized but not reduced.

Example:

Prepare an array of the following set of body temperatures (°F) of 20 individuals.

98.3	98.6	98.6	98.8	98.5
98.6	98.7	98.4	98.5	98.6
98.7	98.4	98.6	98.7	98.6
98.5	99.0	98.9	98.6	98.9

The array is made by listing the body temperatures (°F) from the lowest to the highest.

Temperature (°F)

98.3	98.5	98.6	98.6	98.8
98.4	98.5	98.6	98.7	98.8
98.4	98.6	98.6	98.7	98.9
98.5	98.6	98.6	98.7	99.0

answer.

THE FREQUENCY DISTRIBUTION

A more precise tabulation consists of arranging the given data in classes and listing their frequencies. Such an arrangement is called the *frequency distribution*. In this arrangement, the data are both organized and reduced.

Example:

Prepare a frequency distribution of the body temperatures given in the preceding example.

The frequency distribution of the body temperatures is made by separating the values into classes and listing the number of times a value appears in each class. If 5 classes of 0.2 beginning with 98.15 are chosen, the tabulation is made in the following manner.

Class	Tally	Frequency
98.15–98.35	|	1
98.35–98.55	⧗⧗	5
98.55–98.75	⧗⧗ ⧗⧗	10
98.75–98.95	|||	3
98.95–99.15	|	1
	Total:	20

This tabulation shows a concentration of values in the 98.55 to 98.75 class.

Although there is no definitive number, frequency distributions generally should have not less than 5 classes and not more than 15. The choice of the number of classes depends on the nature of the data and good judgment. Unequal class intervals should be avoided for ease of understanding.

AVERAGES

Mean, Median, and Mode. One of the common summary measures, or measures of central tendency, is the *arithmetic mean* or *average*. This measure is computed by adding the values of all the items in a set of data and dividing by the number of items. The formula for the arithmetic mean or average is:

$$\overline{X} = \frac{\text{Sum of values (X)}}{\text{Number of values}} = \frac{\Sigma X}{n}$$

The notation $\overline{X}$ (read X-bar) is the symbol for the average. The symbol Σ (the Greek capital letter sigma) means the summation of all the items of the variable X, and n refers to the number of values in the given set of data.

Example:

Referring to the array of the set of body temperatures, find the arithmetic mean of the recorded values.

$$\overline{X} = \frac{\Sigma X}{n}$$

$$\frac{1(98.3) + 2(98.4) + 3(98.5) + 7(98.6) + 3(98.7) + 2(98.8) + 1(98.9) + 1(99.0)}{20}$$

$$= \frac{1972.4}{20} = 98.6, \text{ answer.}$$

Another type of average is called the *median*. The median is also the *fiftieth percentile* of a distribution; i.e., the value below which 50% of the data are found. The median is sometimes referred to as the *middle* item in a series; it *is* the middle item given an odd number of items. The median may be considered the average of the two middle items or, if greater precision is desired, it is the *weighted average* of the two middle items (tenth and eleventh).

Example:

Referring to the array of the set of body temperatures, find the median of the recorded values.

Average of the two middle temperatures =

$$\frac{98.6 + 98.6}{2} = \frac{197.2}{2} = 98.6, \textit{answer.}$$

or,

Weighted average of the two middle temperatures =

$$\frac{7(98.6) + 3(98.7)}{10} = \frac{986.3}{10} = 98.63, \text{ or } 98.6, \textit{answer.}$$

A third type of summary measure is the *mode*. It is the item that appears most *frequently* in a set of values. The mode in the array of the set of body temperatures is 98.6 because that temperature appears the greatest number of times in the tabulation. The mode and the median are considered as "positional averages" because they are determined by location. The arithmetic mean is a "computed average."

MEASURES OF VARIATION

Range, Average Deviation, and Standard Deviation. The measures of central tendency that have been discussed offer one characteristic of a distribution. Another characteristic is the measure of variation within the distribution. The simplest measure of variation is the *range,* or the difference between the largest and smallest item in a distribution. The range is symbolized by *R*. For the body temperature distribution previously cited, R = 0.7.

The amount by which a given single item in a set of values differs from the mean of those values is the *deviation*. A deviation is considered positive if the item is larger than the mean, and negative if it is smaller. One of the measures used to describe how much, on average, an item deviates from the mean is called the *average deviation*. It is obtained by summing all the deviations from the mean without regard to algebraic sign and dividing by the number of deviations. The formula for average deviations *(A.D.)* follows:

$$A.D. = \frac{\text{Sum of absolute deviations}}{\text{Number of deviations}} = \frac{\Sigma \mid X - \overline{X} \mid}{n} = \frac{\Sigma d}{n}$$

Example:

Using a micrometer caliper, the diameter of a sample of a nylon suture material at different points on the strand was found to be 0.230 mm, 0.265 mm, 0.225 mm, 0.240 mm, 0.250 mm, 0.240 mm, 0.260 mm, 0.235 mm, 0.225 mm, and 0.270 mm. Calculate the mean and the average deviation.

Diameter (mm)	Absolute Deviation (mm)
0.230	0.014
0.265	0.021
0.225	0.019
0.240	0.004
0.250	0.006
0.240	0.004
0.260	0.016
0.235	0.009
0.225	0.019
0.270	0.026
2.440	0.138

$$\text{Mean} = \frac{2.440}{10} = 0.244 \text{ mm, } and$$

$$\text{A.D.} = \frac{0.138}{10} = 0.0138 \text{ or } 0.014 \text{ mm, } answers.$$

The more common measure of variation is the *standard deviation* of the items in a given set of values. It is a measure of the precision of the mean and is obtained by (1) squaring the deviations, (2) summing the squared deviations and dividing by the number of deviations *minus 1*, and (3) finding the square root of the quotient of the division. The formula for standard deviation (S.D.) follows:

$$\text{S.D.} = \sqrt{\frac{\text{Sum of (deviations)}^2}{\text{Number of deviations minus one}}} = \sqrt{\frac{\Sigma d^2}{n-1}}$$

(The -1 in this formula is referred to as a "degree of freedom.")

Example:

In checking the weights of a set of divided powders, the following values were obtained: 304 mg, 295 mg, 310 mg, 305 mg, 290 mg, 306 mg, 298 mg, 293 mg, 302 mg, and 297 mg. Calculate the mean and the standard deviation.

Weight (mg)	Deviation (mg)	(Deviation)^2
304	+ 4	16
295	− 5	25
310	+ 10	100
305	+ 5	25
290	− 10	100
306	+ 6	36
298	− 2	4
293	− 7	49
302	+ 2	4
297	− 3	9
3000		368

$$\text{Mean} = \frac{3000}{10} = 300 \text{ mg, } and$$

$$\text{S.D.} = \sqrt{\frac{\Sigma d^2}{n-1}} = \sqrt{\frac{368}{9}} = \sqrt{40.9} = 6.4 \text{ mg, } answers.$$

In general, the following approximate relationships may be used to compare the accuracy of measures of variation:

(1) The average deviation is approximately $\frac{4}{5}$ of the standard deviation.

(2) The range is never less than the standard deviation nor more than seven times the standard deviation.

SOME ASPECTS OF PROBABILITY

When you speak of "probability," you should make sure that both you and your listener know the sense in which you are using the word. In our everyday speech, "probability" often expresses merely a hunch about some likelihood or possibility; we may indicate the strength of our hunch in phrases ranging from "extremely probable" to "very unlikely." Sometimes the hunch can be supported—like the predictions of a competent weather prophet—by good evidence. Sometimes, however, we have no other evidence except a vague "feeling," which lacks the degree of reliability sought in the world of mathematics and science.

To the mathematician, "probability", in a usage that has been termed "classical," is a kind of *certainty*. Not certainty that an event E will take place. Certainty, rather, about the *chance* that E will take place, in competition with a number N of alternate events that might happen to take place instead. The mathematician envisions an ideal or abstract world in which the chances of every competing event are *absolutely equal*. This basic premise is called the *Principle of Indifference*. It can claim 100% accuracy in some formulas only when referring imaginatively to an infinite number of cases.

As soon as "classical" probability formulas were devised, they were predictably seized by gamblers and financial speculators, and the literature abounds with references to coin tossing, dice rolling, and card dealing, as well as to expectations of births, deaths, and shipwrecks. But, warn the mathematicians, the rules apply only if we respect the Principle of Indifference: our coins must not be bent, nor our dice loaded, nor our cards marked or stacked.

The statistician, whose research now carries into every field of human interest and activity, has been forced to recognize and overcome a twofold handicap. For one, actual events rarely and perhaps never are patterned by the Principle of Indifference. For another, of equal significance, the statistician deals with a total number of cases (called the "population") that lies a long way this side of infinity.

True, when the "population" is enormous, such as the number of molecules of gas in a chamber or even the far lesser number of fine particles in a powder, you can regard the great postulate of science that *like causes always produce like effects* as a certainty. As a chemist, for example, you may feel certain that your gas laws will not be broken by random molecules, which all at once head toward one end of the chamber; as a pharmacist, you may feel certain that with proper mixing, a small amount of a potent substance like atropine sulfate will be uniformly distributed throughout a larger amount of a diluent such as powdered lactose.

Even when dealing with much smaller "populations," the statistician has found a satisfactory substitute for "classical" probability. "Applied" probability, as indicated in the definition of statistics in the opening paragraph of this chapter, is revealed by the *relative frequency* of an event shown by an *actual survey* of cases.

An extended treatment of the subject is beyond the scope of this book. The odds are you will find delight and profit if you explore this increasingly important area of study.

Meanwhile, the following elementary observations may be of interest, and you may find ways to apply them in your own practice.

1. When an event E is one of a total N of equally likely alternatives, the chance, or probability p, of its occurrence is one in that total number:

$$p = \frac{1}{N} \text{ or 1 chance in N}$$

The fraction $\frac{1}{N}$ may be expressed as a percentage.

The so-called "odds" are 1 to $N - 1$.

Example:

If a question on a multiple-choice examination directs you to underscore one of five alternative answers, what is your chance of guessing the correct answer?

$$\frac{1}{N} = \frac{1}{5} \text{ or 1 chance in 5, or 20\%, } \textit{answer.}$$

What are the odds in favor of a correct guess?

$$1 \text{ to } N - 1 = 1 \text{ to 4, } \textit{answer.}$$

2. The probability q of the nonoccurrence of E in the preceding example is

$$q = \frac{N - 1}{N} = N - 1 \text{ in } N = 4 \text{ in 5, or 80\%}$$

The *odds* in favor of q are $N - 1$ to $1 = 4$ to 1.

3. If E has several (or n) chances of occurring among a given total N of alternatives, its chances are

$$p = \frac{n}{N} \text{ or n chances in N}$$

A "classic" example is the drawing of a playing card from a pack. The chance of drawing the Queen of Spades is 1 in 52, but the chance of drawing any *one* of the *four* queens is

$$\frac{n}{N} = \frac{4}{52} = \frac{1}{13} \text{ or 1 chance in 13}$$

Example:

If you are asked to underscore the two correct answers among six alternatives in a multiple-choice examination, what is your chance of guessing one correct answer?

$$\frac{n}{N} = \frac{2}{6} = \frac{1}{3} \text{ or 1 chance in 3, } \textit{answer.}$$

4. A succession of events may or may not, one by one, exhaust the total or possible alternatives. If you draw a queen from a pack and then restore it before a second drawing, you have restored the $\frac{4}{52}$ or $\frac{1}{13}$ ratio. If you withdraw a queen and then draw again, hoping for another queen, you have a new ratio: three remaining queens among 51 remaining cards gives 3 in 51 or 1 in 17. A third drawing after removal of two queens faces a ratio of

two queens in 50 cards, or 1 in 25, and if this succeeds, a fourth attempt will face 1 in 49. You combine odds by multiplying, and your chances of drawing four queens in succession are only 1 in 270,725. Perhaps you can figure out why your chance of drawing them in the order of spades, hearts, diamonds, clubs is only 1 in 6,497,400.

You must be alert to such shifting odds to avoid one of the most treacherous pitfalls in the game of probability.

Example:

Referring to the multiple-choice question cited in observation 3, what are your chances of guessing both correct answers among the six alternatives?

By analysis of the chances you face in each step of your two-part answer, you may reckon chances of 2 in 6 or 1 in 3 for a correct first step; but then you face a chance of 1 in 5 for a correct second step. Combining the two ratios, you have the following chance of being twice correct:

$$\frac{1}{3} \times \frac{1}{5} = \frac{1}{15} \text{ or 1 chance in 15, } \textit{answer.}$$

A clear proof of this analytic calculation may be charted. Presented with six alternatives—a, b, c, d, e, f—you may pair them in 15 possible ways, and only one pair will contain the two correct answers:

```
a   a   a   a   a
b   c   d   e   f

b   b   b   b   c
c   d   e   f   d

c   c   d   d   e
e   f   e   f   f
```

Therefore, you have only a 1 in 15 chance of guessing the correct pair.

5. Often the probability of the occurrence of an event or the percentage of occurrences in a total number of cases cannot be calculated in advance of research. Recall that the *relative frequency* of the event is the number of times it actually occurs in a total number of *observations. Statistical probability* (in contrast to "classical" probability) may be defined as *the limit of the relative frequency as the number of observations increases.*

To illustrate, consider the extent of your vocabulary. The mean average percentage of words you know on a few representative pages of your dictionary will enable you to calculate roughly, perhaps within a limit of five percentage points more or less, how many words you know in the entire dictionary. Test yourself on several dozen more pages, and your score will approach a limit of one percentage point.

6. When a limited number of samplings is supposed to represent an unattainable whole "population," the selection of samples should be as *random* as possible, so that every member of the whole (in theory at least) has an equal chance of being selected. A survey of public opinion should not be limited to the dwellers on one or two streets in a city, or to people whose names begin with *A*, or to members of a particular club.

Example:

Criticize the procedure of a tablet maker who selected for assay every fiftieth tablet during the first part of a run.

Because a machine might conceivably have regular cycles of varying dependability, the selection of samples should be at random intervals scattered throughout the entire run, *answer.*

7. In any survey-by-sampling, the greater the number of measurements, the greater the probability that their mean average will approach the true one being sought. Therefore, in appraising the value of a statistical report of apparent general reliability, be ready to question any "breakdowns" into components that may be individually unreliable. For example, a survey of the hair-grooming habits of 5000 American males may appear to be representative of American males in general. If, however, the population is "broken down" into special groups (460 lawyers, 57 clergymen, 275 teachers, 13 convicts, etc.), can we fairly generalize about American lawyers, clergymen, teachers, convicts, etc.?

For comparing two surveys of a similar kind, it has been found that *the probability of a truer mean average varies as the square root of the number of measurements.*

Example:

Two groups of researchers made a series of freezing point determinations on an 0.9% solution of sodium chloride, which, theoretically, freezes at $-0.52°C$. Group A made 36 measurements, group B made 16. Assuming equal skill, which group probably found a truer average?

$$\frac{A}{B} = \frac{\sqrt{36}}{\sqrt{16}} = \frac{6}{4} = \frac{3}{2} \text{ or a 3 to 2 probability in favor of Group A, } answer.$$

8. Another means of comparing the reliability of two sets of measurements involves the average deviations from the mean averages. *The reliability varies inversely as the deviations.*

Example:

In the preceding example, if given the average deviation of report A as 0.006°C and of report B as 0.012°C, you could compare their reliability as follows:

$$\frac{A}{B} = \frac{\dfrac{1}{0.006}}{\dfrac{1}{0.012}} = \frac{0.012}{0.006} = \frac{2}{1} \text{ or a 2 to 1 probability in favor of Group A, } answer.$$

9. If the results of two investigations differ in number of measurements and in average deviation from the mean average, you can use both factors together in comparing relative trustworthiness, keeping in mind that this parameter varies *directly with the square root of the number of measurements and inversely as the average deviation from the mean average.*

Example:

Combine the data in the two preceding examples.

$$\frac{A}{B} = \frac{\sqrt{36}}{\sqrt{16}} \times \frac{\dfrac{1}{0.006}}{\dfrac{1}{0.012}} = \frac{0.072}{0.024} = \frac{3}{1} \text{ or 3 to 1 in favor of A, } answer.$$

Or, combining the separate answers in observations 7 and 8:

$$\frac{A}{B} = \frac{3}{2} \times \frac{2}{1} = \frac{6}{2} = \frac{3}{1} \text{ or 3 to 1 in favor of A, } answer.$$

10. In many a survey, particularly if of a social nature, the reliability of some of the measurements may be open to question, or a reported measurement may be irrelevant to the purpose of the survey. Any measurement that is widely out of line with others of its

kind may be rejected, because its inclusion would have a disproportionate and misleading influence on the mean average and other calculations.

For example, a pharmacist in a small isolated town that had lost its only resident physician headed a committee to investigate the possibility of arranging a subsidy to attract a young general practitioner. The inhabitants consisted of several score household-ers, most of whom worked in a mill that was the only local industry. Also included in the committee were an eccentric, uncooperative recluse, rumored to be rich, and the mill owner, a man of known considerable means. The committee decided that its survey to ascertain the average family income need not include the recluse and should not include the mill owner. The latter's income would have raised the mean average significantly.

Practice Problems

1. The blood pressures of a group of 15 individuals were recorded as follows:

125	130	127	136	132
126	134	125	120	125
138	119	130	126	124

    Prepare an array of the data, calculate the mean, and find the median and the mode from the array.

2. A sample of catgut was measured for diameter with a micrometer caliper. The values obtained at 10 different points on the strand were:

0.230 mm	0.225 mm	0.240 mm	0.250 mm
0.225 mm	0.260 mm	0.270 mm	0.265 mm
0.235 mm	0.255 mm		

    Calculate the mean, the range, and the average deviation.

3. In checking the weights of a set of 15 tablets, the following values were obtained:

95 mg	100 mg	98 mg	103 mg	100 mg
102 mg	105 mg	104 mg	97 mg	99 mg
104 mg	101 mg	105 mg	96 mg	101 mg

    Calculate the mean, the average deviation, and the standard deviation for the set of values.

4. In determining the viscosity of a liquid in terms of centipoises, 10 observations were made and the following values were recorded:

10.5 cps	9.6 cps	10.0 cps	9.5 cps
10.0 cps	10.3 cps	9.9 cps	11.0 cps
9.8 cps	10.0 cps		

    Calculate the mean, the average deviation, and the standard deviation for the recorded values.

5. A series of 15 samples of a solution were assayed. The results, in terms of percent of active ingredient, were as follows:

5.05%	4.92%	4.85%	5.23%	5.05%
4.89%	5.05%	5.20%	5.15%	4.96%
4.95%	5.00%	5.02%	5.10%	4.87%

Calculate the mean, and find the median and the mode for the recorded data.

6. During a year-long community centennial celebration, the local pharmacist collaborated by keeping 300 tags identifying his regular customers in a drum. Each week for 50 weeks, a tag was drawn from the drum, a souvenir prize was awarded, and the tag was returned to the drum.
   (a) In any drawing, what was any customer's chance of winning the prize?
   (b) During the series of drawings, what was a customer's chance of winning two prizes?
   (c) What was a customer's chance of winning two prizes in a row?
   (d) If the tags, once drawn, had not been returned to the drum, what would have been a previously unawarded customer's chance of winning in the last drawing?

7. In choosing a sample of 25 subjects for a certain experiment, a researcher has a group of 50 individuals available from which to select the sample. The researcher assigns a number to each of the 50 subjects corresponding to an identical number on each of 50 buttons. He shakes the buttons in a container, draws one button, shakes the remaining buttons, then draws another button, shakes the buttons again, draws a third, and so on until he has 25 buttons. The subjects whose numbers correspond to the numbers on the buttons drawn are chosen for the experiment. Is this a random selection? Justify your answer.

8. Report A on a reduction in absenteeism in an industrial institution attributed to vaccination during an outbreak of influenza: among the 1,952 employees, 183 cases (9.4%) of clinical influenza were noted; in the vaccinated group of 847, only 15 cases (1.77%) appeared.
   Report B on a similar study: in a total of 3,497 employees, of which 1,148 received vaccination, the influenza attack rate was 10.8% as compared with 15.02% in the controls.
   Comparing only the total "population" in these reports, calculate the odds that report B may have produced more reliable percentages.

9. An old-time check of the body temperature of 25 people "in normal health" found an average of 98.4°F with an average deviation of 0.18°F. A later check of 100 people found an average temperature of 98.6°F with an average deviation of 0.12°F. By comparing both "population" and average deviation, calculate the ratio of the reliability of the two checks.

10. An aptitude test devised for undergraduate applicants to graduate school was administered experimentally to 15 subjects. With a possible score of 200, the results were as follows:

141	115	153
119	109	132
108	127	138
69	126	114
157	132	120

Compare the mean averages and average deviations calculated with and without the inclusion of the low 69. Which figures would probably be more reliable?

11. In checking the weight variation of a batch of uncoated tablets formulated to contain 250 mg of a drug substance, 20 tablets were weighed individually and the following values were obtained:

250 mg	260 mg	242 mg	235 mg	239 mg
245 mg	225 mg	267 mg	250 mg	258 mg
230 mg	232 mg	275 mg	248 mg	263 mg
248 mg	256 mg	250 mg	232 mg	250 mg

(a) Calculate the mean or average weight of the tablets sampled.
(b) If the designated weight tolerance, based on average weight, is 7.5%, do all the tablets sampled fall within this limit?

12. A series of belladonna tincture assays yielded the following values in terms of milligrams of total alkaloids per 100 mL:

40 mg	35 mg	28 mg
33 mg	29 mg	32 mg
27 mg	31 mg	27 mg
30 mg	25 mg	30 mg

Calculate the mean, and find the median and the mode for the recorded values.

E Thermometry

A *thermometer* is an instrument for measuring temperature, or intensity of heat. For practical purposes, a liquid such as alcohol or mercury undergoes a constant and measurable expansion or contraction with a rising or lowering of temperature. If contained in a small rigid bulb attached to a hermetically sealed extension tube, the liquid forces a column upward in the tube on expansion and draws the column down again on contraction. If the tube has a uniform bore and it is marked with evenly spaced lines, we have a thermometer.

Any number of degrees of temperature may be marked off between any two fixed points on the tube, and similar degrees can then be uniformly extended above and below them. Late seventeenth-century physicists suggested the constant temperatures of melting ice and of pure water boiling under normal atmospheric pressure as offering the most convenient fixed points (Fig. AE.1).

In 1709, the German scientist Gabriel Fahrenheit (who improved the construction of thermometers and was the first to use mercury instead of alcohol) took for 0° the temperature of a mixture of snow and sal ammoniac (equal parts by weight). He discovered that by the scale he had marked on his thermometer, ice melted at 32° and water boiled at 212°, with a difference of 180° between these two points. The *Fahrenheit thermometer* is still commonly used in the United States.

In 1742, Anders Celsius, a Swedish astronomer, suggested the convenience of a thermometer with a scale having a difference of 100° between two fixed points, and the *centigrade thermometer* was devised, with 0° for the freezing and 100° for the boiling points of water.

On each thermometer, negative numbers are used to designate degrees "below" the arbitrarily selected zero.

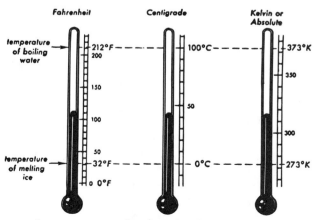

Fig. AE.I. Mercury thermometers showing the Fahrenheit, Centigrade, and Kelvin scales (White's *Modern College Physics*, Princeton, N.J., D. Van Nostrand Company, Inc., 1962).

Because 100 centigrade degrees (100° to 0°) measure the same difference in temperature that is measured by 180 Fahrenheit degrees (212° to 32°), each centigrade degree is the equivalent of 1.8 or $\frac{9}{5}$ the size of each Fahrenheit degree; therefore, any given rise or fall in temperature is measured by $\frac{9}{5}$ as many Fahrenheit degrees as centigrade degrees. So, we may construct a general formula for converting from one system to the other:

$$\frac{\text{Number of centigrade degrees above or below any degree centigrade}}{\text{Number of Fahrenheit degrees above or below an equivalent degree Fahrenheit}} = \frac{5}{9}$$

In other words, every 5° change in temperature as measured by the centigrade thermometer is a 9° change as measured by the Fahrenheit thermometer.

To derive a specific working proportion, it remains for us only to select points on the two thermometers that are known to be equivalent, are easy to remember, and are convenient to use in calculations.

Some equivalent readings above and below the melting point of ice follow:

0°C =	32°F	0°C =	32°F
5°C =	41°F	−5°C =	23°F
10°C =	50°F	−10°C =	14°F
15°C =	59°F	−5°C =	5°F
20°C =	68°F	−20°C =	− 4°F
30°C =	86°F	−30°C =	− 22°F
40°C =	104°F	−40°C =	− 40°F
50°C =	122°F	−50°C =	− 58°F
75°C =	167°F	−75°C =	−103°F
100°C =	212°F	−100°C =	−148°F
and so on.		and so on.	

First or Fundamental Method. Modern physicists not only have verified the hypothesis that "cold" is lower "heat" activity, but also found the point at which no such activity would be present, called *absolute zero*. Temperatures measured from this point are called *absolute temperatures* or temperatures on the *Kelvin scale*. Absolute zero has been computed as approximately −273° centigrade or −459.4° Fahrenheit. Consequently, this temperature may be considered the basic point of equivalence in the two systems:

$$-273°C = -459.4°F$$

Subtracting −273 from any given number of degrees centigrade yields the number of centigrade degrees above absolute zero. But subtracting a negative number is the same as adding its positive counterpart, so we may express this operation as C + 273. Similarly, any number of Fahrenheit degrees above absolute zero may be expressed as F + 459.4.

Our general proportion can now be specifically revised:

$$\frac{C + 273}{F + 459.4} = \frac{5}{9}$$

Using this proportion, if given the value of C, we could compute the corresponding value of F, and vice versa.

This can scarcely be called a working formula, however, because the numbers involved would not permit swift calculation. At least two other points of equivalence are both easy to remember and easy to use: (1) the temperature at which both thermometers happen to register the same number of degrees, and (2) the temperature of melting ice.

Second Method. The temperature registered as −40° centigrade happens also to be −40° Fahrenheit. The difference between any number of degrees centigrade and −40°C may be expressed as C + 40, and the difference between any number of degrees Fahrenheit and −40°F may be expressed as F + 40. By our general proportion, then,

$$\frac{C + 40}{F + 40} = \frac{5}{9}$$

Because this proportion is easy to remember, it is favored by many students, who usually sum up a working procedure as follows:

1. To convert centigrade to Fahrenheit, *add 40 to the given number of centigrade degrees, multiply by $\frac{9}{5}$ (or by 1.8), and subtract 40.*
2. To convert Fahrenheit to centigrade, *add 40 to the given number of Fahrenheit degrees, multiply by $\frac{5}{9}$ (or divide by 1.8), and subtract 40.*

These rules interpret the following derived equations:

$$1.\ F = \tfrac{9}{5}\,(C + 40) - 40 \text{ or } F = 1.8\,(C + 40) - 40$$

$$2.\ C = \tfrac{5}{9}\,(F + 40) - 40 \text{ or } C = \left(\frac{F + 40}{1.8}\right) - 40$$

Third or Standard Method. The method of conversion that is most common, because its calculations are simplest, is based on the fact that 0° centigrade is equivalent to 32° Fahrenheit. Any number of centigrade degrees above or below 0°C may be expressed as C − 0, or simply C. Any number of Fahrenheit degrees above or below 32° Fahrenheit may be expressed as F − 32. Hence:

$$1.\ \frac{C}{F - 32} = \frac{5}{9}$$

$$2.\ C = \tfrac{5}{9}\,(F - 32) \text{ or } C = (F - 32) \div 1.8$$

$$3.\ F = 32 + \tfrac{9}{5}\,C \text{ or } F = 32 + (1.8 \times C)$$

Perhaps a majority of scientists use equations 2 and 3, depending on the direction of conversion, and resolve them by simple arithmetic.

Fourth and Easiest Method. Here is a noteworthy fact: *no matter what specific proportion we select, if we multiply means and extremes and simplify the result, we get the same working equation.*

$$1.\quad \frac{C + 273}{F + 459.4} = \frac{5}{9}$$

$$9\,C + 2457 = 5\,F + 2297$$

$$9\,C = 5\,F - 160$$

$$2.\quad \frac{C + 40}{F + 40} = \frac{5}{9}$$

$$9\,C + 360 = 5\,F + 200$$

$$9\,C = 5\,F - 160$$

$$3.\quad \frac{C}{F - 32} = \frac{5}{9}$$

$$9\,C = 5\,F - 160$$

Once the principle is understood, therefore, it would seem advisable to use this equation (by the rules of elementary algebra) for conversion in either direction. It is easy to remember; it is convenient to use; it prevents the errors that frequently arise from careless interchange of $\frac{5}{9}$ and $\frac{9}{5}$ or confusion of the minus and plus signs in the other equations.

Examples:

Convert 26 °C to Fahrenheit.

$$
\begin{aligned}
9\ C &= 5\ F\ -\ 160 \\
9 \times 26 &= 5\ F\ -\ 160 \\
234\ +\ 160 &= 5\ F \\
5\ F &= 394 \\
F &= 78.8°,\ answer.^{1}
\end{aligned}
$$

Convert −12 °C to Fahrenheit.

$$
\begin{aligned}
9\ C &= 5\ F\ -\ 160 \\
9 \times -12 &= 5\ F\ -\ 160 \\
-108\ +\ 160 &= 5\ F \\
5\ F &= 52 \\
F &= 10.4°,\ answer.
\end{aligned}
$$

Convert 162 °F to centigrade.

$$
\begin{aligned}
9\ C &= 5\ F\ -\ 160 \\
9\ C &= (5 \times -162)\ -\ 160 \\
9\ C &= 650 \\
C &= 72\tfrac{2}{9}°,\ answer.
\end{aligned}
$$

Convert −62 °F to centigrade.

$$
\begin{aligned}
9\ C &= 5\ F\ -\ 160 \\
9\ C &= (5 \times -62)\ -\ 160 \\
9\ C &= -470 \\
C &= -52\tfrac{2}{9}°,\ answer.
\end{aligned}
$$

The instrument used to measure body temperature is termed the clinical or *fever thermometer.* The difference between this type and an ordinary thermometer (such as those used in the laboratory or to register air temperature) is that the mercury column in a clinical thermometer rises to the maximum temperature and remains at that point until shaken back into the reservoir at the bottom of the instrument. Clinical thermometers are of three general types: (1) the *oral thermometer,* slender in the design of stem and bulb reservoir; (2) the *rectal thermometer,* having a blunt, pear-shaped thick bulb reservoir for both safety and to ensure retention in the rectum; and (3) a small "universal" or "security" thermometer, which is stubby in design, for both oral or rectal use. These thermometers are available in both Fahrenheit and centigrade scales. Taking temperatures rectally in infants is a common practice and one that may be applied in older pediatric and in adult patients as the circumstances warrant. In addition to standard mercury thermometers, oral electronic digital fever thermometers are commonly used in the institutional and home setting. Both of these types of instruments work by the absorption of heat from the point of body contact. Heat causes the expansion and rise of mercury in the glass thermometer and the

---

[1] When centigrade degrees are converted to Fahrenheit, fractions are fifths and are customarily expressed as decimals; when Fahrenheit degrees are converted to centigrade, fractions are ninths.

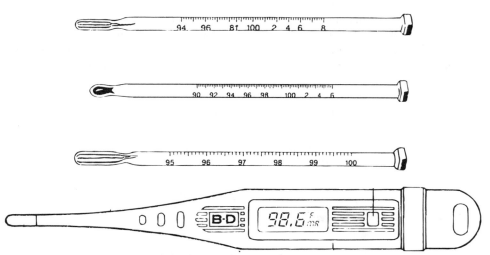

Fig. AE.2. Examples of various clinical thermometers. From top to bottom: oral fever thermometer; rectal thermometer; basal thermometer; oral digital fever thermometer. (Courtesy of Becton Dickinson and Company.)

response of the thermocouple in the electronic device. The new *infrared emission detection (IRED) ear thermometer* instantly (1 to 2 seconds) measures heat *radiated* from the tympanic membrane without actually touching the membrane.

Other specialized thermometers are available, including *basal thermometers* and *low-reading thermometers.* The *basal temperature* is the body's normal resting temperature, generally taken immediately on awakening in the morning. In women, body temperature normally rises slightly because of hormonal changes associated with ovulation. Basal thermometers, calibrated in tenths of a degree, are designed to measure these slight changes in temperature. When charted over the course of a month, these changes are useful in assessing optimal times for conception.

Low-reading thermometers are required in diagnosing hypothermia. The standard clinical thermometer reads from 34.4°C (94°F) to 42.2°C (108°F), which is not fully satisfactory in measuring hypothermia, which may involve body temperatures of 35°C (95°F) or lower. A low-reading thermometer registers temperatures between 28.9°C (84°F) to 42.2°C (108°F). Examples of various thermometers are shown in Figure AE.2.

Until recently, the *normal* body temperature for healthy adults was accepted to be 37°C (98.6°F) based on studies performed over a century ago.[2] The recent use of advanced electronic digital thermometers, however, has shown that normal adult temperature may vary widely between individuals (from 96.3°F to 99.9°F in one study).[3] Lowest body temperatures generally occur in the early morning and peak high temperatures in the late afternoon, with an average diurnal variation of approximately 0.9°F.

Practice Problems

1. Convert 10°C to Fahrenheit.

2. Convert −30°C to Fahrenheit.

---

[2] Wunderlich, C.A. and Sequin, E.: *Medical Thermometry and Human Temperature*, New York, William Wood & Co., 1871.

[3] Mackowiak, P.A., Wasserman, S.S., and Levine, M.M.: A critical appraisal of 98.6°F, the upper limit of the normal body temperature and other legacies of Carl Reinhold August Wunderlich. JAMA, *268*:1578, 1992.

3. Convert 4°C to Fahrenheit.

4. Convert −173°C to Fahrenheit.

5. Convert 77°F to centigrade.

6. Convert 240°F to centigrade.

7. The "normal" temperature of a patient is 98.6°F. Express this temperature on the centigrade scale.

8. A saturated solution of sodium chloride boils at 227.1°F. What is its boiling point on the centigrade scale?

9. The range of a centigrade thermometer is −5° to 300°. What is this range on the Fahrenheit scale?

10. Liquid petrolatum has a kinematic viscosity of 38.1 centistokes at 37.8°C. Express this temperature on the Fahrenheit scale.

11. The USP expression *"excessive heat"* refers to any temperature above 104°F. Express this temperature on the centigrade scale.

12. If a person shows a temperature of 102.5°F on a clinical thermometer, what would the temperature be on the centigrade scale?

13. If mercury freezes at −40°F, what is its freezing point on the centigrade scale?

14. The USP defines a *refrigerator* as a cold place in which the temperature is maintained thermostatically between 2° and 8°C. Express this temperature range on the Fahrenheit scale.

15. Theobroma oil melts between 30° and 35°C. What is the range of its melting point on the Fahrenheit scale?

16. If the maximum density of water is reached at 4°C, what would this point be on the Fahrenheit scale?

17. A specific gravity determination was made at 20°C. What was the temperature on the Fahrenheit scale?

18. Oxygen can be liquefied at −119°C. Express this temperature on (*a*) the Fahrenheit scale and (*b*) the absolute scale.

19. The USP defines a *freezer* as a cold place in which the temperature is maintained thermostatically between −20° and −10°C. Express this temperature range on the Fahrenheit scale.

20. A table of specifications states that a certain substance must congeal at −34.6°F. Express this temperature on the centigrade scale.

21. In preparing a vanishing cream, you are directed to heat the oil phase to 80°C and the aqueous phase to 82°C. Express these temperatures on the Fahrenheit scale.

22. The directions for the preparation of a certain formulation specified that the ingredients were to be heated for 15 minutes at 70°F. This instruction included a typographical error; it should have read 70°C. What is the difference in centigrade degrees between these two readings?

23. The critical temperature of a certain aerosol propellant is 388.4°F and its freezing point is − 168°F. Express these temperatures on the centigrade scale.

24. Dry ice vaporizes at − 112°F. What is the corresponding temperature on (a) the centigrade scale and (b) the Kelvin scale?

25. A pharmacist purchased a biologic refrigerator that is equipped with a centigrade thermometer. At what temperature should the refrigerator be set for storing insulin that is directed to be kept at 40°F?

26. Rubber closures for containers for injections are sterilized preferably with moist heat in an autoclave at 121°C for 15 to 20 minutes. Express this temperature using the Fahrenheit scale.

27. A patient's rectal temperature reading is frequently 1°F higher than the oral temperature reading. Express this difference in degrees centigrade.

28. A woman charting her basal temperature finds that her body temperature on day 14 is 97.7°F and on day 18 is 98.6°F. Express this temperature range and the difference in degrees centigrade.

F

Proof Strength

In the *United States Pharmacopeia*, all alcohol concentrations are expressed in percent volume-in-volume, based on the quantity of absolute alcohol (pure ethyl alcohol) present as determined at 15.56°C. In commerce, additional expressions of alcohol strength apply as follows.

Proof spirit is an aqueous solution containing 50% (v/v) of absolute alcohol. Alcohols of other percentage strengths are said to be *above proof* or *below proof*, depending on whether they contain more or less than 50% (v/v) of absolute alcohol.

Proof strength of alcohol is expressed by taking 50% alcohol, or proof spirit, as *100 proof*. Then, 100% or *absolute* alcohol is twice as strong, or 200 proof; 25% alcohol is half as strong, or 50 proof; and, inevitably, proof strength is always numerically twice as great as percentage strength (v/v). Hence, if percentage strength (v/v) is multiplied by 2, we have the corresponding proof strength: 35% alcohol is 70 proof, 95% alcohol is 190 proof, and so on. Conversely, if proof strength is divided by 2, we have percentage strength (v/v): 160 proof alcohol is 80% (v/v) strength, 90 proof alcohol is of 45% (v/v) strength, and so on.

Alcohol and alcoholic beverages are generally measured in gallons, for purposes of taxation, whatever their percentage strengths. For this and other reasons, a unit called the *proof gallon* is frequently used to measure, or evaluate, alcohols of given quantities and strengths. The tax on alcohol or alcoholic liquors is quoted at a definite figure per proof gallon. A *drawback* or refund of the tax paid on distilled spirits used in the manufacture of pharmaceutical preparations is allowed by the government and may be obtained by eligible claimants. Like the tax on distilled spirits, the drawback is quoted at a definite rate per proof gallon. Some hospital pharmacists and pharmaceutical manufacturers obtain a federal permit that allows the purchase of tax-free alcohol for use in the preparation of pharmaceuticals.

A *proof gallon* is 1 wine gallon (a gallon by measure) of proof spirit. In other words, 1 proof gallon = 1 wine gallon of an alcohol solution containing $\frac{1}{2}$ wine gallon of absolute alcohol and having, therefore, a strength of 100 proof or 50% (v/v). Any quantity of alcohol containing $\frac{1}{2}$ wine gallon of absolute alcohol is said "to be the equivalent of" or "to contain" 1 proof gallon. So, 2 wine gallons of 50 proof or 25% (v/v) alcohol would contain $\frac{1}{2}$ wine gallon of absolute alcohol, and would therefore be the equivalent of 1 proof gallon; however, 3 wine gallons of such a solution would contain $1\frac{1}{2}$ proof gallons.

Number of Proof Gallons in a Given Quantity of Alcohol of Specified Strength. To calculate the number of proof gallons contained in a given quantity of alcohol of specified strength, observe the following. Because a proof gallon has a percentage strength of 50% (v/v), the equivalent number of proof gallons may be calculated by the formula:

$$\text{Proof gallons} = \frac{\text{Wine gallons} \times \text{Percentage strength of solution}}{50\ (\%)}$$

Because proof strength is twice percentage strength, the formula may be revised as follows:

$$\text{Proof gallons} = \frac{\text{Wine gallons} \times \text{Proof strength of solution}}{100\ (\text{proof})}$$

Example:

How many proof gallons are contained in 5 wine gallons of 75% (v/v) alcohol?

First method:
1 proof gallon = 1 wine gallon of 50% (v/v) strength

$$\frac{5 \ (\text{wine gallons}) \times 75 \ (\%)}{50 \ (\%)} = 7.5 \text{ proof gallons, } answer.$$

Second method:
75% (v/v) = 150 proof

$$\frac{5 \ (\text{wine gallons}) \times 150 \ (\text{proof})}{100 \ (\text{proof})} = 7.5 \text{ proof gallons, } answer.$$

Number of Wine Gallons of Alcohol Equivalent to Number of Proof Gallons. To calculate the number of wine gallons of alcohol of specified strength equivalent to a given number of proof gallons, observe the following.

$$\text{Wine gallons} = \frac{\text{Proof gallons} \times 50 \ (\%)}{\text{Percentage strength of solution}}$$

or,

$$\text{Wine gallons} = \frac{\text{Proof gallons} \times 100 \ (\text{proof})}{\text{Proof strength of solution}}$$

Example:

How many wine gallons of 20% (v/v) alcohol would be the equivalent of 20 proof gallons?

First method:
1 proof gallon = 1 wine gallon of 50% (v/v) strength

$$\frac{20 \ (\text{proof gallons}) \times 50 \ (\%)}{20 \ (\%)} = 50 \text{ wine gallons, } answer.$$

Second method:
20% (v/v) = 40 proof

$$\frac{20 \ (\text{proof gallons}) \times 100 \ (\text{proof})}{40 \ (\text{proof})} = 50 \text{ wine gallons, } answer.$$

Tax on a Quantity of Alcohol of Specified Strength. To calculate the tax on a given quantity of alcohol of a specified strength, observe the following.

Example:

If the tax on alcohol is quoted at $13.50 per proof gallon, how much tax would be collected on 10 wine gallons of alcohol marked "190 proof"?

$$\frac{10 \ (\text{wine gallons}) \times 190 \ (\text{proof})}{100 \ (\text{proof})} = 19 \text{ proof gallons}$$

$$\$13.50 \times 19 \ (\text{proof gallons}) = \$256.50, \ answer.$$

Practice Problems

1. How many proof gallons are represented by 54 wine gallons of 95% (v/v) alcohol?

2. How many gallons of proof spirit are in 25 wine gallons of a sample that contains 70% (v/v) of pure alcohol?

3. How many proof gallons are contained in 500 wine gallons of Diluted Alcohol, NF, that contain 49% (v/v) of pure alcohol?

4. During a certain month, a hospital pharmacist used 54 gallons of 95% alcohol and 5 gallons of absolute (100%) alcohol. How many proof gallons were used during the month?

5. A pharmaceutical manufacturer has 4,500 gallons of 95% (v/v) alcohol. How many proof gallons are represented by this quantity?

6. How many wine gallons of 95% (v/v) alcohol would contain 91.2 proof gallons?

7. Calculate the volume, in wine gallons, represented by 175 proof gallons of 70% (v/v) alcohol.

8. If a drum contains 54 wine gallons of 95% (v/v) alcohol, how much tax must be paid on it at the rate of $13.50 per proof gallon?

9. If the tax on alcohol is $13.50 per proof gallon, how much tax must be paid on 5 wine gallons of Alcohol, USP, that contain 94.9% (v/v) of pure alcohol?

10. If alcohol is taxed at the rate of $13.50 per proof gallon, compute the tax on 6 wine gallons of 65% (v/v) alcohol.

11. The drawback on alcohol is $12.50 per proof gallon. If an eligible claimant used 18 gallons of 95% alcohol, how much drawback will be allowed?

12. A manufacturing pharmacist received a drawback of $1500 on the alcohol that was used during a certain period. If the drawback on alcohol is $12.50 per proof gallon, how many wine gallons of 95% alcohol were used during the period?

13. The formula for an elixir calls for 4 gallons of 95% alcohol. Alcohol (95%) costs $35.00 per gallon and the drawback is $12.50 per proof gallon. Calculate the net cost of the alcohol in the formula.

14. The drawback on a quantity of 95% alcohol used in the manufacture of a certain medicinal preparation was $237.50, and the net cost of the alcohol was $106.50. If the rate of drawback is $12.50 per proof gallon, what was the original purchase price per gallon of the alcohol?

15. On the first of the month, a hospital pharmacist had on hand a drum containing 54 gallons of 95% alcohol. During the month, the following amounts were used:
    (*a*) 10 gallons in the manufacture of bathing lotion
    (*b*) 20 gallons in the manufacture of medicated alcohol
    (*c*) 5 gallons in the manufacture of soap solution
    How many proof gallons of alcohol were on hand at the end of the month?

16. A hospital pharmacist had two drums (108 gallons) of 95% alcohol and 10 pints of absolute (100%) alcohol on hand on the first of the month. During the month, 20 gallons of 70% (v/v) alcohol and 30 gallons of 50% (v/v) alcohol were prepared. Two pints of absolute alcohol were also dispensed. How many proof gallons did the alcohol inventory show at the end of the month?

G

Solubility Ratios

The *solubility* of a substance is the ratio between the amount of it contained in a given amount of saturated solution (at a given temperature) and the amount of solvent therein. For instance, if 400 g of saturated solution contain 100 g of solute and 300 g of solvent, the solubility of the active ingredient (at that temperature) is 100:300 and may be expressed as 1:3. The relative amounts of solute and solvent may be calculated from various data, such as the ratio or percentage strength of the saturated solution.

The *Reference Tables* of the *United States Pharmacopeia* give approximate solubilities of USP and NF articles as 1 g of solute in so many milliliters of solvent (for example, *1 g of sodium chloride is soluble in 2.8 mL of water*). Solubilities may also be expressed as so many grams of solute in 100 mL of a saturated solution.

Solubility of a Substance. Calculating the solubility of a substance for any kind of solution involves the following procedure: (1) use the data to set up a proportion including the ratio *1:x*, *x* being the number of parts by weight containing 1 part by weight of active ingredient, and (2) if required, calculate the *volume* of *x* weight parts of solvent.

Examples:

What is the solubility of an anhydrous chemical if 100 g of a saturated aqueous solution leave a residue of 25 g after evaporation?

100 g − 25 g = 75 g of water

$$\frac{25 \ (g)}{75 \ (g)} = \frac{1 \ (part)}{x \ (parts)}$$

x = 3 parts of water, indicating a solubility of

1:3, or 1 g in 3 g or mL of water, *answer*.

What is the solubility of an anhydrous chemical if 100 g of a saturated alcoholic solution leave a residue of 20 g after evaporation? (The specific gravity of the alcohol is 0.80.)

100 g − 20 g = 80 g of alcohol

$$\frac{20 \ (g)}{80 \ (g)} = \frac{1 \ (part)}{x \ (parts)}$$

x = 4 parts of alcohol, indicating a solubility of 1:4,

or 1 g in 4 g of alcohol 4 g of water measure 4 mL

$\dfrac{4 \ mL}{0.80}$ = 5 mL, indicating a solubility of 1 g in 5 mL of alcohol, *answer*.

Each 100 mL of a saturated aqueous solution contain 25 g of a substance. The specific gravity of the solution is 1.15. Calculate the solubility of the substance.

100 mL of water weigh 100 g

100 mL × 1.15 = 115 g (weight of 110 mL of saturated solution)

115 g − 25 g = 90 g of water

$$\frac{25\ (g)}{90\ (g)} = \frac{1\ (part)}{x\ (parts)}$$

x = 3.6 parts of water, indicating a solubility of 1 : 3.6, or 1 g in 3.6 g

or mL of water, *answer.*

What is the solubility of the active ingredient if a saturated aqueous solution has a strength of 20% (w/w)?

100 parts − 20 parts = 80 parts of solvent in every 100 parts of solution

$$\frac{20\ (parts)}{80\ (parts)} = \frac{1\ (part)}{x\ (parts)}$$

x = 4 parts of solvent, indicating a solubility of 1 : 4,

or 1 g in 4 g or mL of water, *answer.*

Percentage Strength (w/w) of Saturated Solution with Given Solubility. To determine the percentage strength (w/w) of a saturated solution when the solubility is given, observe the following.

Examples:

One gram of boric acid is soluble in 18 mL of water. What is the percentage strength (w/w) of a saturated aqueous solution?

1 g + 18 g (18 mL of water) = 19 g

$$\frac{19\ (g)}{1\ (g)} = \frac{100\ (\%)}{x\ (\%)}$$

x = 5.26%, *answer.*

One gram of boric acid is soluble in 18 mL of alcohol. What is the percentage strength (w/w) of a saturated alcoholic solution? (The specific gravity of the alcohol is 0.80.)

18 mL of water weigh 18 g

18 g × 0.80 = 14.4 g, weight of 18 mL of alcohol

1 g + 14.4 g = 15.4 g of solution

$$\frac{15.4\ (g)}{1\ (g)} = \frac{100\ (\%)}{x\ (\%)}$$

x = 6.49%, *answer.*

Practice Problems

1. What is the solubility of a substance in water if 125 g of a saturated aqueous solution yield a 20-g residue on evaporation?

2. What is the solubility of a chemical if a saturated aqueous solution has a strength of 15% (w/w)?

3. A saturated aqueous solution contains 30 g of a substance in each 100 mL. The specific gravity of the solution is 1.10. Calculate the solubility of the substance.

4. One gram of calcium hydroxide is soluble in 630 mL of water at 25°C. What is the percentage strength (w/w) of a saturated solution?

5. The solubility of sodium borate is 1 g in 16 mL of water at 25°C. What is the percentage strength (w/w) of a saturated solution?

6. Each 500 mL of a saturated aqueous solution contain 400 g of a substance. The specific gravity of the solution is 1.30. What is the solubility of the substance?

7. The solubility of a substance is 1 g in 3 mL of water. When 5 g of it are dissolved in 15 mL of water, the volume of the resulting solution is 16.8 mL. How many grams of the substance and how many milliliters of water should be used to make 200 mL of a saturated solution?

8. One gram of a substance is soluble in 0.55 mL of water. When 20 g of it are dissolved in 11 mL of water, the volume of the resulting solution is 23.5 mL.
   (a) How many grams of the substance and how many milliliters of water should be used in preparing 1000 mL of a saturated solution?
   (b) Calculate the percentage strength (w/w) of the solution.
   (c) Calculate the percentage strength (w/v) of the solution.
   (d) What is the specific gravity of the saturated solution?

9. Each 100 mL of a saturated solution of potassium iodide contain 100 g of potassium iodide. The specific gravity of the solution is 1.7. Calculate the solubility of potassium iodide.

10. The solubility of magnesium sulfate is 1 g in 0.8 mL of water at 25°C. How many grams of magnesium sulfate should be used in preparing a liter of a saturated solution? Assume a specific gravity of 1.30 for the saturated solution at 25°C.

11. If the percentage strength (w/v) of a saturated aqueous solution of sucrose is 85% and the specific gravity of the solution is 1.313, what is the solubility of sucrose in water?

H Emulsion Nucleus

In the preparation of emulsions by the *Continental Method* ("4-2-1 Method"), the proportions for the *nucleus* or *primary emulsions* are "fixed oil 4 parts by volume, water 2 parts by volume, and acacia 1 part by corresponding weight." The mixture therefore contains one half as much water by volume as oil and one quarter as much acacia by "corresponding" weight.

When emulsions of volatile oils are prepared by this method, the proportions are "volatile oil 2 parts by volume, water 2 parts by volume, and acacia 1 part by corresponding weight."

Quantities of Ingredients for Nucleus or Primary Emulsion. To calculate the quantities of ingredients required for a nucleus or primary emulsion, observe the following:

Examples:

A castor oil emulsion contains 30% of castor oil. How much castor oil, water, and acacia are required to prepare the primary emulsion in the formulation of a liter of the emulsion?

$$1 \text{ liter} \qquad = 1000 \text{ mL}$$
$$1000 \text{ mL} \times 30\% \quad = 300 \text{ mL of castor oil required}$$

Because castor oil is a *fixed* oil, the ratio *4-2-1* is used.

4	—	2	—	1
300 mL		150 mL		75 g, *answers.*
oil		water		acacia

In preparing the emulsion, the castor oil and acacia are mixed, the water is added, and the mixture is emulsified, forming the primary emulsion, which is then diluted to the required volume.

A mineral oil emulsion contains 25% of mineral oil. How much mineral oil, water, and acacia are required to prepare the primary emulsion in the formulation of a gallon of the emulsion?

$$1 \text{ gallon} \qquad = 3785 \text{ mL}$$
$$3785 \times 25\% \quad = 946 \text{ mL of mineral oil required}$$

Because mineral oil is a *fixed* oil, the ratio *4-2-1* is used.

4	—	2	—	1
946 mL		473		236.5 g, *answers.*
oil		water		acacia

A turpentine emulsion contains 15% of turpentine oil. How much turpentine oil, water, and acacia are required to prepare the primary emulsion in the formulation of 4 liters of the emulsion:

$$4 \text{ liters} \qquad = 4000 \text{ mL}$$
$$4000 \text{ mL} \times 15\% \quad = 600 \text{ mL of turpentine oil required}$$

Because turpentine oil is a *volatile* oil, the ratio *2-2-1* is used.

2	—	2	—	1
600 mL		600 mL		300 g, *answers.*
oil		water		acacia

Practice Problems

In each of the following formulas, calculate (*a*) the amount of acacia and (*b*) the amount of water to be used in preparing the nucleus or primary emulsion.

1. Mineral Oil   500 mL   (A *fixed* oil.)
    Acacia   q.s.
    Syrup   100 mL
    Vanillin   40 mg
    Alcohol   60 mL
    Purified Water, to make   1000 mL
    Label: Mineral Oil Emulsion.

2. Castor Oil   (A *fixed* oil.)
    Syrup   aa   25%
    Acacia   q.s.
    Purified Water, to make   2000 mL
    Label: Cod Liver Oil Emulsion.

3. Cod Liver Oil   50%   (A *fixed* oil.)
    Acacia   q.s.
    Syrup   10%
    Peppermint Water, to make   5000 mL
    Label: Cod Liver Oil Emulsion.

4. Turpentine Oil   150 mL   (A *volatile* oil.)
    Syrup   100 mL
    Acacia   q.s.
    Purified Water, to make   1000 mL
    Label: Turpentine Oil Emulsion.

I

HLB System: Problems Involving HLB Values

The systematic choice of emulsifying agents in the formulation of many emulsion systems depends on their HLB (Hydrophile-Lipophile-Balance) values. These values form the basis of the so-called HLB System, which was developed by Griffin.[1] The system presupposes a scale of HLB numbers and is based on the facts (1) that every surfactant or emulsifier molecule is in part hydrophilic and in part lipophilic, and (2) that a certain balance between these two parts is necessary for various types of surfactant functions. In this scheme, each surfactant or emulsifying agent is assigned a number that varies from 1 to 20. The lower values are assigned to substances that are predominantly lipophilic (oil-loving) and have a tendency to form water-in-oil (w/o) emulsions. The higher values are given to those materials that show hydrophilic (water-loving) characteristics and favor the formation of oil-in-water (o/w) emulsions. Consequently, the HLB number of an emulsifying agent is an index of the type of emulsion that has the greatest tendency to form. The HLB values of a few selected surfactants are given in Table AI.1.

Just as surfactants and emulsifiers are assigned HLB numbers, so, too, the ingredients to be emulsified have been given certain "required HLB" numbers. These designations have been determined experimentally and are necessary for the proper emulsification of the dispersed phase. The "required HLB" values for some of the more commonly used ingredients in emulsion formulation are given in Table AI.2.

HLB of a Blend of Emulsifying Agents. When two or more emulsifiers are combined, the HLB of the combination is determined arithmetically by adding the contribution that each makes to the HLB total of the mixture.

Example:

What is the HLB of a mixture of 40% of Span 60 and 60% of Tween 60?

$$\text{HLB of Span 60} \quad = \quad 4.7$$
$$\text{HLB of Tween 60} \quad = 14.9$$

	HLB		% of mixture		
Span	60 4.7	$\times$	40%	=	1.9
Tween	60 14.9	$\times$	60%	=	8.9

$$\text{HLB of mixture} \quad = 10.8, \textit{answer.}$$

"Required HLB" of a Combination of Ingredients to be Emulsified. The "required HLB" of each ingredient is multiplied by the percentage or the fraction of the oil phase that the ingredient represents; the products are then added to give the "required HLB" for emulsification of the oil phase.

Example:

Calculate the "required HLB" for the oil phase of the following o/w emulsion.

Cetyl Alcohol	15.0 g
White Wax	1.0 g
Lanolin, Anhydrous	2.0 g

---

[1] Griffin, W.C.: Calculation of HLB values of non-ionic surfactants. *J. Soc. Cos. Chem.*, 5:249, 1954.

Emulsifier		q.s.
Glycerin		5.0 g
Distilled Water	ad	100.0 g

The oil phase represents *18 parts* of the entire formula.

Cetyl Alcohol $\quad = \quad {}^{15}\!/_{18}$ of the oil phase

White Wax $\quad\quad = \quad {}^{1}\!/_{18}$ of the oil phase

Lanolin, Anhydrous $\quad = \quad {}^{2}\!/_{18}$ of the oil phase

	Required *HLB*		*Fraction of* *oil phase*	
Cetyl Alcohol	15	×	${}^{15}\!/_{18}$	= 12.5
White Wax	12	×	${}^{1}\!/_{18}$	= 0.7
Lanolin, Anhydrous	10	×	${}^{2}\!/_{18}$	= <u>1.1</u>

"Required HLB" of the oil phase = 14.3, *answer.*

Table AI.1. HLB Values of Some Surfactants

Surfactant	*HLB*
Sorbitan trioleate (Span 85)*	1.8
Sorbitan tristearate (Span 65)*	2.1
Sorbitan sesquioleate (Arlacel 83)*	3.7
Glyceryl monostereate, NF	3.8
Sorbitan monooleate, NF, (Span 80)*	4.3
Sorbitan monostearate, NF, (Span 60)*	4.7
Sorbitan monopalmitate, NF, (Span 40)*	6.7
Sorbitan monolaurate, NF, (Span 20)*	8.6
Polyoxyethylene sorbitan tristearate (Tween 65)*	10.5
Polyoxyethylene sorbitan trioleate (Tween 85)*	11.0
Polyethylene glycol 400 monosterate	11.6
Polysorbate 60, NF, (Tween 60)*	14.9
Polyoxyethylene monostearate (Myrj 49)*	15.0
Polysorbate 80, NF, (Tween 80)*	15.0
Polysorbate 40, NF, (Tween 40)*	15.6
Polysorbate 20, NF, (Tween 20)*	16.7

* ICI Americas, Inc., Wilmington, Delaware.

Table AI.2. "Required HLB" Values of Some Ingredients

	"Required HLB" for	
	w/o	*o/w*
Ingredient	*Emulsion*	
Acid, Stearic	6	15
Alcohol, Cetyl	—	15
Alcohol, Stearyl	—	14
Lanolin, Anhydrous	8	10
Oil, Cottonseed	5	10
Oil, Mineral	5	12
Petrolatum	5	12
Wax, Beeswax	4	12

Relative Amounts of Emulsifiers to Obtain "Required HLB". Problems of this type are conveniently solved by alligation alternate (see Chapter 8).

Examples:

In what proportion should Tween 80 and Span 80 be blended to obtain a "required HLB" of 12.0?

$$\text{HLB of Tween 80} \quad = \; 15.0$$
$$\text{HLB of Span 80} \quad = \quad 4.3$$

By alligation,

15.0		7.7 parts of Tween 80
	12.0	
4.3		3.0 parts of Span 80

Relative amounts: 7.7:3.0 or 72%:28%, *answer.*

A formula for a cosmetic cream calls for 35 g of an emulsifier blend consisting of Tween 40 and Span 20. If the "required HLB" is 12.6, how many grams of each emulsifier should be used in preparing the cream?

$$\text{HLB of Tween 40} \quad = \; 15.6$$
$$\text{HLB of Span 20} \quad = \quad 8.6$$

By alligation,

15.6		4.0 parts of Tween 40
	12.6	
8.6		3.0 parts of Span 20

Relative amounts 4:3 with a total of 7 parts

$$\frac{4 \text{ (parts)}}{7 \text{ (parts)}} = \frac{x \text{ (g)}}{35 \text{ (g)}}$$

$$x = 20 \text{ g of Tween 40, } and$$

$$\frac{3 \text{ (parts)}}{7 \text{ (parts)}} = \frac{y \text{ (g)}}{35 \text{ (g)}}$$

$$y = 15 \text{ g of Span 20, } answers.$$

Practice Problems

1. What is the HLB of an emulsifier blend consisting of 25% of Span 20 and 75% of Tween 20?

2. Calculate the HLB of a mixture of 45 g of Span 80 and 55 g of Polysorbate 80.

3. What is the HLB of an emulsifier blend consisting of 20% of Span 60, 20% of Span 80, and 60% of Tween 60?

4. Calculate the "required HLB" for the oil phase of the following oil-in-water type lotion.

Stearyl Alcohol		250 g
White Petrolatum		250 g
Propylene Glycol		120 g
Emulsifier		q.s.
Preserved Water	ad	1000 g

5. Calculate the "required HLB" for the oil phase of the following oil-in-water type lotion.

Mineral Oil		30%
Lanolin, Anhydrous		2%
Cetyl Alcohol		3%
Emulsifier		q.s.
Preserved Water	ad	100%

6. In what proportion should Tween 60 and Arlacel 83 be blended to obtain a "required HLB" of 11.5?

7. The "required HLB" of an oil phase is 13.2. What percentage of Tween 40 and of Span 40 should be used to give the "required HLB"?

8. The formula for a greaseless ointment calls for 100 g of an emulsifier blend consisting of Polysorbate 80 and Span 80. If the "required HLB" of the oil phase is 11.5, how many grams of each emulsifier should be used in preparing the ointment?

9. The formula for a cosmetic cream calls for 5% of an emulsifier blend consisting of Span 60 and Tween 20. If the "required HLB" of the oil phase is 14.0, how many grams of each emulsifier should be used in preparing 500 g of the cream?

10.

Stearic Acid		8.0%
Cetyl Alcohol		1.0%
Lanolin, Anhydrous		1.0%
Emulsifier		4.0%
Glycerin		10.0%
Preserved Water	ad	100.0%

(*a*) Calculate the "required HLB" of the oil phase.

(*b*) How many grams of Span 80 and how many grams of Tween 60 should be used in formulating 1000 g of the product?

J Exponential and Logarithmic Notation

EXPONENTIAL NOTATION

Many physical and chemical measurements deal with either very large or very small numbers. Because it often is difficult to handle conveniently numbers of such magnitude in performing even the simplest arithmetic operations, it is best to use exponential notation or *powers of 10* to express them. Thus, we may express *121* as *1.21×10^2*, *1210* as *1.21×10^3*, and *1,210,000* as *1.21×10^6*. Likewise, we may express *0.0121* as *1.21×10^{-2}*, *0.00121* as *1.21×10^{-3}*, and *0.00000121* as *1.21×10^{-6}*.

When numbers are written in this manner, the first part is called the *coefficient*, customarily written with one figure to the left of the decimal point. The second part is the *exponential factor* or *power of 10*.

The exponent represents the number of places that the decimal point has been moved—positive to the left and negative to the right—to form the exponential. Thus, when we convert *19000* to *1.9×10^4*, we move the decimal point 4 places to the left; hence the exponent 4. And when we convert *0.0000019* to *1.9×10^{-6}*, we move the decimal point 6 places to the right; hence the *negative* exponent $^{-6}$.

FUNDAMENTAL ARITHMETIC OPERATIONS WITH EXPONENTIALS

In the *multiplication* of exponentials, the exponents are *added*. For example, $10^2 \times 10^4 = 10^6$. In the multiplication of numbers that are expressed in exponential form, the *coefficients* are multiplied together in the usual manner, and this product is then multiplied by the power of *10* found by algebraically *adding* the exponents.

Examples:

$$(2.5 \times 10^2) \times (2.5 \times 10^4) \quad = 6.25 \times 10^6, \text{ or } 6.3 \times 10^6$$
$$(2.5 \times 10^2) \times (2.5 \times 10^{-4}) \quad = 6.25 \times 10^{-2}, \text{ or } 6.3 \times 10^{-2}$$
$$(5.4 \times 10^2) \times (4.5 \times 10^3) \quad = 24.3 \times 10^5 = 2.4 \times 10^6$$

In the *division* of exponentials, the exponents are *subtracted*. For example, $10^2 \div 10^5 = 10^{-3}$. In the division of numbers that are expressed in exponential form, the *coefficients* are divided in the usual way and the result is multiplied by the power of *10* found by algebraically *subtracting* the exponents.

Examples:

$$(7.5 \times 10^5) \div (2.5 \times 10^3) \quad = 3.0 \times 10^2$$
$$(7.5 \times 10^{-4}) \div (2.5 \times 10^6) \quad = 3.0 \times 10^{-10}$$
$$(2.8 \times 10^{-2}) \div (8.0 \times 10^{-6}) \quad = 0.35 \times 10^4 = 3.5 \times 10^3$$

Note that in each of these examples, the result is rounded off to the number of *significant figures* contained in the *least* accurate factor, and it is expressed with only one figure to the left of the decimal point.

In the *addition* and *subtraction* of exponentials, the expressions must be changed (by moving the decimal points) to forms having any common power of 10, and then the coefficients only are added or subtracted. The result should be rounded off to the number of *decimal places* contained in the *least* precise component, and it should be expressed with only one figure to the left of the decimal point.

Examples:

$$(1.4 \times 10^4) + (5.1 \times 10^3)$$

$$
\begin{array}{rccl}
 & 1.4 & \times & 10^4 \\
5.1 \times 10^3 = & \underline{0.51} & \times & 10^4 \\
\text{Total:} & 1.91 & \times & 10^4, \text{ or } 1.9 \times 10^4, \text{ \textit{answer.}}
\end{array}
$$

$$(1.4 \times 10^4) - (5.1 \times 10^3)$$

$$
\begin{array}{rccl}
1.4 \times 10^4 = & 14.0 & \times & 10^3 \\
 & \underline{-5.1} & \times & 10^3 \\
\text{Difference:} & 8.9 & \times & 10^3, \text{ \textit{answer.}}
\end{array}
$$

$$(9.83 \times 10^3) + (4.1 \times 10^1) + (2.6 \times 10^3)$$

$$
\begin{array}{rccl}
 & 9.83 & \times & 10^3 \\
4.1 \times 10^1 = & 0.041 & \times & 10^3 \\
 & \underline{2.6} & \times & \underline{10^3} \\
\text{Total:} & 12.471 & \times & 10^3, \text{ or} \\
 & 12.5 & \times & 10^3 = 1.25 \times 10^4, \text{ \textit{answer.}}
\end{array}
$$

Practice Problems

1. Write each of the following in exponential form:
    (a) 12,650
    (b) 0.0000000055
    (c) 451
    (d) 0.065
    (e) 625,000,000

2. Write each of the following in the usual numeric form:
    (a) 4.1×10^6
    (b) 3.65×10^{-2}
    (c) 5.13×10^{-6}
    (d) 2.5×10^5
    (e) 8.6956×10^3

3. Find the product:
    (a) $(3.5 \times 10^3) \times (5.0 \times 10^4)$
    (b) $(8.2 \times 10^2) \times (2.0 \times 10^{-6})$
    (c) $(1.5 \times 10^{-6}) \times (4.0 \times 10^6)$
    (d) $(1.5 \times 10^3) \times (8.0 \times 10^4)$
    (e) $(7.2 \times 10^5) \times (5.0 \times 10^{-3})$

4. Find the quotient:
    (a) $(9.3 \times 10^5) \div (3.1 \times 10^2)$
    (b) $(3.6 \times 10^{-4}) \div (1.2 \times 10^6)$
    (c) $(3.3 \times 10^7) \div (1.1 \times 10^{-2})$

5. Find the sum:
    (a) $(9.2 \times 10^3) + (7.6 \times 10^4)$
    (b) $(1.8 \times 10^{-6}) + (3.4 \times 10^{-5})$
    (c) $(4.9 \times 10^2) + (2.5 \times 10^3)$

6. Find the difference:
    (a) $(6.5 \times 10^6) - (5.9 \times 10^4)$
    (b) $(8.2 \times 10^{-3}) - (1.6 \times 10^{-3})$
    (c) $(7.4 \times 10^3) - (4.6 \times 10^2)$

COMMON LOGARITHMIC NOTATION

We have seen that exponential notation allows us to express any number as a *coefficient times a whole number power of 10*—as when we interpret *150* to mean *1.5 $\times 10^2$*—and that this system of notation offers us a convenient shorthand, as it were, for expressing and manipulating very large or very small numbers.

Still another system, called *common logarithmic notation*, goes the exponential system one better. In common logarithmic notation, *every number is expressed simply as a power of 10*—not with absolute precision, but with sufficient accuracy for any given purpose—and we may multiply any two numbers so expressed, or divide one by the other, by the simple process of adding or subtracting their exponents.

The *exponent* that indicates *to what power 10 must be raised to equal approximately a given number* is called the *common logarithm* of that number. It follows that the logarithm of *10* or of any integral power of *10* is always a positive or negative integer:

$$\log 10 \text{ (or } 1 \times 10^1) \quad = 1$$
$$\log 100 \text{ (or } 1 \times 10^2) \quad = 2$$
$$\log 1000 \text{ (or } 1 \times 10^3) \quad = 3$$

and so on; and

$$\log 1 \text{ (or } 1 \times 10^0) \quad = 0$$
$$\log 0.1 \text{ (or } 1 \times 10^{-1}) \quad = \text{-}1$$
$$\log 0.01 \text{ (or } 1 \times 10^{-2}) \quad = \text{-}2$$

and so on. If these were the only numbers in existence, no table of logarithms would be needed; for a given number, say *1,000,000* (or 1×10^6), if we know the system, we can readily supply its logarithm: 6; or, given the logarithm 6, we can readily reconstruct the number it represents: *1,000,000*.

Any number *not* in the *10's* series, however, must contain a certain *excess* over some power of *10*—as *150* contains 10^2 plus an excess of *50*. Therefore, the logarithm of such a number always consists of a positive or negative whole-numbered exponent *plus* a positive decimal-fraction exponent (carried to as many decimal places as suit our purposes). As it turns out, the power of *10* that approximates *150* (or *1.5 $\times 10^2$*) is $10^{2.1761}$, and therefore *log 150 = 2.1761.*

The *whole-number exponent* is called the *characteristic*. It accounts for the integral power of *10* contained in the given number and hence serves to locate the *decimal point* in that number. If a number is given in ordinary notation, you can find the characteristic by converting it to exponential notation, in which the characteristic appears as a power of *10*.

The *decimal-fraction exponent* is called the *mantissa*, which you can find in a table of logarithms. The mantissa represents the *significant figures* in a given number, regardless of the location of the decimal point. In other words, given the sequence *610*, a four-place table will tell you the mantissa is *7853*, whether the number *is 61.0*, or *6.10*, or *0.00610*.

Compare this series of logarithms with the logarithms of the 10's series given previously:

$$\log 6.10 \ (\text{or } 6.10 \times 10^0) \quad = 0.7853$$
$$\log 61.0 \ (\text{or } 6.10 \times 10^1) \quad = 1.7853$$
$$\log 610 \ (\text{or } 6.10 \times 10^2) \quad = 2.7853$$
$$\log 6100 \ (\text{or } 6.10 \times 10^3) \quad = 3.7853$$

and so on; and

$$\log 0.610 \ (\text{or } 6.10 \times 10^{-1}) \quad = \bar{1}.7853$$
$$\log 0.0610 \ (\text{or } 6.10 \times 10^{-2}) \quad = \bar{2}.7853$$
$$\log 0.00610 \ (\text{or } 6.10 \times 10^{-3}) \quad = \bar{3}.7853$$

and so on. Note that putting the minus sign *over* the characteristic indicates it alone is negative, and that the mantissa, as always, is positive.

NATURAL LOGARITHMS

The base of the *natural* or *Naperian* system of logarithms is *e*, which is the irrational number 2.71828 . . . . When it is necessary to change from a natural logarithm to a common logarithm, the computation may be performed by using the following relationship:

$$\log_e n = 2.303 \log_{10} n$$

in which 2.303 is the logarithm of 10 to the base 2.71828.

USE OF LOGARITHM TABLES

Logarithm tables give mantissas calculated to four-place, five-place accuracy, and upward, depending on the table and its purpose. A four-place table ensures an accuracy within 0.5% when we work with three-figure numbers.

Table AJ.1 has typical features. It contains (1) a column to the left and a row at the top to guide us in locating the mantissas of three-figure numbers; (2) the four-place mantissa of all three-figure numbers, and (3) columns of proportional parts providing us with a quick means of calculating more accurate mantissas when given numbers of four-figure accuracy, a process called *interpolation*.

Finding the Logarithm of a Number. To find the logarithm of a number, determine the characteristic, then find the mantissa in the log table.

Examples:

Find the log of 262.

$262 = 2.62 \times 10^2$
By inspection of the ten factor, the characteristic = 2.
To find the mantissa, focus attention on the digits *262*.
In the left-hand column in the log table, find *26*; opposite it and in the column numbered *2* is the desired mantissa 0.4183.
(The table omits the 0.)
Therefore, log 262 = 2.4183, *answer.*

Find the log of 2627.

$2627 = 2.627 \times 10^3$
By inspection of the ten factor, the characteristic = 3.
In the left-hand column in the table, find *26*; opposite it and in the column numbered *2*, find the mantissa 0.4183; opposite *26* and in column 7 under proportional parts, find 11 (meaning 0.0011 but written without zeros) and add it to 0.4183 to obtain the desired mantissa 0.4194.
Therefore, log 2627 = 3.4194, *answer.*

Find the log of 0.002627.

$0.002627 = 2.627 \times 10^{-3}$
By inspection of the ten factor, the characteristic = $\bar{3}$.
The mantissa is determined as in the preceding example.
Therefore, log 0.002627 = $\bar{3}$.4194, *answer.*

Finding the Antilogarithm of a Logarithm. When a problem is solved by logarithms, the result is expressed as the *logarithm* of the answer. Therefore, it is necessary to find the *antilogarithm* or *the number corresponding to the logarithm.* If the mantissa of a logarithm is known, its antilogarithm can be found by a *reverse reading* of the log table.

Examples:

Find the antilogarithm of the logarithm 1.7604.

The mantissa 0.7604 is found in the column numbered 6 opposite *57,* and the resulting figure is *576.*
The characteristic is 1 and the required number is
5.76×10^1 or 57.6, *answer.*

Find the antilogarithm of the logarithm 3.7607.

Because the mantissa 0.7607 is not found in the log table, interpolation must be used.
In the log table, 0.7607 falls *between* 0.7604 and *0.7612;* therefore, the resulting figure must be between *576* and *577.*
The *given* mantissa is 0.0003 (or 3 units) more than the mantissa 0.7604.
Therefore, opposite 0.7604, find 3 in column 4 of proportional parts.
The required figure is *5764.*
The characteristic is 3 and the required number is
$5.764 \times 10^3 = 5764$, *answer.*

Table AJ.1. Logarithms

Natural Numbers	0	1	2	3	4	5	6	7	8	9	Proportional Parts								
											1	2	3	4	5	6	7	8	9
10	0000	0043	0086	0128	0170	0212	0253	0294	0334	0374	4	8	12	17	21	25	29	33	37
11	0414	0453	0492	0531	0569	0607	0645	0682	0719	0755	4	8	11	15	19	23	26	30	31
12	0792	0828	0864	0899	0934	0969	1004	1038	1072	1106	3	7	10	14	17	21	24	28	31
13	1139	1173	1206	1239	1271	1303	1335	1367	1399	1430	3	6	10	13	16	19	23	26	29
14	1461	1492	1523	1553	1584	1614	1644	1673	1703	1732	3	6	9	12	15	18	21	24	27
15	1761	1790	1818	1847	1875	1903	1931	1959	1987	2014	3	6	8	11	14	17	20	22	25
16	2041	2068	2095	2122	2148	2175	2201	2227	2253	2279	3	5	8	11	13	16	18	21	24
17	2304	2330	2355	2380	2405	2430	2455	2480	2504	2529	2	5	7	10	12	15	17	20	22
18	2553	2577	2601	2625	2648	2672	2695	2718	2742	2765	2	5	7	9	12	14	16	19	21
19	2788	2810	2833	2856	2878	2900	2923	2945	2967	2989	2	4	7	9	11	13	16	18	20
20	3010	3032	3054	3075	3096	3118	3139	3160	3181	3201	2	4	6	8	11	13	15	17	19
21	3222	3243	3263	3284	3304	3324	3345	3365	3385	3404	2	4	6	8	10	12	14	16	18
22	3424	3444	3464	3483	3502	3522	3541	3560	3579	3598	2	4	6	8	10	12	14	15	17
23	3617	3636	3655	3674	3692	3711	3729	3747	3766	3784	2	4	6	7	9	11	13	15	17
24	3802	3820	3838	3856	3874	3892	3909	3927	3945	3962	2	4	5	7	9	11	12	14	16
25	3979	3997	4014	4031	4048	4065	4082	4099	4116	4133	2	3	5	7	9	10	12	14	15
26	4150	4166	4183	4200	4216	4232	4249	4265	4281	4298	2	3	5	7	8	10	11	13	15
27	4314	4330	4346	4362	4378	4393	4409	4425	4440	4456	2	3	5	6	8	9	11	13	14
28	4472	4487	4502	4518	4533	4548	4564	4579	4594	4609	2	3	5	6	8	9	11	12	14
29	4624	4639	4654	4669	4683	4698	4713	4728	4742	4757	1	3	4	6	7	9	10	12	13
30	4771	4786	4800	4814	4829	4843	4857	4871	4886	4900	1	3	4	6	7	9	10	11	13
31	4914	4928	4942	4955	4969	4983	4997	5011	5024	5038	1	3	4	6	7	8	10	11	12
32	5051	5065	5079	5092	5105	5119	5132	5145	5159	5172	1	3	4	5	7	8	9	11	12
33	5185	5198	5211	5224	5237	5250	5263	5276	5289	5302	1	3	4	5	6	8	9	10	12
34	5315	5328	5340	5353	5366	5378	5391	5403	5416	5428	1	3	4	5	6	8	9	10	11
35	5441	5453	5465	5478	5490	5502	5514	5527	5539	5551	1	2	4	5	6	7	9	10	11
36	5563	5575	5587	5599	5611	5623	5635	5647	5658	5670	1	2	4	5	6	7	8	10	11
37	5682	5694	5705	5717	5729	5740	5752	5763	5775	5786	1	2	3	5	6	7	8	9	10
38	5798	5809	5821	5832	5843	5855	5866	5877	5888	5899	1	2	3	5	6	7	8	9	10
39	5911	5922	5933	5944	5955	5966	5977	5988	5999	6010	1	2	2	4	5	7	8	9	10
40	6021	6031	6042	6053	6064	6075	6085	6096	6107	6117	1	2	3	4	5	6	8	9	10
41	6128	6138	6149	6160	6170	6180	6191	6201	6212	6222	1	2	3	4	5	6	7	8	9
42	6232	6243	6253	6263	6274	6284	6294	6304	6314	6325	1	2	3	4	5	6	7	8	9
43	6335	6345	6355	6365	6375	6385	6395	6405	6415	6425	1	2	3	4	5	6	7	8	9
44	6435	6444	6454	6464	6474	6484	6493	6503	6513	6522	1	2	3	4	5	6	7	8	9
45	6532	6542	6551	6561	6571	6580	6590	6599	6609	6618	1	2	3	4	5	6	7	8	9
46	6628	6637	6646	6656	6665	6675	6684	6693	6702	6712	1	2	3	4	5	6	7	7	8
47	6721	6730	6739	6749	6758	6767	6776	6785	6794	6803	1	2	3	4	5	5	6	7	8
48	6812	6821	6830	6839	6848	6857	6866	6875	6884	6893	1	2	3	4	4	5	6	7	8
49	6902	6911	6920	6928	6937	6946	6955	6964	6972	6981	1	2	3	4	4	5	6	7	8
50	6990	6998	7007	7016	7024	7033	7042	7050	7059	7067	1	2	3	3	4	5	6	7	8
51	7076	7084	7093	7101	7110	7118	7126	7135	7143	7152	1	2	3	3	4	5	6	7	8
52	7160	7168	7177	7185	7193	7202	7210	7218	7226	7235	1	2	2	3	4	5	6	7	7
53	7243	7251	7259	7267	7275	7284	7292	7300	7308	7316	1	2	2	3	4	5	6	6	7
54	7324	7332	7340	7348	7356	7364	7372	7380	7388	7396	1	2	2	3	4	5	6	6	7

(continued)

SOME LOGARITHMIC COMPUTATIONS

As shown in the first of the subsequent examples, when a negative number is "added", it is actually *subtracted*; and as shown in the third example, when a negative number is "subtracted," it is actually *added*.

The fourth example shows the curious but consistent fact, when subtracting one logarithm from another, that if you *borrow* from a negative characteristic (as 1 is borrowed from the − 1 of the minuend), you *increase* the value of the negative characteristic (as

Table AJ.I. *(Continued)*

Natural Numbers	0	1	2	3	4	5	6	7	8	9	Proportional Parts								
											1	2	3	4	5	6	7	8	9
55	7404	7412	7419	7427	7435	7443	7451	7459	7466	7474	1	2	2	3	4	5	5	6	7
56	7482	7490	7497	7505	7513	7520	7528	7536	7543	7551	1	2	2	3	4	5	5	6	7
57	7559	7566	7574	7582	7589	7597	7604	7612	7619	7627	1	2	2	3	4	5	5	6	7
58	7634	7642	7649	7657	7664	7672	7679	7686	7694	7701	1	1	2	3	4	4	5	6	7
59	7709	7716	7723	7731	7738	7745	7752	7760	7767	7774	1	1	2	3	4	4	5	6	7
60	7782	7789	7796	7803	7810	7818	7825	7832	7839	7846	1	1	2	3	4	4	5	6	6
61	7853	7860	7868	7875	7882	7889	7896	7903	7910	7917	1	1	2	3	4	4	5	6	6
62	7924	7931	7938	7945	7952	7959	7966	7973	7980	7987	1	1	2	3	3	4	5	6	6
63	7993	8000	8007	8014	8021	8028	8035	8041	8048	8055	1	1	2	3	3	4	5	5	6
64	8062	8069	8075	8082	8089	8096	8102	8109	8116	8122	1	1	2	3	3	4	5	5	6
65	8129	8136	8142	8149	8156	8162	8169	8176	8182	8189	1	1	2	3	3	4	5	5	6
66	8195	8202	8209	8215	8222	8228	8235	8241	8248	8254	1	1	2	3	3	4	5	5	6
67	8261	8267	8274	8280	8287	8293	8299	8306	8312	8319	1	1	2	3	3	4	5	5	6
68	8325	8331	8338	8344	8351	8357	8363	8370	8376	8382	1	1	2	3	3	4	4	5	6
69	8388	8395	8401	8407	8414	8420	8426	8432	8439	8445	1	1	2	3	3	4	4	5	6
70	8451	8457	8463	8470	8476	8482	8488	8494	8500	8506	1	1	2	2	3	4	4	5	6
71	8513	8519	8525	8531	8537	8543	8549	8555	8561	8567	1	1	2	2	3	4	4	5	5
72	8573	8579	8585	8591	8597	8603	8609	8615	8621	8627	1	1	2	2	3	4	4	5	5
73	8633	8639	8645	8651	8657	8663	8669	8675	8681	8686	1	1	2	2	3	4	4	5	5
74	8692	8698	8704	8710	8716	8722	8727	8733	8739	8745	1	1	2	2	3	4	4	5	5
75	8751	8756	8762	8768	8774	8779	8785	8791	8797	8802	1	1	2	2	3	3	4	5	5
76	8808	8814	8820	8825	8831	8837	8842	8848	8854	8859	1	1	2	2	3	3	4	5	5
77	8865	8871	8876	8882	8887	8893	8899	8904	8910	8915	1	1	2	2	3	3	4	4	5
78	8921	8927	8932	8938	8943	8949	8954	8960	8965	8971	1	1	2	2	3	3	4	4	5
79	8976	8982	8987	8993	8998	9004	9009	9015	9020	9026	1	1	2	2	3	3	4	4	5
80	9031	9036	9042	9047	9053	9058	9063	9069	9074	9079	1	1	2	2	3	3	4	4	5
81	9085	9090	9096	9101	9106	9112	9117	9122	9128	9133	1	1	2	2	3	3	4	4	5
82	9138	9143	9149	9154	9159	9165	9170	9175	9180	9186	1	1	2	2	3	3	4	4	5
83	9191	9196	9201	9206	9212	9217	9222	9227	9232	9238	1	1	2	2	3	3	4	4	5
84	9243	9248	9253	9258	9263	9269	9274	9279	9284	9289	1	1	2	2	3	3	4	4	5
85	9294	9299	9304	9309	9315	9320	9325	9330	9335	9340	1	1	2	2	3	3	4	4	5
86	9345	9350	9355	9360	9365	9370	9375	9380	9385	9390	1	1	2	2	3	3	4	4	5
87	9395	9400	9405	9410	9415	9420	9425	9430	9435	9440	0	1	1	2	2	3	3	4	4
88	9445	9450	9455	9460	9465	9469	9474	9479	9484	9489	0	1	1	2	2	3	3	4	4
89	9494	9499	9504	9509	9513	9518	9523	9528	9533	9538	0	1	1	2	2	3	3	4	4
90	9542	9547	9552	9557	9562	9566	9571	9576	9581	9586	0	1	1	2	2	3	3	4	4
91	9590	9595	9600	9605	9609	9614	9619	9624	9628	9633	0	1	1	2	2	3	3	4	4
92	9638	9643	9647	9652	9657	9661	9666	9671	9675	9680	0	1	1	2	2	3	3	4	4
93	9685	9689	9694	9699	9703	9708	9713	9717	9722	9727	0	1	1	2	2	3	3	4	4
94	9731	9736	9741	9745	9750	9754	9759	9763	9768	9773	0	1	1	2	2	3	3	4	4
95	9777	9782	9786	9791	9795	9800	9805	9809	9814	9818	0	1	1	2	2	3	3	4	4
96	9823	9827	9832	9836	9841	9845	9850	9854	9859	9863	0	1	1	2	2	3	3	4	4
97	9868	9872	9877	9881	9886	9890	9894	9899	9903	9908	0	1	1	2	2	3	3	4	4
98	9912	9917	9921	9926	9930	9934	9939	9943	9948	9952	0	1	1	2	2	3	3	4	4
99	9956	9961	9965	9969	9974	9978	9983	9987	9991	9996	0	1	1	2	2	3	3	3	4

the -1 becomes -2, which is canceled out when the 2 of the subtrahend is "subtracted" from it).

Examples:

Multiply (5.25×10^3) *by* (8.92×10^{-6}) *by* (7.56×10^5).

$$\log (5.25 \times 10^3) = 3.7202$$
$$\log (8.92 \times 10^{-6}) = \bar{6}.9504$$
$$\log (7.56 \times 10^5) = \underline{5.8785}$$
$$\text{Total:} \qquad\qquad 4.5491$$

Antilogarithm of $4.5491 = 3.541 \times 10^4 = 35410$, or (retaining only three significant figures), 35400, *answer.*

Divide 29600 by 5.544.

$$29600 = 2.96 \times 10^4$$
$$5.544 = 5.544 \times 10^0$$
$$\log (2.96 \times 10^4) \quad = 4.4713$$
$$\log (5.544 \times 10^0) \quad = \underline{0.7438}$$
$$\text{Difference:} \qquad\qquad 3.7275$$

Antilogarithm of $3.7275 = 5.34 \times 10^3 = 5340$, *answer.*

Divide 7500 by 0.627.

$$7500 = 7.50 \times 10^3$$
$$0.627 = 6.27 \times 10^{-1}$$
$$\log (7.50 \times 10^3) \quad = 3.8751$$
$$\log (6.27 \times 10^{-1}) \quad = \underline{\bar{1}.7973}$$
$$\text{Difference:} \qquad\qquad 4.0778$$

Antilogarithm of $4.0778 = 1.196 \times 10^4 = 11960$, or (retaining only three significant figures), 12000, *answer.*

Divide 0.191 by 0.0452.

$$0.191 = 1.91 \times 10^{-1}$$
$$0.0452 = 4.52 \times 10^{-2}$$
$$\log (1.91 \times 10^{-1}) \quad = \bar{1}.2810$$
$$\log (4.52 \times 10^{-2}) \quad = \underline{\bar{2}.6551}$$
$$\text{Difference:} \qquad\qquad 0.6259$$

Antilogarithm of $0.6259 = 4.226 \times 10^0 = 4.226$, or (retaining only three significant figures), 4.23, *answer.*

Find the value of

$$\frac{(4.54 \times 10^6) \times (3.25 \times 10^3)}{(1.21 \times 10^8)}$$

$$\log (4.54 \times 10^6) \quad = \quad 6.6571$$
$$\log (3.25 \times 10^3) \quad = \quad \underline{3.5119}$$
$$\text{Total:} \qquad\qquad\qquad 10.1690 = log\ of\ numerator$$

$$\log (1.21 \times 10^8) \quad = \quad \underline{8.0282} = log\ of\ denominator$$
$$\text{Difference:} \qquad\qquad 2.0862$$

Antilogarithm of $2.0862 = 1.219$ or $1.22 \times 10^2 = 122$, *answer.*

Practice Problems

1. Find the logarithm of each of the following numbers.
    (a) 2245   (f) 0.7245
    (b) 5.265   (g) 215000

(c) 7000   (h) 0.0001372
(d) 187.9   (i) 63.78
(e) 0.002934   (j) 6.2×10^6

2. Find the antilogarithm corresponding to each of the following logarithms.
    (a) 4.4512   (f) 2.1668
    (b) 1.1523   (g) 0.0261
    (c) 0.3302   (h) $\bar{3}.8902$
    (d) $\bar{1}.1105$ (i) 1.9234
    (e) 2.7892   (j) $\bar{2}.1234$

3. Compute each of the following by means of logarithms.
    (a) 23.87×954.6
    (b) 8542×0.8562
    (c) 655.7×0.02253
    (d) $(8.235 \times 10^2) \times (4.296 \times 10^{-4}) \times (2.325 \times 10^3)$
    (e) $26.74 \times 5.987 \times 106.7$

4. Compute each of the following by means of logarithms.
    (a) $9525 \div 1.267$
    (b) $2500 \div 12.65$
    (c) $0.2925 \div 56.85$
    (d) $(1.658 \times 10^4) \div (4.689 \times 10^2)$
    (e) $0.491 \div 0.0357$

5. Find the value of each of the following by means of logarithms.

    (a) $\dfrac{(6.29 \times 10^2) \times (1.23 \times 10^4)}{(9.75 \times 10^4)} =$

    (b) $\dfrac{1{,}667{,}000 \times 0.4101}{(6.31 \times 10^3)} =$

    (c) $\dfrac{(7.32 \times 10^2)}{(4.315 \times 10^{-4}) \times (5.795 \times 10^3)} =$

K

Some Calculations Involving Buffer Solutions

BUFFERS AND BUFFER SOLUTIONS

When a minute trace of hydrochloric acid is added to pure water, a significant increase in *hydrogen-ion* concentration occurs immediately. In a similar manner, when a minute trace of sodium hydroxide is added to pure water, it causes a correspondingly large increase in the *hydroxyl-ion* concentration. These changes take place because water alone cannot neutralize even traces of acid or base, i.e., it has no ability to resist changes in hydrogen-ion concentration or pH. A solution of a neutral salt, such as sodium chloride, also lacks this ability. Therefore, it is said to be *unbuffered.*

The presence of certain substances or combinations of substances in aqueous solution imparts to the system the ability to maintain a desired pH at a relatively constant level, even with the addition of materials that may be expected to change the hydrogen-ion concentration. These substances or combinations of substances are called *buffers*; their ability to resist changes in pH is referred to as *buffer action*; their efficiency is measured by the function known as *buffer capacity*; and solutions of them are called *buffer solutions*. By definition, then, a *buffer solution* is a system, usually an aqueous solution, that possesses the property of resisting changes in pH with the addition of small amounts of a strong acid or base.

Buffers are used to establish and maintain an ion activity within rather narrow limits. In pharmacy, the most common buffer systems are used (1) in the preparation of such dosage forms as injections and ophthalmic solutions, which are placed directly into pH-sensitive body fluids; (2) in the manufacture of formulations in which the pH must be maintained at a relatively constant level to ensure maximum product stability; and (3) in pharmaceutical tests and assays requiring adjustment to or maintenance of a specific pH for analytic purposes.

Buffer solutions are usually composed of a *weak acid and a salt of the acid,* as for example, acetic acid and sodium acetate, or a *weak base and a salt of the base,* such as ammonium hydroxide and ammonium chloride. Typical buffer systems that may be used in pharmaceutical formulations include the following pairs: acetic acid and sodium acetate, boric acid and sodium borate, and disodium phosphate and sodium acid phosphate. Formulas for standard buffer solutions for pharmaceutical analysis are given in the *United States Pharmacopeia.*

In the selection of a buffer system, due consideration must be given to the dissociation constant of the weak acid or base to ensure maximum buffer capacity. This dissociation constant, in the case of an acid, is a measure of the strength of the acid; the more readily the acid dissociates, the higher its dissociation constant and the stronger the acid. Selected dissociation constants or K_a values are given in Table AK.1.

The dissociation constant or K_a value of a weak acid is given by the equation:

$$K_a = \frac{(H^+)(A^-)}{(HA)} \qquad \text{where } A^- = \text{salt}$$
$$HA = \text{acid}$$

Table AK.1. Dissociation Constants of Some Weak Acids at 25°C

Acid	K_a
Acetic	1.75×10^{-5}
Barbituric	1.05×10^{-4}
Benzoic	6.30×10^{-5}
Boric	6.4×10^{-10}
Formic	1.76×10^{-4}
Lactic	1.38×10^{-4}
Mandelic	4.29×10^{-4}
Salicylic	1.06×10^{-3}

Because the numeric values of most dissociation constants are small numbers and may vary over many powers of 10, it is more convenient to express them as negative logarithms, i.e.,

$$pK_a = -\log K_a$$

When equation $K_a = \dfrac{(H^+)(A^-)}{(HA)}$ is expressed in logarithmic form, it is written:

$$pK_a = -\log (H^+) - \log \frac{salt}{acid}$$

and because $pH = -\log (H^+)$

then

$$pK_a = pH - \log \frac{salt}{acid}$$

and

$$pH = pK_a + \log \frac{salt}{acid}$$

BUFFER EQUATION

The equation just derived is the Henderson-Hasselbalch equation for weak acids, commonly known as the *buffer equation*.

Similarly, the dissociation constant or K_b value of a weak base is given by the equation:

$$K_b = \frac{(B^+)(OH^-)}{(BOH)} \qquad \begin{array}{l} \text{in which } B^+ = salt \\ \text{and BOH} = base \end{array}$$

and the buffer equation for weak bases, which is derived from this relationship, may be expressed as:

$$pH = pK_w - pK_b + \log \frac{base}{salt}$$

The buffer equation is useful (1) for calculating the pH of a buffer system if its composition is known, and (2) for calculating the molar ratio of the components of a buffer system required to give a solution of a desired pH. The equation may also be used to calculate the change in pH of a buffered solution with the addition of a given amount of acid or base.

pK$_a$ Value of a Weak Acid with Known Dissociation Constant. Calculating the pK$_a$ value of a weak acid, given its dissociation constant, K$_a$, involves the following.

Example:

> *The dissociation constant of acetic acid is 1.75×10^{-5} at 25°C. Calculate its pK$_a$ value.*

$$K_a = 1.75 \times 10^{-5}$$

and
$$\log K_a = \log 1.75 + \log 10^{-5}$$

$$= 0.2430 - 5 = -4.757 \text{ or } -4.76$$

Because
$$pK_a = -\log K_a$$

$$pK_a = -(-4.76) = 4.76, \text{ } answer.$$

pH Value of a Salt/Acid Buffer System. Calculating the pH value of this type of system involves the following.

Example:

> *What is the pH of a buffer solution prepared with 0.05 M sodium borate and 0.005 M boric acid? The pK$_a$ value of boric acid is 9.24 at 25°C.*

Note that the ratio of the components of the buffer solution is given in molar concentrations.

Using the buffer equation for weak acids,

$$pH = pK_a + \log \frac{salt}{acid}$$

$$= 9.24 + \log \frac{0.05}{0.005}$$

$$= 9.24 + \log 10$$

$$= 9.24 + 1$$

$$= 10.24, \text{ } answer.$$

pH Value of a Base/Salt Buffer System. Calculating the pH value of this type of system involves the following.

Example:

> *What is the pH of a buffer solution prepared with 0.05 M ammonia and 0.05 M ammonium chloride? The K$_b$ value of ammonia is 1.80×10^{-5} at 25°C.*

Using the buffer equation for weak bases,

$$pH = pK_w - pK_b + \log \frac{base}{salt}$$

Because the K$_w$ value for water is 10^{-14} at 25°C, pK$_w$ = 14.

$$K_b \; = \; 1.80 \times 10^{-5}$$

and $\quad\quad\quad \log K_b \; = \; \log 1.8 + \log 10^{-5}$

$$= \; 0.2553 - 5 \; = \; -4.7447 \; \text{or} \; -4.74$$

$$pK_b \; = \; -\log K_b$$

$$= \; -(-4.74) \; = \; 4.74$$

and $\quad\quad\quad\quad pH \; = \; 14 - 4.74 + \log \dfrac{0.05}{0.05}$

$$= \; 9.26 + \log 1$$

$$= \; 9.26, \; answer.$$

Molar Ratio of Salt/Acid for a Buffer System of Desired pH. Calculating the molar ratio of salt/acid required to prepare a buffer system with a desired pH value involves the following.

Example:

What molar ratio of salt/acid is required to prepare a sodium acetate-acetic acid buffer solution with a pH of 5.76? The pK_a value of acetic acid is 4.76 at 25°C.

Using the buffer equation,

$$pH \; = \; pK_a + \log \dfrac{salt}{acid}$$

$$\log \dfrac{salt}{acid} \; = \; pH - pK_a$$

$$= \; 5.76 - 4.76 \; = \; 1$$

antilog of $1 \; = \; 10$

ratio $\quad\quad\quad = \; 10/1 \; \text{or} \; 10:1, \; answer.$

Quantity of Components in a Buffer Solution to Yield a Specific Volume. Calculating the amounts of the components of a buffer solution required to prepare a desired volume, given the molar ratio of the components and the total buffer concentration, involves the following.

Example:

The molar ratio of sodium acetate to acetic acid in a buffer solution with a pH of 5.76 is 10:1. Assuming the total buffer concentration is 2.2×10^{-2} mol/L, how many grams of sodium acetate (m.w.-82) and how many grams of acetic acid (m.w.-60) should be used in preparing a liter of the solution?

Because the molar ratio of sodium acetate to acetic acid is 10:1.

the mole fraction of sodium acetate $= \; \dfrac{10}{1 + 10} \; \text{or} \; \dfrac{10}{11}$

and the mole fraction of acetic acid $= \; \dfrac{1}{1 + 10} \; \text{or} \; \dfrac{1}{11}$

If the total buffer concentration $= \; 2.2 \times 10^{-2}$ mol/L,

$$\text{the concentration of sodium acetate} = \frac{10}{11} \times (2.2 \times 10^{-2})$$

$$= 2.0 \times 10^{-2} \text{ mol/L}$$

$$\text{and the concentration of acetic acid} = \frac{1}{11} \times (2.2 \times 10^{-2})$$

$$= 0.2 \times 10^{-2} \text{ mol/L}$$

then 2.0×10^{-2} or $0.02 \times 82 = 1.64$ g of sodium acetate per liter of solution, *and*

0.2×10^{-2} or $0.002 \times 60 = 0.120$ g of acetic acid per liter of solution, *answers.*

The efficiency of buffer solutions, i.e., their specific ability to resist changes in pH, is measured in terms of *buffer capacity*; the *smaller* the pH change with the addition of a given amount of acid or base, the *greater* the buffer capacity of the system. Among other factors, the buffer capacity of a system depends on (1) the relative concentration of the buffer components and (2) the ratio of the components. For example, a 0.5 M acetate buffer at a pH of 4.76 would have a higher buffer capacity than a 0.05 M buffer.

If a strong base such as sodium hydroxide is added to a buffer system consisting of equimolar concentrations of sodium acetate and acetic acid, the base is neutralized by the acetic acid forming more sodium acetate, and the resulting *increase* in pH is slight. Actually, the addition of the base increases the concentration of sodium acetate and decreases *by an equal amount* the concentration of acetic acid. In a similar manner, the addition of a strong acid to a buffer system consisting of a weak base and its salt would produce only a small *decrease* in pH.

Change in pH with Addition of an Acid or Base. Calculating the change in pH of a buffer solution with the addition of a given amount of acid or base involves the following.

Example:

Calculate the change in pH after adding 0.04 mol of sodium hydroxide to a liter of a buffer solution containing 0.2 M concentrations of sodium acetate and acetic acid. The pK_a value of acetic acid is 4.76 at 25°C.

The pH of the buffer solution is calculated by using the buffer equation as follows:

$$pH = pK_a + \log \frac{\text{salt}}{\text{acid}}$$

$$= 4.76 + \log \frac{0.2}{0.2}$$

$$= 4.76 + \log 1$$

$$= 4.76$$

The addition of 0.04 mol of sodium hydroxide converts 0.04 mol of acetic acid to 0.04 mol of sodium acetate. Consequently, the concentration of acetic acid is *decreased* and the concentration of sodium acetate is *increased* by equal amounts, according to the following equation:

$$pH = pK_a + \log \frac{salt + base}{acid - base}$$

and $$pH = pK_a + \log \frac{0.2 + 0.04}{0.2 - 0.04}$$

$$= pK_a + \log \frac{0.24}{0.16}$$

$$= 4.76 + 0.1761 = 4.9361 \text{ or } 4.94$$

Because the pH before the addition of the sodium hydroxide was 4.76, the change in pH = 4.94 − 4.76 = 0.18 unit, *answer*.

Practice Problems

1. The dissociation constant of lactic acid is 1.38×10^{-4} at 25°C. Calculate its pK_a value.

2. Calculate the pK_a value of an acid having a dissociation constant of 1.75×10^{-10} at 25°C.

3. The dissociation constant of ethanolamine is 2.77×10^{-5} at 25°C. Calculate its pK_b value.

4. Calculate the pK_b value of urea, which has a dissociation constant of 1.5×10^{-14} at 25°C.

5. What is the pH of a buffer solution prepared with 0.055 M sodium acetate and 0.01 M acetic acid? The pK_a value of acetic acid is 4.76 at 25°C.

6. Calculate the pH of a buffer solution containing 0.1 mol of acetic acid and 0.2 mol of sodium acetate per liter. The pK_a value of acetic acid is 4.76 at 25°C.

7. What is the pH of a buffer solution prepared with 0.5 M disodium phosphate and 1 M sodium acid phosphate? The pK_a value of sodium acid phosphate is 7.21 at 25°C.

8. What is the pH of a buffer solution prepared by using 0.001 molar sodium benzoate and 0.01 molar benzoic acid? The pK_a value of benzoic acid is 4.20 at 25°C.

9. What molar ratio of salt to acid would be required to prepare a buffer solution with a pH of 4.5? The pK_a value of the acid is 4.05 at 25°C.

10. What molar ratio of base to salt would be required to prepare a buffer solution of pH 6.8? The dissociation constant of the base is 4.47×10^{-5} at 25°C.

11. What is the change in pH on adding 0.02 mol of sodium hydroxide to a liter of a buffer solution containing 0.5 M of sodium acetate and 0.5 M acetic acid? The pK_a value of acetic acid is 4.76 at 25°C.

12. What molar ratio of salt/acid is required to prepare a sodium borate-boric acid buffer solution with a pH of 9.44? The pK_a value of boric acid is 9.24 at 25°C.

13. The molar ratio of salt to acid needed to prepare a sodium acetate-acetic acid buffer

solution is $1:1$. Assuming that the total buffer concentration is 0.1 mol/L, how many grams of sodium acetate (m.w.-60) should be used in preparing 2 liters of the solution?

14. What is the change in pH with the addition of 0.01 hydrochloric acid to a liter of a buffer solution containing 0.05 M of ammonia and 0.05 M of ammonium chloride? The K_b value of ammonia is 1.80×10^{-5} at 25°C.

L

Chemical Problems

ATOMIC AND MOLECULAR WEIGHTS

Most chemical problems involve the use of *atomic* or *combining weights* of the elements, and the validity of their solutions depends on the *Law of Definite Proportions.*

The *atomic weight* of an element is the ratio of the weight of its atom to the weight of an atom of another element taken as a standard. Long ago, hydrogen, with a weight taken as 1, was used as the standard. For many years, the weight of oxygen, taken as 16, proved a more convenient standard. In 1961, however, the International Union of Pure and Applied Chemistry (following similar action by the International Union of Pure and Applied Physics) released the most up-to-date table of atomic weights based on carbon, taking 12 as the relative nuclidic mass of the isotope ^{12}C. The rounded-off *approximate* atomic weights in the table given on the inside back cover and those based on the long-familiar oxygen table are identical and continue to be sufficiently accurate for most chemical calculations likely to be encountered by pharmacists.

The *combining* or *equivalent weight* of an *element* is that weight of the given element that will combine with (or displace) 1 g atomic weight of hydrogen (or the equivalent weight of some other element). For example, when hydrogen and chlorine react to form HCl, 1.008 g of hydrogen react with 35.45 g of chlorine; therefore, the equivalent weight of chlorine is 35.45.

The *equivalent weight* of a *compound* is that weight of a given compound that is chemically equivalent to 1.008 g of hydrogen. Thus, 1 mol or 36.46 g of HCl contains 1.008 g of hydrogen and this amount is displaceable by one equivalent weight of a metal; hence, its equivalent weight is 36.46. Also, 1 mol or 40.00 g of NaOH are capable of neutralizing 1.008 g of hydrogen; therefore, its equivalent weight is 40.00. One mol or 98.09 of H_2SO_4, however, contains 2.016 g of hydrogen, which is displaceable by *two* equivalent weights of a metal; consequently, its equivalent weight is 98.08/2 or 49.04.

The *Law of Definite Proportions* states that elements invariably combine in the same proportion by weight to form a given compound.

Percentage Composition. Calculating the percentage composition of a compound involves the following.

Example:

Calculate the percentage composition of anhydrous dextrose, $C_6H_{12}O_6$.

$$\begin{array}{ccccccc}
C_6 & & H_{12} & & O_6 & & \\
(6 \times 12.01) & + & (12 \times 1.008) & + & (6 \times 16.00) & = & \\
72.06 & + & 12.096 & + & 96.00 & = & 180.16
\end{array}$$

$$\frac{180.16}{72.06} = \frac{100\ (\%)}{x\ (\%)}$$

$$x = 40.00\% \text{ of carbon, } and$$

$$\frac{180.16}{12.096} = \frac{100\ (\%)}{y\ (\%)}$$

$$y = 6.71\% \text{ of hydrogen, } and$$

$$\frac{180.16}{96.00} = \frac{100\ (\%)}{z\ (\%)}$$

$$z = 53.29\% \text{ of oxygen, } answers.$$

Check: $40.00\% + 6.71\% + 53.29\% = 100\%$

Percentage of a Constituent. Calculating the percentage of a constituent in a compound involves the following. Approximate atomic weights may ordinarily be used in solving problems of this kind.

Example:

Calculate the percentage of lithium (Li) in lithium carbonate, Li_2CO_3.

Molecular weight of lithium carbonate $= 74$
Atomic weight of lithium $= 7$

$$\frac{74}{2 \times 7} = \frac{100\ (\%)}{x\ (\%)}$$

$$x = 18.9\%, answer.$$

Weight of Constituent Given Weight of Compound. Calculating the weight of a constituent, given the weight of a compound, involves the following. Approximate atomic weights may ordinarily be used in solving problems of this kind.

Example:

A ferrous sulfate elixir contains 220 mg of ferrous sulfate ($FeSO_4 \cdot 7H_2O$) per teaspoonful dose. How many milligrams of elemental iron are represented in the dose?

Molecular weight of $FeSO_4 \cdot 7H_2O = 278$
Atomic weight of Fe $= 56$

$$\frac{278}{56} = \frac{220\ (mg)}{x\ (mg)}$$

$$x = 44.3 \text{ or } 44 \text{ mg}, answer.$$

Weight of Compound Given Weight of Constituent. Calculating the weight of a compound, given the weight of a constituent, involves the following. Approximate atomic weights may ordinarily be used in solving problems of this kind.

Example:

How many milligrams of sodium fluoride will provide 500 μg of fluoride ion?

$$\text{Na} \quad \text{F}$$

$$23 + 19 = 42$$

$$\frac{19}{42} = \frac{500\ (\mu g)}{x\ (\mu g)}$$

$$x = 1105\ \mu g\ or\ 1.1\ mg,\ answer.$$

CHEMICALLY EQUIVALENT QUANTITIES

Solving Problems. Approximate atomic weights may ordinarily be used in solving problems of this kind.

Examples:

The formula for 1000 g of a cosmetic cream calls for 14.7 g of potassium carbonate ($K_2CO_3 \cdot 1\frac{1}{2}H_2O$). How many grams of 85% potassium hydroxide (KOH) could be used to replace the potassium carbonate in formulating the cream?

	Molecular weights:	Equivalent weights:
$K_2CO_3 \cdot 1\frac{1}{2}H_2O$	165	82.5
KOH	56	56

$$\frac{82.5}{56} = \frac{14.7\ (g)}{x\ (g)}$$

$$x = 9.98\ g\ of\ 100\%\ KOH$$

$$and\ \frac{85\ (\%)}{100\ (\%)} = \frac{9.98\ (g)}{x\ (g)}$$

$$x = 11.74\ g\ of\ 85\%\ KOH,\ answer.$$

The formula for Magnesium Citrate Oral Solution calls for 27.4 g of anhydrous citric acid ($C_6H_8O_7$) in 350 ml of the product. How many grams of citric acid monohydrate ($C_6H_8O_7 \cdot H_2O$) may be used in place of the anhydrous salt?

Molecular weights:

$$C_6H_8O_7 \cdot H_2O = 210 \qquad C_6H_8O_7 = 192$$

$$\frac{192}{210} = \frac{27.4\ (g)}{x\ (g)}$$

$$x = 29.97\ or\ 30\ g,\ answer.$$

Practice Problems

1. Calculate the percentage composition of ether, $(C_2H_5)_2O$.

2. What is the percentage composition of Dibasic Sodium Phosphate, USP, $Na_2HPO_4 \cdot 7H_2O$?

3. What is the percentage composition of Monobasic Sodium Phosphate, USP, $NaH_2PO_4 \cdot H_2O$?

4. Calculate the percentage of water in dextrose, $C_6H_{12}O_6 \cdot H_2O$.

5. How many grams of water are represented in 2000 g of magnesium sulfate, $MgSO_4 \cdot 7H_2O$?

6. What is the percentage of calcium in calcium gluconate, $C_{12}H_{22}CaO_{14}$?

7. A commercially available tablet contains 0.2 g of $FeSO_4 \cdot 2H_2O$. How many milligrams of elemental iron are represented in a daily dose of three tablets?

8. A certain solution contains 110 mg of sodium fluoride, NaF, in each 1000 mL. How many milligrams of fluoride ion are represented in each 2 mL of the solution?

9. How many milliliters of a solution containing 0.275 mg of histamine acid phosphate (m.w.-307) per milliliter should be used in preparing 30 mL of a solution that is to contain the equivalent of 1:10,000 of histamine (m.w.-111)?

10. ℞   Sodium Fluoride   q.s.
          Multiple Vitamin Drops   ad   60.0 mL
          (Five drops = 1 mg of fluoride ion)
          Sig. Five drops in orange juice daily.
    The dispensing dropper calibrates 20 drops/mL. How many milligrams of sodium fluoride should be used in preparing the prescription?

11. In preparing magnesium citrate oral solution, 2.5 g of potassium bicarbonate ($KHCO_3$) are needed to charge each bottle. If no potassium bicarbonate is available, how much sodium bicarbonate ($NaHCO_3$) should be used?

12. The formula for Albright's solution "M" calls for 8.84 g of anhydrous sodium carbonate (Na_2CO_3) per 1000 mL. How many grams of 95% sodium hydroxide (NaOH) should be used to replace the anhydrous sodium carbonate in preparing 5 liters of the solution?

13. Ferrous sulfate syrup contains 40 g of ferrous sulfate ($FeSO_4 \cdot 7H_2O$) per 1000 mL. How many milligrams of iron (Fe) are represented in the usual dose of 10 mL of the syrup?

14. How many grams of 42% (MgO equivalent) magnesium carbonate are required to prepare 14 liters of magnesium citrate oral solution so that 350 mL contain the equivalent of 6.0 g of MgO?

15. Five hundred grams of effervescent sodium phosphate contain 100 g of anhydrous dibasic sodium phosphate (Na_2HPO_4). How many grams of Dibasic Sodium Phosphate, USP, ($Na_2HPO_4 \cdot 7H_2O$) are represented in each 10-g dose of effervescent sodium phosphate?

16. How many grams of epinephrine bitartrate (m.w.−333) should be used in preparing 500 mL of an ophthalmic solution containing the equivalent of 2% of epinephrine (m.w.−183)?

M Glossary Of Pharmaceutical Dosage Forms and Drug Delivery Systems[1]

Aerosols

Pharmaceutical aerosols are products packaged under pressure that contain therapeutically active ingredients that are released as a fine mist, spray, or foam on actuation of the valve assembly. The pressure within the aerosol container that forces the product out of the valve is provided by an inert compressed or liquefied gas, termed the *propellant*. The product formulation and the type of valve used determine the emission; i.e., fine mist, coarse spray, foam, etc. Some aerosol emissions are intended to be inhaled deep into the lungs (**inhalation aerosol**) and must be of finer particles (less than 10 μm) than those intended for topical application to the skin or the mucous membranes of the nose, mouth, vagina, or rectum. Some aerosols have *metered valve* assemblies that permit a specific quantity of emission on valve actuation for dosage regulation.

Aromatic Waters

Aromatic waters are clear, saturated solutions of volatile oils or other aromatic substances in water. They are used orally, topically, or pharmaceutically for the characteristics of the aromatic material they contain.

Capsules

Capsules are solid dosage forms in which one or more medicinal and/or inert substances are enclosed within small shells of gelatin. Capsule shells are produced in varying sizes, shapes, thickness, softness, and color. Hard shell capsules, which have two telescoping parts—the body and the cap—are commonly used in extemporaneous hand-filling operations as well as in small and large scale manufacture of commercial capsules. They usually are filled with powder mixtures and granules. After filling, the two capsule parts are joined for tight closure. They may also be sealed and bonded through a variety of special processes for added quality assurance and capsule integrity.

Soft-shell gelatin capsules, which are unibodied, are formed, filled, and sealed in the same process. Highly specialized and large-scale equipment is required, and thus soft gelatin capsules are only prepared commercially. They are rendered soft through the addition of a plasticizer to the capsule shell formulation. Soft gelatin capsules may be filled with powders, semisolids, or liquids.

Capsules are intended to contain a specific quantity of fill, with the capsule size selected to accommodate that quantity most closely. In addition to their medication content, capsules usually contain inert pharmaceutical substances, such as fillers, disintegrants, solubilizers, etc. When swallowed, the gelatin shell is dissolved by the gastrointestinal fluids, releasing the contents. Capsules containing only nontherapeutic materials are termed *placebos* and are used widely in controlled clinical studies to evaluate the activity of a drug compared to nondrug in a group of human subjects.

---

[1] Some portions of this *Glossary* have been abstracted from the *United States Pharmacopeia* 23 and the *National Formulary* 18, pp. 1940-1986. Copyright 1994, The USP Convention, Inc., with permission.

Some capsules and tablets, or their granulated contents, may be *enteric coated*, i.e., coated with special materials to resist the release of the medication in the gastric fluid of the stomach to prevent either drug inactivation or gastric irritation. Drugs in enteric coated products are intended to be released after transit through the stomach into the intestines.

Extended-release capsules are formulated in such a manner to provide the active release of the medication from the dosage form over an extended period of time, such as 12 hours. The purpose is to provide constant drug release and sustained drug-blood levels of the drug for steady-state therapy and/or to enhance patient compliance by reducing the need for more frequent dosing.

Collodions

Collodions are liquid preparations composed of pyroxylin dissolved in a solvent mixture usually composed of alcohol and ether with or without added medicinal substances. They are intended for external application to the skin. The solvent rapidly evaporates, leaving a thin protective film of pyroxylin (and medication, such as salicylic acid as a corn remover) as an occlusive coating.

Creams

Creams are semisolid preparations containing one or more drug substances dissolved or dispersed in a suitable base. Many creams are either oil-in-water emulsions or aqueous microcrystalline dispersions of long chain fatty acids or alcohols in a water-washable base. Compared to ointments, creams are easier to spread and considered by many patients to be more aesthetically appealing in the topical delivery of medications. Creams are used primarily for administering drugs to the skin, although some are prepared for vaginal use.

Drug Delivery Systems

Various physical carriers are used to deliver medications to site-specific areas in various drug delivery systems, among which are transdermal, ocular, and intrauterine systems.

Transdermal drug delivery systems are designed to support the passage of drug substances from the surface of the skin, through its various layers, and into the systemic circulation. The systems are highly sophisticated skin patches containing the drug formulation within a reservoir as part of the device for the controlled delivery of drug into the skin.

Ocular drug delivery systems consist of drug-impregnated membranes, which when placed in the lower conjunctival sac, release medication over an extended period.

Intrauterine drug delivery systems consist of a drug-containing intrauterine device that releases medication over an extended period after insertion.

Elixirs

Elixirs are sweetened, flavored, hydroalcoholic solutions intended for oral administration. They may be *nonmedicated* or *medicated* and are used in the same manner as syrups. Compared to syrups, elixirs are usually less sweet and less viscous because they contain a lesser amount of sugar. Because of their hydroalcoholic character, elixirs are better able than are syrups to maintain both water-soluble and alcohol-soluble components in solution. Additional co-solvents, such as glycerin or propylene glycol, also may be used. The proportion of alcohol present in elixirs varies widely with the formulation and the requirements for solution. Elixirs of high alcoholic content generally include artificial sweeteners rather than sucrose as the sweetener. Because of their alcoholic content, elixirs generally are not administered to infants, young children, or other persons following alcohol-restricted diets.

Emulsions

An emulsion is a type of disperse system in which one liquid is dispersed throughout another liquid in the form of fine droplets. The two liquids, generally an oil and water, are immiscible and constitute two phases that tend to separate into layers unless a third agent, an *emulsifier* or *emulsifying agent*, is added to facilitate the emulsification process and to provide stability to the system.

In emulsions, the disperse phase is referred to as the *internal phase,* and the dispersing phase is termed the *external phase.* When the oil is the internal phase, the emulsion is called an oil-in-water or "o/w" emulsion. If water is the internal phase, the emulsion is called a water-in-oil or "w/o" emulsion. The type of emulsion produced is largely determined by the hydrophilicity or lipophilicity of the emulsifying agent. Emulsifying agents that are more hydrophilic generally produce oil-in-water emulsions, whereas emulsifying agents that are more lipophilic generally produce water-in-oil emulsions. Emulsifying agents may have both hydrophilic and lipophilic characteristics. The term hydrophile-lipophile balance ("HLB") quantifies this characteristic and is used in formulating and preparing emulsions of the desired type.

Calculations are used to determine the quantities of oil, water, and emulsifying agent to use in preparing a stable emulsion. Emulsions are most frequently prepared and administered orally for the medicinal benefit of the oil (e.g., mineral oil, oleaginous vitamins A and D). The taste and oleaginous feel of the oil is masked when administered in the form of an oil-in-water emulsion with a flavored aqueous external phase. In addition to oral emulsions, some emulsions are prepared for topical administration (such as some lotions, foams, and creams) and for intravenous injection, for the nutritional benefit of the oil (usually soybean oil).

Implants or Pellets

Implants or pellets are small, sterile, solid dosage forms containing concentrated drug for implantation in the body where they continuously release their medication over prolonged periods. Pellets generally are prepared by compression and implanted subcutaneously by means of a special injector or by surgical incision.

Inhalations

Inhalations are finely powdered drug substances, solutions, or suspensions of drug substances administered by the nasal or oral respiratory route for local or systemic effects. Special devices are used to facilitate administration.

Injections

Injections are sterile preparations intended for parenteral administration by needle or pressure syringe. Drugs may be injected into most any vessel or tissue of the body, but the most common routes are intravenous (IV), intramuscular (IM), and subcutaneous (SC). Injections may be solutions or suspensions of a drug substance in an aqueous or nonaqueous vehicle. They may be *small volume injections*, packaged in ampuls for single-dose administration, or vials for multiple dose injections. *Large volume parenterals,* containing 100-mL to 1 liter of fluid, are intended for the slow intravenous administration (or *infusion*) of medications and/or nutrients in the institutional or home-care setting. Calculations with regard to injections include a number of special aspects: the relation of the injection volume to drug dosage and patient factors such as weight, body surface area, or disease state; the relation of the dosing regimen to the flow rate of the parenteral; and formulation calculations related to isotonicity, osmolality, or milliequivalent content.

Some injections are available to the pharmacist in the dry state, requiring *constitution* with a prescribed liquid immediately before use to render the product suitable for injection. In these instances, calculations may be used to determine the quantity of liquid needed to prepare a product of desired concentration. A similar circumstance applies when the pharmacist is called on to place a drug "additive" (as an antibiotic) in a large-volume parenteral fluid to achieve a specified concentration of drug. The source of the additive may be an ampul or vial of the desired drug, requiring the pharmacist to calculate the volume of injection to add to the parenteral fluid.

Liniments

Liniments are alcoholic or oleaginous solutions, suspensions, or emulsions of medicinal agents intended for external application to the skin, generally by rubbing.

Lotions

Lotions are liquid preparations intended for external application to the skin. They are generally suspensions or emulsions of dispersed solid or liquid materials in an aqueous vehicle. Their fluidity allows rapid and uniform application over a wide skin surface. Lotions are intended to soften the skin and leave a thin coat of their components on the skin's surface as they dry.

Lozenges

Lozenges are solid preparations containing one or more medicinal agents in a flavored, sweetened base intended to dissolve or disintegrate slowly in the mouth, releasing medication generally for localized effects. Lozenges are prepared by molding or compression.

Magmas and Gels

Magmas and gels are examples of fine pharmaceutical suspensions in which the suspensoid has a high degree of physical attraction to the aqueous vehicle, forming a gelatinous mixture that maintains the uniformity and stability of the suspension. Magmas and gels are administered orally.

Ointments

Ointments are semisolid preparations intended for topical application. Most ointments are applied to the skin, although they may also be administered ophthalmically, nasally, aurally, rectally, or vaginally. With few exceptions, ointments are applied for their local effects on the tissue membrane rather than for systemic effects.

It is possible for systemic effects to occur after the topical application of medications. Systemic absorption, which takes place through the skin's surface, is referred to as *percutaneous absorption*. Percutaneous absorption may be enhanced by many factors, including the hydration of the skin, a concentrated (rather than dilute) application of preparation over a large surface area, application to thin rather than thick skin, through the hydrophilic-lipophilic nature of the drug, and by virtue of the occlusive features of the topical preparation and/or dressing.

Nonmedicated ointments serve as the vehicles, or *ointment bases*, for the addition of medication. Ointment bases are usually of four general types: (1) hydrocarbon or oleaginous bases (such as petrolatum), which do not mix well with aqueous preparations and provide an occlusive barrier to the skin; (2) absorption bases (such as lanolin), which permit the absorption of aqueous solutions, usually resulting in water-in-oil emulsions; and, (3) water-removable bases (such as hydrophilic ointment), which are oil-in-water emulsions, or,

(4) water-soluble bases (such as polyethylene glycol ointment), both of which are water washable.

In preparing a *medicated ointment*, the appropriate ointment base is selected to which the medication is added. The solid and semisolid materials in ointments are generally weighed in preparing a prescription or product. Liquid components may be measured volumetrically or converted by calculation to corresponding weight and then weighed. Because ointments are semisolid preparations, they are also prepared, packaged, and dispensed on a weight basis. Special care must be taken in the preparation of ophthalmic ointments to render them free from microorganisms and to assure that the powders used in the formulation are either dissolved in the ointment base or micronized to a state of powder fineness to reduce or eliminate grittiness that could cause eye irritation.

Pastes

Pastes are semisolid dosage forms that contain one or more drug substances intended for topical application. Generally, pastes contain a higher proportion of solid materials than ointments and thus are more stiff, less greasy, and more absorptive of serous secretions when used on the skin. Medicated dental pastes are also prepared for adhesion to the mucous membranes for local effect.

Plasters

Plasters are solid or semisolid adhesive masses spread across a suitable backing material and intended for external application to a part of the body for protection or for the medicinal benefit of added agents.

Powders

Powders are dry mixtures of finely divided medicinal and nonmedicinal agents intended for internal or external use. Powders may be dispensed to a patient and used in bulk form (such as powders measured by the spoonful to make a douche solution) or they may be divided into single dosage units and packaged in folded papers or unit-of-use envelopes.

Solutions

Solutions are liquid preparations that contain one or more chemical substances (solute/s) dissolved in a solvent or mixture of solvents. The solutes may be active or inactive ingredients and may be solids, liquids, or gases in their natural undissolved state. The most common solvent used in pharmaceuticals is water; however, such liquids as alcohol, glycerin, and propylene glycol are used as solvents or co-solvents depending on the product requirements for stability and use.

Solutions are formulated for administration by various routes, such as *oral solutions* (mouth), *ophthalmic solutions* (eye), *otic solutions* (ear), *nasal solutions* (nose), *rectal solutions, urethral solutions, epicutaneous solutions* (skin), and those administered by *injection*. Solutions used to bathe or flush open wounds or body cavities are termed *irrigations*. Certain solutions have special requirements, such as sterility (e.g., injections, irrigations, and ophthalmic solutions).

The concentration of active ingredients in solutions varies greatly. Some solutions are very dilute, whereas others are highly concentrated, depending on the nature of the therapeutic agent and its intended use. The concentration of a given solution may be expressed in molar strength, milliequivalent strength, percentage strength, ratio strength, or other expression (e.g., milligrams per milliliter) describing the amount of active ingredient per unit of volume. Knowledge of the content or concentration of a solution is critical in calculating the volume required to administer a desired dose of drug.

Spirits

Spirits are alcoholic or hydroalcoholic solutions of volatile substances. Depending on their contents, some spirits are used orally for medicinal purposes and others as flavoring agents.

Suspensions

Suspensions are preparations containing finely divided, undissolved drug particles dispersed throughout a liquid vehicle. Because the drug particles are not dissolved, suspensions assume a degree of opacity depending on the concentration and size of the suspended particles.

Suspensions are one type of *disperse systems*, common among pharmaceutical preparations. Other types include emulsions, lotions, magmas, and gels. In these preparations, the suspended particles are referred to as the *suspensoid*, the *disperse*, or *dispersed phase*, and the vehicle is termed the *dispersion* or *dispersing phase*. The particles of the disperse phase may be colloidal (about 1 mμ or less), fine (about 1 μm), or coarse (100 μm). Particles of greater density have a tendency to settle and form a sediment. The addition of suspending agents, which add viscosity to the vehicle, is one method of maintaining the dispersed phase in suspension. Before administration, it is essential to redistribute any settled particles to assure uniform dosing.

Suspensions are formulated for administration by a number of routes, including oral, otic, ophthalmic, epidermal, parenteral (by injection), and others, each with its own requisite characteristics. For example, ophthalmic suspensions must be sterile and the suspensoid must be micronized or very finely reduced to eliminate any grittiness that might cause irritation.

Suppositories

Suppositories are solid dosage forms intended for insertion into body orifices where they melt, soften, or dissolve and exert localized or systemic effects. They are commonly used rectally and vaginally, and occasionally urethrally. Suppositories are prepared in various weights, sizes, and shapes depending on their intended use. Rectal suppositories intended for adults usually weigh about 2 g, measure about $1\frac{1}{2}$ in. in length, and are cylindric or bullet-shaped. Rectal suppositories for infants and children are proportionately smaller. Vaginal suppositories commonly weigh about 5 g and are globular, oviform, or conical. Urethral suppositories are thin and pencil-shaped, weighing approximately 4 g and measuring about 140 mm when intended for males and half the weight and length when intended for females.

Bases of various types are used for suppositories as vehicles for the medication, including cocoa butter (theobroma oil), glycerinated gelatin, polyethylene glycols of various molecular weights, hydrogenated vegetable oils, and fatty acid esters of polyethylene glycol. Depending on the base used, the suppository either softens, melts, or dissolves after insertion, releasing its medication for the intended local action or for absorption and systemic effects.

In addition to suppositories, especially prepared and shaped tablets, capsules, aerosol foams, ointments, creams, jellies, and solutions are designed for vaginal use. Rectal ointments, creams, foams, and enema solutions are also available.

Syrups

Syrups are concentrated, aqueous solutions of a sugar or sugar substitute. *Nonmedicated* syrups are sweet, pleasant-tasting vehicles for medicinal substances to be added later, either in the extemporaneous compounding of prescriptions or in the preparation of a standard formula for a *medicated syrup*. Among the nonmedicated ingredients in syrups, other than the sugar or sugar substitute, are flavoring agents, colorants, co-solvents, and antimicrobial preservatives to prevent microbial growth. Syrups are administered orally for the therapeutic value of the medicinal agent(s).

Tablets

Tablets are solid dosage forms containing one or more medicinal substances with or without added pharmaceutical ingredients. Among the pharmaceutical agents used are diluents, disintegrants, colorants, binders, solubilizers, and coatings. Tablets may be coated for appearance, for stability, to mask the bitter taste of the medication, or to provide controlled drug release. Most tablets are manufactured on the industrial scale by compression, using highly sophisticated machinery. Punches and dies of various shapes and sizes enable the preparation of a wide variety of tablets of distinctive shapes, sizes, and surface markings.

Most tablets are intended to be swallowed whole. Some, however, are prepared to be "chewable," and produce a pleasant taste and feel with mastication. Other tablets are intended to be dissolved in the mouth (buccal tablets) or under the tongue (sublingual tablets), whereas effervescent tablets are intended to be dissolved in water before taking.

Tablets are formulated to contain a specific quantity of drug substance. To enable flexibility in dosing, manufacturers commonly make available various tablet or capsule strengths of a given medication. As required, a tablet may also be broken in half (many tablets are "scored" or grooved for this purpose), or, more than a single tablet may be taken as a prescribed dose.

Tinctures

Tinctures are alcoholic or hydroalcoholic solutions of either pure chemical substances or of plant extractions. Most chemical tinctures are applied topically (e.g., Iodine Tincture). Plant extractions are used for their content of active pharmacologic agents. Some extractions are administered as standardized preparations (e.g., Belladonna Tincture), whereas other types, such as fluidextracts and extracts, are mostly used to prepare other dosage forms. *Fluidextracts* are liquid preparations of plant extractives, each milliliter containing the active constituents from 1 g of the standard drug that it represents. *Extracts* are highly concentrated powdered or pilular (ointment-like) extractives of plant constituents prepared by the reduction of fluidextracts through evaporation.

Review Problems

1. In preparing a cough syrup containing 0.030 g of hydromorphone hydrochloride, a pharmacist weighed the hydromorphone hydrochloride on a torsion balance with a sensitivity requirement of 4 mg. Calculate the percentage of error that may have been incurred by the pharmacist.

2. ℞ Atropine Sulfate   0.5 mg
       Bismuth Subgallate   0.3 g
       Carbowax Base   q.s.
       Make 10 such suppositories
       Sig. One at night.

   Using a torsion prescription balance with a sensitivity requirement of 6 mg, explain how you would obtain the correct amount of atropine sulfate with an error not greater than 5%. Use bismuth subgallate as the diluent.

3. A vitamin liquid contains, in each 0.5 mL, the following:

Thiamine Hydrochloride	1 mg
Riboflavin	400 μg
Ascorbic Acid	50 mg
Nicotinamide	2 mg

   Calculate the quantity, expressed in grams, of each ingredient in 30 mL of the liquid.

4. A certain injectable solution contains 30 mg of a drug substance in 30 mL. How many milliliters of the solution should be administered to provide a weekly dose of 100 μg of the drug substance?

5. The prophylactic dose of riboflavin is 2 mg. How many micrograms of riboflavin are in a capsule containing three times the prophylactic dose?

6. How many grams of codeine phosphate are left in an original 5-g bottle after the amount required to prepare 100 capsules, each containing 15 mg of codeine phosphate as one of the ingredients, is used?

7. ℞ Cyanocobalamin   10 μg per mL
       Disp. 10-mL sterile vial.
       Sig. 1.5 mL every other week.

   (*a*) How many micrograms of cyanocobalamin will be administered over 12 weeks?
   (*b*) How many milligrams of cyanocobalamin are in 10 mL of this preparation?

8. A pharmacist purchased 5 gallons of alcohol. At different times 2 pints, 2 gallons, 8 fluidounces, and ½ gallon were used by the pharmacist. What volume, in fluidounces, remained?

9. A prescription call for 750 mg of tetracaine hydrochloride. If the tetracaine hydro-

chloride costs $14.50 per 5 g, what is the cost of the amount needed for the prescription?

10. If homatropine hydrobromide costs $27.50 per 10 g, what is the cost of 18 gr?

11. A pharmacist purchased 5 g of codeine phosphate. It was used by the pharmacist in preparing 50 capsules, each containing 30 mg of codeine phosphate, and in formulating 1 pint of a cough syrup containing 60 mg of codeine phosphate per fluidounce. For purposes of inventory, how many grams of codeine phosphate remained?

12. How many micrograms of nitroglycerin are contained in a $\frac{1}{200}$-gr tablet?

13. If iodine costs $41.65 per 500 g, and iodine tincture contains 20 g of iodine in a liter, what will be the cost of the iodine in 1 pint of the tincture?

14. ℞   Podophyllum Resin   25%
         Compound Benzoin Tincture   ad   30 mL
         Sig. Apply locally for venereal warts.
   At $36.50 per 30 g, what is the cost of podophyllum resin needed in preparing the prescription?

15. The dose of a certain antibiotic is 5 mg/kg of body weight. How many milligrams should be used for a person weighing 145 lb?

16. If chloral hydrate costs $26.75 per 500 g, what is the cost of the amount needed to prepare a liter of a solution containing 300 mg per teaspoonful?

17. An elixir is to contain 250 μg of an alkaloid in each teaspoonful dose. How many grams of the alkaloid will be required to prepare 5 liters of the elixir?

18. The dose of a drug is 15 mg/m^2 b.i.d. for 1 week. How many milligrams of the drug would be required for a full course of therapy for a child 42 in. tall and weighing 50 lb?

19. The initial dose of a drug is 0.25 mg/kg of body weight. How many milligrams should be prescribed for a person weighing 154 lb?

20. ℞   Lugol's Solution   30 mL
         Sig. Ten drops in water once a day.
   Lugol's solution contains 5% of iodine. If the dispensing dropper calibrates 25 drops/mL, calculate the amount, in milligrams, of iodine in each dose of the solution.

21. The dose of methotrexate for meningeal leukemia in children is 12 mg/m^2 by the intrathecal route. Calculate the dose, in milligrams, for a child 28 in. tall and weighing 52 lb.

22. The pediatric dose of chloral hydrate may be determined on the basis of 8 mg/kg of body weight or on the basis of a pediatric dose of 250 mg/m^2. Calculate the dose on each basis for a child weighing 44 lb and measuring 36 in. in height.

23. The rectal dose of sodium thiopental is 45 mg/kg of body weight. How many milliliters of a 10% solution should be used for a person weighing 150 lb?

24. ℞   Penicillin G Procaine   300,000 units
         Buffered Crystalline Penicillin G   100,000 units
         Crystalline Dihydrostreptomycin   1 g
         Sterile Water for Injection   ad   3 mL
         Make a multiple-dose vial containing 5 doses.
         Sig. For intramuscular use only. Sterile.
    To permit withdrawal of the five doses prescribed, an excess volume of 0.80
    mL must be present in the 15-mL vial. How much of each of the three antibiotics
    should be used in compounding the prescription?

25. ℞   Sodium Fluoride   q.s.
         Vitamin Drops   ad   50 mL
         (10 drops = 2.2 mg NaF)
         Sig. Ten (10) drops in orange juice.

    Assuming that the dispensing dropper calibrates 25 drops/mL, how many milli-
    grams of sodium fluoride should be used in preparing the prescription?

26. How many chloramphenicol capsules, each containing 250 mg, are needed to
    provide 25 mg/kg per day for 1 week for a person weighing 175 lb?

27. The dose of piperazine citrate is 50 mg/kg of body weight once daily for seven
    consecutive days. How many milliliters of piperazine citrate syrup containing 500
    mg per teaspoonful should be prescribed for a child weighing 66 lb?

28. A physician prescribed 5 mg of a drug per kilogram of body weight once daily
    for a patient weighing 132 lb. How many 100-mg tablets of the drug are required
    for a dosage regimen of 2 weeks?

29. ℞   Morphine Sulfate
         Cocaine Hydrochloride   aa   10 mg/30 mL
         Compazine®   5 mg/30 mL
         Aromatic Elixir   q.s. ad   480 mL
         Sig. Tsp. ii p.r.n. pain.
    (a) How many milligrams of morphine sulfate would be contained per dose?
    (b) How many milligrams of cocaine hydrochloride would be used in filling the
        prescription?
    (c) How many milliliters of a solution containing 5 mg of Compazine® per millili-
        ter would be used in filling the prescription?

30. If 240 mL of a cough mixture contain 0.6 g of diphenhydramine hydrochloride,
    how many milligrams are contained in each teaspoonful of the mixture?

31. ℞   Dextromethorphan   15 mg/5 mL
         Guaifenesin Syrup   ad   240 mL
         Sig. 5 mL q. 4 h. p.r.n. cough.
    How many milligrams of dextromethorphan should be used in filling the pre-
    scription?

32. Kaopectate® Concentrate contains 1.2 g of attapulgite per 30 mL. How many
    milligrams of attapulgite are contained in a tablespoonful dose of a mixture contain-
    ing 120 mL of paregoric and 240 mL of Kaopectate® Concentrate?

33. If a dosage table for a prefabricated drug product indicates the dose for a patient weighing 110 lb is 0.4 mg/kg of body weight, taken three times a day for 10 days, how many 10-mg tablets of the product should be dispensed?

34. The child's dose of gentamicin for a urinary tract infection is 1 mg/kg administered every 8 hours for 10 days. What would be (*a*) the single dose and (*b*) the total dose for a 15-year-old child weighing 110 lb?

35. ℞   Noscapine   0.72 g
        Guaifenesin   4.80 g
        Alcohol   15.0 mL
        Cherry Syrup   ad   120.0 mL
        Sig. 5 mL t.i.d. p.r.n. cough.

    How many milligrams each of noscapine and guaifenesin would be contained in each dose?

36. Naldecon® Pediatric Drops contain 270 mg of phenylpropanolamine per 30 mL. How many milligrams of the drug would be administered to a child on delivery of a 0.25-mL dose?

37. The maintenance dose of choledyl is 13.2 mg/kg/day or 800 mg, whichever is less, in q.i.d. dosing. How many 100-mg tablets of the drug should a 200-lb patient take at each dosing interval?

38. A medication order calls for 6 μg/kg of body weight of pentagastrin to be administered subcutaneously to a patient weighing 154 lb. The source of the drug is an ampul containing 0.5 mg in each 2 mL of the solution. How many milliliters of the solution should be injected?

39. If the loading dose of kanamycin is 7 mg/kg of body weight, how many grams should be administered to a patient weighing 165 lb?

40. The usual pediatric dose of a drug is 300 mg/m². Using the nomogram in Chapter 4, calculate the dose for a child weighing 20 kg and measuring 90 cm in height.

41. A beclomethasone diproprionate inhaler contains 10 mg of active ingredient and delivers 200 doses. How many micrograms of beclomethasone diproprionate are delivered per dose?

42. A medication order calls for 0.1 mg/kg of albuterol to be administered to a 23-lb child. The source of the drug is a solution containing 0.5 g of albuterol in 100 mL. How many milliliters of the solution should be used in filling the order?

43. If a physician prescribed V-Cillin K®, 500 mg q.i.d. × 10 days, how many milliliters of a product containing 500 mg of V-Cillin K® per 5 mL should be dispensed?

44. ℞   Codeine Phosphate   30 mg/5 mL
        Robitussin® Syrup   30 mL
        Elixophyllin®   ad   240 mL
        Sig. _____ gtts as directed.

    If a dropper delivers 20 drops/mL, and the dose of codeine phosphate is 0.5 mg/kg of body weight, how many drops of the prescription should be administered as a dose to a 22-lb child?

45. From Figure 4.2, determine the duration (number of hours) that the serum concentration of a hypothetic drug is at or above its minimum effective concentration.

46. The pediatric dose of acyclovir for aplastic anemia is given as 15 mg/kg/day for 10 days. Using the nomogram in Figure 4.5, give the corresponding dose on a "_____ mg/m^2" basis for a child measuring 55 cm in height and weighing 10 kg.

47. If the recommended dose of gentamicin sulfate for a patient with normal kidney function is 3 mg/kg/day, divided into three equal doses given every 8 hours, how many milligrams should be administered per dose to a patient weighing 182 lb?

48. Plasma protein fraction (PPF) is available as a 5% (w/v) solution. If the dose of the solution for a child is given as 5 mL/lb, how many grams of PPF would be administered to a child weighing 20 kg?

49. The fatal dose of cocaine has been approximated at 1.2 g for a 150-lb person. Express this effect on a milligram per kilogram basis.

50. Milk of Magnesia chewable tablets contain 311 mg of magnesium hydroxide per tablet. How many pounds of magnesium hydroxide are needed to manufacture 50,000 tablets?

51.
Coal Tar	50 g
Bentonite	80 g
Water	300 mL
Hydrophilic Ointment	80 g
Zinc Oxide Paste, to make	1000 g

How much of each ingredient should be used in preparing 5 lb of the ointment?

52.
Aminophylline	250 mg
Phenobarbital Sodium	50 mg
Benzocaine	20 mg
Carbowax Base	2 g

Calculate the quantity of each ingredient to be used in preparing 250 suppositories.

53. The following formula for glycerin suppositories is sufficient to prepare 50 suppositories. Calculate the amount of each ingredient needed to prepare 300 suppositories.

Glycerin	91 g
Sodium Stearate	9 g
Purified Water, to make	100 g

54.
Coal Tar	10 g
Polysorbate 80	5 g
Zinc Oxide Paste	985 g

Calculate the quantity of each ingredient required to prepare 10 lb of the ointment.

55.
Menthol	0.2	g
Hexachlorophene	0.1	g
Glycerin	10	mL
Isopropyl Alcohol	35	mL
Purified Water ad	100	mL

Calculate the quantity of each ingredient required to prepare 1 gallon of the lotion.

56. Set up a formula for 5 lb of glycerogelatin containing 10 parts, by weight, of zinc oxide, 15 parts, by weight, of gelatin, 40 parts, by weight, of glycerin, and 35 parts, by weight, of water.

57. Furosemide injection contains 10 mg of furosemide in each milliliter, packaged in prefilled 2-mL syringes. Calculate the amount, in grams, of furosemide required to manufacture 4000 such syringes.

58. A chocolated laxative contains 90 mg of phenolphthalein per tablet. Calculate the amount, in grams, of phenolphthalein needed to manufacture 1000 packages of the product, each containing 24 tablets.

59. If 5000 mL of a syrup weigh 6565 g, calculate (*a*) its specific gravity and (*b*) its specific volume.

60. A saturated solution contains, in each 100 mL, 100 g of a substance. If the solubility of the substance is 1 g in 0.7 mL of water, what is the specific gravity of the saturated solution?

61. In making a certain syrup, 6800 g of sucrose were dissolved in enough water to make 8 liters. Assuming the specific gravity of the syrup to be 1.313, how many milliliters of water were used?

62. A certain liniment is prepared by mixing 2 lb of methyl salicylate (sp. gr. 1.18), 1 liter of alcohol (sp. gr. 0.8), and 1 lb of chloroform (sp. gr. 1.475). What is the volume, in milliliters, of the mixture?

63. A formula for 200 g of an ointment contains 10 g of glycerin. How many milliliters of glycerin having a specific gravity of 1.25 should be used in preparing 1 lb of the ointment?

64.

White Wax	12.5 g
Mineral Oil	60.0 g
Lanolin	2.5 g
Sodium Borate	1.0 g
Rose Water	24.0 g

Label: Cold Cream.

How many milliliters of mineral oil having a specific gravity of 0.900 should be used in preparing 10 lb of the cream?

65. How many milliliters of a commercially available 50% (v/v) solution of glycerin should be used to provide 2 g of glycerin per kilogram of body weight for a person weighing 110 lb? The specific gravity of glycerin is 1.25.

66. A perfume oil has a specific gravity of 0.960 and costs $28.75 per kg. What is the cost of 120 mL?

67. A formula for a mouth rinse contains 1.6 mL of cinnamon oil per 1000 mL. If the cinnamon oil (sp. gr. 1.050) is bought at $27.00 per 120 g, calculate the cost of the oil required to prepare 20,000 mL of the mouth rinse.

68. Cocaine hydrochloride topical solution for local anesthesia of mucous membranes

of the nose, mouth, and throat is available in concentrations of 40 mg/mL and 100 mg/mL. Express these concentrations in terms of percentage strength.

69. Given a solution of potassium permanganate prepared by dissolving sixteen 0.2-g tablets in enough purified water to make 1600 mL,
    (a) What is the percentage strength of the solution?
    (b) What is the ratio strength of the solution?

70. Given a salt solution of 1:1500 concentration, what is:
    (a) the percentage strength?
    (b) the weight, in micrograms, of the salt per milliliter?
    (c) the number of milliliters required to prepare 2 liters of a 1:2500 solution?

71. The manufacturer specifies that one Domeboro® tablet dissolved in 1 pint of water makes a modified Burow's Solution approximately equivalent to a 1:40 dilution. How many tablets should be used in preparing ½ gallon of a 1:10 dilution?

72. ℞   Potassium Iodide
             (50 mg per tsp)
             Ephedrine Sulfate Syrup   ad   240 mL
             Sig. Teaspoonful as directed.
    Potassium Iodide Oral Solution, USP, contains 1 g/mL of potassium iodide.
    How many milliliters of the solution should be used to obtain the potassium iodide required in compounding the prescription?

73. Eight hundred and seventy grams of sucrose are dissolved in 470 mL of water, and the resulting volume is 1010 mL. Calculate (a) the percentage strength (w/v) of the solution, (b) the percentage strength (w/w) of the solution, and (c) the specific gravity of the solution.

74. A formula for a cosmetic cream calls for 0.04% of a mixture of 65 parts of methylparaben and 35 parts of propylparaben. How many grams of each should be used in formulating 10 lb of the cream?

75. On June 1st, a pharmacist purchased 5 g of cocaine hydrochloride. During the month the following were dispensed:

    30 g of an ointment containing 3% of cocaine hydrochloride
    60 mL of a solution containing 1% of cocaine hydrochloride
    15 mL of a solution containing 4% of cocaine hydrochloride

    How many grams of cocaine hydrochloride were left in stock for the July 1st narcotic inventory?

76. Thiamylal sodium is an intravenous anesthetic agent. How many milliliters of a 2.5% solution and how many milliliters of normal saline (0.9%) are required to prepare 500 mL of a 0.3% solution of thiamylal sodium?

77. ℞   Clindamycin Hydrochloride   0.6 g
             Propylene Glycol   6.0 mL
             Purified Water   8.0 mL
             Isopropyl Alcohol   ad   60.0 mL
             Sig. Apply b.i.d.
    How many capsules, each containing 150 mg of clindamycin hydrochloride, would be used in preparing the prescription? Also, what would be the percentage concentration (w/v) of clindamycin hydrochloride in the prescription?

78. ℞   Ephedrine Sulfate   0.4%
           Benzocaine   1 : 1000
           Cocoa Butter   ad   2 g
           M. ft. suppos. DTD no. 24
           Sig. Insert at night.
    To prepare the prescription, (*a*) how many milligrams of ephedrine sulfate are
    needed and (*b*) how many grams of a 10% (w/w) benzocaine ointment would
    supply the proper amount of benzocaine?

79. ℞   Hydrocortisone   1%
           Precip. Sulfur   20%
           Zinc Oxide Paste   ad   60 g
           Sig. Apply.
    How many grams each of (*a*) hydrocortisone and (*b*) precipitated sulfur are
    needed to prepare the prescription?

80. ℞   Lincomycin Hydrochloride   1.2 g
           Propylene Glycol   4.0 mL
           Purified Water   24.0 mL
           Isopropyl Alcohol (70%)   ad   60.0 mL
           Sig. Apply b.i.d. for acne.
    How many milliliters of a vial containing 300 mg of lincomycin hydrochloride
    per milliliter would be used in preparing the prescription? Also, what would be the
    percentage concentration (w/v) of lincomycin hydrochloride in the prescription?

81. ℞   Triamcinolone Cream (0.1% w/w)
           Aquaphor Unibase   aa   30 g
           M. ft. ungt.
           Sig. Apply t.i.d.
    Calculate the percentage strength (w/w) of triamcinolone in the prescription.

82. Polyethylene glycol ointment contains 60% (w/w) of polyethylene glycol 400.
    How many milliliters of polyethylene glycol 400 having a specific gravity of 1.135
    are required to make 10 lb of the ointment?

83. The product Haley's M-O contains 304 mg of magnesium hydroxide and 1.25
    mL of mineral oil per teaspoonful. Express the amounts of these ingredients in
    terms of percentage.

84. Insulin Injection is preserved with 0.25% (w/v) of metacresol.
    (*a*) Express this concentration as a ratio strength.
    (*b*) Calculate the quantity, in milligrams, of metacresol in a 20-mL vial of the
         injection.

85. Paregoric contains the equivalent of 0.4% of opium. How many milligrams of
    opium are represented in a tablespoonful dose of a mixture of equal parts of parego-
    ric and Kaopectate®?

86. If a dry powder mixture of the antibiotic amoxicillin is diluted with water to 80
    mL by a pharmacist to prepare a prescription containing 125 mg of amoxicillin
    per 5 mL, (*a*) how many grams of amoxicillin are in the dry mixture, and (*b*) what
    is the percentage strength of amoxicillin in the prepared prescription?

87.   A prefilled syringe of lidocaine hydrochloride contains 100 mg per 5 mL of the injection. Express the concentration of lidocaine hydrochloride as a percentage strength (w/v).

88.   If 10 mL of a nitroglycerin injection (5 mg of nitroglycerin per milliliter) are added to make a liter of intravenous fluid, what is the percentage strength (w/v) of nitroglycerin in the finished product?

89.   A cupric chloride injection (0.4 mg of copper per milliliter) is used as an additive to intravenous solutions for total parenteral nutrition (TPN). What is the final ratio strength of copper in the TPN solution if 2.5 mL of the cupric chloride injection is added to enough of the intravenous solution to prepare 500 mL?

90.   Phenobarbital elixir contains 400 mg of phenobarbital in each 100 mL. A physician wants to increase the phenobarbital content to 30 mg per teaspoonful and to prescribe the dose twice a day for 24 days. How many milligrams of phenobarbital should be added to the prescribed volume of the prescription to provide the amount needed for the dosage regimen?

91.   How many grams of hydrocortisone should be used in preparing 2 lb of a $\frac{1}{4}$% hydrocortisone cream?

92.   How many fluidounces of a commercially available 17% solution of benzalkonium chloride should be used to prepare 1 gallon of a 1:750 solution?

93.   You are directed to prepare 10 liters of a 1:5000 solution of potassium permanganate. If the potassium permanganate is available only in the form of tablets, each containing 0.2 g, how many tablets should be used in preparing the solution?

94.   How many milliliters of 85% (w/w) phosphoric acid with a specific gravity of 1.71 should be used in preparing 10 liters of a 1:2000 solution of phosphoric acid for bladder irrigation?

95.   How many grams of coal tar should be added to 1 lb of Coal Tar Ointment, USP, to increase the strength to 2%? Coal Tar Ointment, USP, contains 1% of coal tar.

96.   A manufacturing pharmacist has on hand four lots of belladonna tincture, containing 25 mg, 27 mg, 33 mg, and 35 mg of alkaloids per 100 mL. How many gallons of each lot should be used to prepare 16 gallons of belladonna tincture containing 30 mg of alkaloids per 100 mL?

97.   ℞   Codeine Sulfate   15 mg/tsp
             Robitussin®   ad   120 mL
             Sig. Two (2) teaspoonfuls q. 6h for cough.
         How many 30-mg tablets of codeine sulfate should be used in preparing the prescription?

98.   How many grams of silver nitrate should be used in preparing 500 mL of a solution such that 10 mL diluted to a liter will yield a 1:5000 solution?

99.   How many milliliters of 95% (v/v) alcohol and of 30% (v/v) alcohol should be mixed to make 4000 mL of 50% (v/v) alcohol?

100. How many grams of benzethonium chloride and how many milliliters of 95% (v/v) alcohol should be used in preparing 1 gallon of a 1:1000 solution of benzethonium chloride in 70% (v/v) alcohol?

101. How many grams of talc should be added to 1 lb of a powder containing 20 g of zinc undecylenate per 100 g to reduce the concentration of zinc undecylenate to 3%?

102. A hospital pharmacist has on hand 14 liters of iodine tincture (2%). How many milliliters of strong iodine tincture (7%) should be mixed with it to yield a product that will contain 3.5% of iodine?

103. How many milliliters of 36% (w/w) hydrochloric acid with a specific gravity of 1.18 are required to prepare 5 gallons of 10% (w/v) hydrochloric acid?

104. A formula for an ophthalmic solution calls for 500 mL of a 0.02% solution of benzalkonium chloride. How many milliliters of a 1:750 solution should be used to obtain the amount of benzalkonium chloride needed in preparing the ophthalmic solution?

105. Express a patient's uric acid level of 5.0 mg/dL in terms of milligrams percent.

106. If a 10-mL serum sample is determined to contain 8 mg of glucose, express the concentration of glucose as (*a*) mg% and (*b*) mg/dL.

107. If a patient's blood urea nitrogen is determined to be 15 mg/dL, what is the equivalent percent concentration?

108. If a patient is determined to have 100 mg% of blood glucose, what is the equivalent concentration in terms of mg/dL?

109. ℞   Potassium Permanganate   q.s.
         Purified Water   ad   500 mL
         Sig. 5 mL diluted to a liter equals a 1:8000 solution.
     How many 0.2-g tablets of potassium permanganate should be used in compounding the prescription?

110. How many milliliters of each of two liquids with specific gravities of 0.950 and 0.875 should be used to prepare 12 liters of a liquid with a specific gravity of 0.925?

111. ℞   Sodium Fluoride   q.s.
         Purified Water   ad   60.0
         Sig. Five drops added to a liter of drinking water.
     The prescriber informs you that the drinking water contains 0.4 ppm of fluoride ion. How many milligrams of sodium fluoride should be used in preparing the solution so that five drops of it diluted to 1 liter with the drinking water will yield a solution containing 1 ppm of fluoride ion? The dispensing dropper calibrates 20 drops/mL.

112. ℞   Epinephrine Bitartrate   2.0 g
         Chlorobutanol   0.3 g
         Sodium Chloride   0.7 g
         Purified Water   ad   100.0 mL
         Sig. Use in the eyes.
     How many milliliters of a 0.9% sodium chloride solution should be used to obtain the sodium chloride for the prescription?

113. ℞   Ephedrine Sulfate   0.5%
         Tetracaine Hydrochloride   0.5%
         Dextrose   q.s.
         Purified Water   ad   30.0
         Make isotonic sol.
         Sig. Nasal spray.
     How many grams of dextrose should be used in preparing the prescription?

114. ℞   Phenobarbital Sodium   15 mg per mL
         Sodium Chloride   q.s.
         Sterile Water for Injection   ad   20 mL
         Make isotonic sol. and sterilize.
         Sig. For office use.
     How many grams of sodium chloride should be used in preparing the prescrip-
tion?

115. ℞   Atropine Sulfate   2%
         Boric Acid   q.s.
         Purified Water   ad   100.0 mL
         Make isotonic sol.
         Sig. For the eyes.
     (a) How many grams of boric acid should be used?
     (b) How many milliliters of a 5% boric acid solution should be used to obtain
         the amount of boric acid needed in the prescription?
     (c) You are directed to sterilize this prescription at a temperature not exceeding
         105°C. Calculate the corresponding F temperature.

116. ℞   Epinephrine   1.0%
         Chlorobutanol   0.5%
         Sodium Chloride   q.s.
         Sterile Water for Injection   ad   15.0 mL
         Make isotonic sol.
         Sig. For the eye.
     (a) How many grams of epinephrine bitartrate (m.w. 333) should be used to obtain
         the amount of epinephrine (m.w. 183) needed in preparing the prescription?
     (b) Starting with epinephrine bitartrate, how many milligrams of sodium chloride
         should be used in preparing the prescription?

117. The formula for Albright's solution "G" calls for 4.37 g of anhydrous sodium
     carbonate (Na_2CO_3, m.w.-106) in 1000 mL of finished product. In preparing
     5 gallons of the solution, how many grams of monohydrated sodium carbonate
     ($Na_2CO_3 \cdot H_2O$, m.w.-124) should be used?

118. In the monograph on Ferrous Sulfate Tablets, the USP states that an "equivalent
     amount of dried ferrous sulfate may be used in place of $FeSO_4 \cdot 7H_2O$ in preparing
     Ferrous Sulfate Tablets." How many grams of dried ferrous sulfate (m.w.-179)
     could be used to replace the $FeSO_4 \cdot 7H_2O$ (m.w.-278) in preparing 10,000 tablets,
     each containing 0.3 g of the hydrated salt?

119. Sodium phosphates oral solution contains, in each 100 mL, 18 g of dibasic sodium
     phosphate ($Na_2HPO_4 \cdot 7H_2O$, m.w.-268) and 48 g of monobasic sodium phosphate
     ($NaH_2PO_4 \cdot H_2O$, m.w.-138). How many grams of dried dibasic sodium phosphate

(Na$_2$PO$_4$, m.w.−142) and of anhydrous monobasic sodium phosphate (NaH$_2$PO$_4$, m.w.−120) should be used in preparing 1 gallon of the solution?

120. If a diabetic patient injects 50 units of NPH Insulin (100 units/mL) twice daily, how many days will a 10-mL vial of the product last the patient?

121. A commercial vial contains 20 million units of penicillin. The label directions state that when 32.4 mL of sterile water for injection are added, an injection containing 500,000 units of penicillin per milliliter results. If a physician prescribes 1 million units of penicillin per milliliter, how many milliliters of sterile water for injection should be used to prepare the product?

122. A physician prescribes 1.6 million units of penicillin G potassium daily for 7 days. If 1 mg of penicillin G potassium is equal to 1595 penicillin G units, how many 250-mg tablets of penicillin G potassium should be dispensed for the prescribed dosage regimen?

123. Rabies vaccine contains 1.25 I.U. per 0.5 mL. The post-exposure dose is 2.5 I.U. administered the day of the exposure and then an additional 2.5 I.U. on days 3, 7, 14, and 28 after exposure. How many milliliters of vaccine are needed for the full course of treatment?

124. It is estimated that an adult with an average daily diet has a salt (sodium chloride) intake of 15 g per day.
    (*a*) How many milliequivalents of sodium (Na$^+$) are represented in the daily salt intake?
    (*b*) How many millimoles of sodium chloride (NaCl, m.w.−58.5) are represented in the daily salt intake?

125. How many grams of potassium chloride should be used in making a liter of a solution containing 5 mEq of potassium per milliliter?

126. What is the percent (w/v) concentration of a solution containing 100 mEq of ammonium chloride per liter?

127. Convert 20 mg% of calcium to milliequivalents of calcium.

128. One liter of blood plasma contains 5 mEq of Ca^{++}. How many millimoles of calcium are represented in this concentration?

129. One hundred (100) mL of blood plasma normally contain 3 mg% of Mg^{++}. Express this concentration in terms of milliequivalents per liter.

130. How many milliequivalents of potassium are contained in each 10-mL dose of a 5% (w/v) solution of potassium chloride (KCl)?

131. ℞   Potassium Chloride   125 g
         Peppermint Water   ad   500 mL
         Sig. 5 mL as directed.
    How many milliequivalents of potassium are represented in the prescribed dose?

132. A patient has been using one 1-g tablet of potassium chloride twice a day. His physician now wishes to change the medication to a liquid dosage form containing 134 mEq of potassium per 100 mL. What dose of the liquid preparation should be prescribed to provide the same amount of potassium as that represented by the tablets?

133. How many grams of sodium bicarbonate should be used in preparing a liter of a solution that is to contain 8 mEq of sodium bicarbonate in each 10 mL?

134. How many milliequivalents of potassium are represented in 5 million units of penicillin G potassium ($C_{16}H_{17}KN_2O_4S$, m.w.–372)? One milligram of penicillin G potassium represents 1595 Penicillin G Units.

135. The formula for a potassium ion elixir is as follows:
    Potassium Chloride   5 mEq/tsp
    Elixir Base   q.s.
    How many grams of potassium chloride are needed to prepare 5 gallons of the elixir?

136. An iron complex with vitamin D tablet contains 540 mg of calcium gluconate ($C_{12}H_{22}CaO_{14}\cdot H_2O$, m.w.–448) and 500 mg of calcium carbonate ($CaCO_3$, m.w.–100). How many milliequivalents of calcium are supplied in the daily prophylactic dose of three tablets?

137. How many grams of calcium chloride ($CaCl_2\cdot 2H_2O$, m.w.–147) are required to prepare half a liter of a solution containing 5 mEq of calcium chloride per milliliter?

138. How many milliosmoles of sodium chloride are represented in 1 liter of a 3% hypertonic sodium chloride solution? Assume complete dissociation.

139. The dissociation constant of benzoic acid is 6.30×10^{-5} at 25°C. Calculate the pK_a value of benzoic acid.

140. Calculate the pH of a buffer solution containing 0.8 mol of sodium acetate and 0.5 mol of acetic acid per liter. The pK_a value of acetic acid is 4.76 at 25°C.

141. What molar ratio of sodium acetate to acetic acid is required to prepare an acetate buffer solution with a pH of 5.0? The K_a value of acetic acid is 1.75×10^{-5} at 25°C.

142. Calculate the molar ratio of dibasic sodium phosphate and monobasic sodium phosphate required to prepare a buffer system with a pH of 7.9. The pK_a value of monobasic sodium phosphate is 7.21 at 25°C.

143. What molar ratio of sodium borate to boric acid should be used in preparing a borate buffer with a pH of 8.8? The K_a value of boric acid is 6.4×10^{-10} at 25°C.

144. Calculate the half-life (years) of ^{60}Co, which has a disintegration constant of 0.01096 $month^{-1}$.

145. A sodium iodide I 131 solution has a labeled activity of 1 mCi/mL as of 12:00 noon on November 17. How many milliliters of the solution should be administered at 12:00 noon on December 1 to provide an activity of 250 μCi? The half-life of ^{131}I is 8.08 days.

146. The blood hemoglobin levels, in grams per 100 mL, for a group of 25 individuals were recorded as follows:

14.0	14.6	15.8	14.5	16.0
16.2	15.0	15.7	15.4	13.5
13.3	13.4	16.1	14.8	14.8
14.7	14.5	15.6	13.9	15.1
15.9	13.3	13.2	15.7	14.5

Prepare an array of the data, calculate the mean, and find the median and the mode from the array.

147. In determining the weight variation of 20 tablets taken at random from a manufacturer's lot, the following weights, in milligrams, were recorded:

325 mg	320 mg	317 mg	315 mg
315 mg	335 mg	340 mg	325 mg
324 mg	340 mg	325 mg	330 mg
330 mg	325 mg	318 mg	323 mg
328 mg	322 mg	322 mg	325 mg

Calculate the mean, the average deviation, and the standard deviation for the recorded weights.

148. A manufacturer recommends that a product be stored at a temperature not exceeding 40°F. Express this temperature on the centigrade scale.

149. A table of specifications states that a certain substance must congeal at $-30 \pm$ 5°C. A sample of the substance was found to congeal at -37°F. Did the sample conform to specifications?

150. A hospital pharmacist has in stock 24 pints of 90 proof brandy and 10 fifths of 88 proof whisky. How many proof gallons are represented by this inventory?

151. A manufacturing pharmacist bought 50 proof gallons of spirits. How many wine gallons does this represent if the purchase was 70% (v/v) alcohol?

152. An alcohol inventory shows 27 gallons of 95% alcohol and 8 pints of absolute (100%) alcohol. How many proof gallons of alcohol are represented by this inventory?

153. If alcohol is taxed at $13.50 per proof gallon, what is the tax on 30 wine gallons of 95% (v/v) alcohol?

154. A blood sample is taken from a 150-lb person. Chemical examination shows the sample contains 0.2% of ethyl alcohol. Assuming that the alcohol is carried in the body fluids and that 70% of the body weight consists of fluids, how many fluid-ounces of 100 proof whisky would have to be absorbed to produce this blood level?

155. A medication order calls for a 1-liter bottle of acetic acid irrigation solution 0.25% (w/v). How many grams of acetic acid are contained in each irrigation dose of 30 mL?

156. A medication order calls for 500 mL of an intravenous solution to contain 0.25 mg of isoproterenol in each 100 mL. How many milliliters of a 1:5000 isoproterenol solution should be used in preparing the intravenous solution?

157. The solubility of magnesium sulfate is 1 g in 1 mL of water at 25°C, and the volume of the resulting solution is 1.5 mL. How many grams of magnesium sulfate and how many milliliters of water should be used in preparing 1 gallon of a saturated solution of magnesium sulfate?

158. The solubility of salicylic acid in water is 1 g in 460 mL. Calculate the percentage strength (w/w) of a saturated solution of salicylic acid.

159. What is the solubility of a chemical if 1200 g of a saturated alcohol solution yield a residue of 75 g on evaporation? The specific gravity of alcohol is 0.8.

160. You are directed to prepare 5 liters of a 50% emulsion of mineral oil. How many grams of acacia and how many milliliters of water should be used in preparing the nucleus or primary emulsion?

161. The formula for a castor oil emulsion calls for 25% of castor oil. In formulating 1 gallon of the emulsion, how many grams of acacia and how many milliliters of water should be used in preparing the nucleus or primary emulsion?

162. Mineral Oil   30%
      Cetyl Alcohol   2%
      Lanolin, Anhydrous   3%
      Emulsifier   5%
      Propylene Glycol   10%
      Preserved Water   ad   100%
      (*a*) Calculate the "required HLB" of the oil phase.
      (*b*) How many grams of Span 60 and how many grams of Tween 20 should be used in formulating 5 lb of the product?

163. Stearic Acid   10.0%
      Lanolin   2.0%
      Mineral Oil   3.0%
      Emulsifier   5.0%
      Propylene Glycol   10.0%
      Purified Water   ad   100.0%
      The emulsifier blend is to consist of Span 80 and Tween 20. How many grams of each should be used in formulating 5 lb of the product?

164. A medication order calls for triamcinolone acetonide suspension to be diluted with normal saline solution to provide 3 mg/mL of triamcinolone acetonide for injection into a lesion. If each 5 mL of the suspension contains 125 mg of triamcinolone acetonide, how many milliliters should be used to prepare 10 mL of the prescribed dilution?

165. ℞   Belladonna Extract   10 mg
              Phenobarbital   30 mg
              Meperidine Hydrochloride   75 mg
              Make 20 such capsules
              Sig. One for pain.
      How many tablets, each containing 100 mg of meperidine hydrochloride, should be used to provide the meperidine hydrochloride needed in preparing the prescription?

166. ℞   Atropine Sulfate   300 μg
              Phenobarbital   30 mg
              Dextroamphetamine Sulfate   3 mg
              Make 20 such capsules
              Sig. One capsule as directed.
      If the dextroamphetamine sulfate is available only in the form of tablets, each containing 15 mg, how many tablets should be used to obtain the dextroamphetamine sulfate needed in preparing the prescription?

167. ℞   Hycodan®   2 mg
             Colchicine   gr $\frac{1}{100}$
             Aspirin   300 mg
             Make 24 such capsules
             Sig. One capsule t.i.d.

        Only colchicine granules, each containing $\frac{1}{120}$ gr, are available. Explain how you would obtain the colchicine needed in preparing the prescription?

168. ℞   Hydrocortisone   1.5%
             Neomycin Ointment
             Emulsion Base   aa ad   30 g
             Sig. Apply.

        If the hydrocortisone is available only in the form of 20-mg tablets, how many tablets should be used to obtain the hydrocortisone needed in preparing the prescription?

169. ℞   Penicillin G Potassium   10,000 units per mL
             Isotonic Sodium Chloride Solution   ad   15 mL
             Sig. For the nose. Store in the refrigerator.

        Only soluble penicillin tablets, each containing 400,000 units of penicillin G potassium, are available. Explain how you would obtain the penicillin G potassium needed in preparing the prescription?

170. A hyperalimentation solution includes 500 mL of D50W. If each gram of dextrose supplies 3.4 kcal, how many kilocalories would the hyperalimentation solution provide?

171. Tobramycin is available in 2-mL prefilled syringes containing 80 mg of tobramycin and 1.5-mL prefilled syringes containing 60 mg of tobramycin. The syringes are calibrated in 0.25-mL units. Explain how you would prepare a medication order calling for 110 mg of tobramycin to be added to 100 mL of D5W for intravenous infusion.

172. Using prefilled tobramycin syringes as described in the preceding problem and with a minimum of waste, explain how you would prepare a medication order calling for three piggy-back infusions, each containing 110 mg of tobramycin in 100 mL of D5W.

173. Calculate the osmolarity, in milliosmoles per liter, of a sodium chloride parenteral additive solution containing 2.5 mEq of sodium chloride per milliliter.

174. A medication order calls for the addition of 25 mEq of sodium bicarbonate to a hyperalimentation formula. How many milliliters of an 8.4% solution should be added to the hyperalimentation formula? (You have on hand a 50-mL ampul of 8.4% sodium bicarbonate solution.)

175. If a liter of an intravenous solution of potassium chloride is to be administered over 5 hours and the dropper in the venoclysis set calibrates 25 drops/ml. What is the required rate of flow in drops per minute?

176. A large-volume parenteral fluid contains 20 mg of a drug per liter. If the desired drug delivery rate is 1 mg per hour and the venoclysis set calibrates 25 drops/mL, what should be the rate of flow in drops per minute?

177. If a physician prescribes a 5 μg/kg/min IV drip of dopamine for a 175-lb patient, and the pharmacist adds an ampul of dopamine (200 mg/5 mL) to a 250-mL bottle of D5W, what drip rate should be run, in drops per minute, using a minidrip set that delivers 60 drops/mL?

178. A medication order calls for 1 liter of a TPN solution to be administered over 6 hours. If the venoclysis set calibrates 20 drops/mL, at what rate of flow, in drops per minute, should the set be adjusted to administer the solution in the designated time interval?

179. A certain hyperalimentation solution contains 600 mL of a 5% protein hydrolysate, 400 mL of 50% dextrose injection, 35 mL of a 20% sterile potassium chloride solution, 100 mL of sodium chloride injection, and 10 mL of a 10% calcium gluconate injection. The solution is to be administered over 6 hours. If the dropper in the venoclysis set calibrates 20 drops/mL, at what rate, in drops per minute, should the flow be adjusted to administer the solution during the designated time interval?

180. A phosphate solution for intravenous infusion contains 40 mmol of sodium phosphate (Na_2HPO_4) and 10 mmol of potassium acid phosphate (KH_2PO_4) per liter. Calculate:
      (*a*) The amount, expressed as milliequivalents, of sodium ion.
      (*b*) The amount, expressed as milliequivalents, of potassium ion.
      (*c*) The amount, in grams, of phosphate represented in the infusion.

181. A solution prepared by dissolving 500,000 units of polymyxin B sulfate in 10 mL of water for injection is added to 250 mL of 5% dextrose injection. The infusion is to be administered over 2 hours. If the dropper in the venoclysis set calibrates 25 drops/mL, at what rate, in drops per minute, should the flow be adjusted to administer the total volume over the designated time interval?

182. A physician orders an intravenous solution to contain 10,000 units of heparin in 1 liter of 5% dextrose solution to be infused at such a rate that the patient will receive 500 units per hour. If the intravenous set delivers 10 drops/mL, how many drops per minute should be infused to deliver the desired dose?

183. An Isuprel Mistometer contains 15 mL of a 1:400 solution of isoproterenol hydrochloride and permits the delivery of 300 single oral inhalations. If each actuation delivers 0.05 mL, how many micrograms of the active ingredient are received in a single oral inhalation?

184. A physician orders 20 mL of 10% magnesium sulfate ($MgSO_4 \cdot 7H_2O$, m.w.-262) to be given as an anticonvulsant. How many milliosmoles of magnesium sulfate will the patient receive?

185. A medication order calls for 20 mEq of potassium chloride in 500 mL of D5W/ 0.45 NSS to be administered at the rate of 125 mL per hour. If the intravenous set is calibrated at 12 drops/mL, what should be the infusion rate in drops per minute?

186. For control of pinworm infections in children and adults, pyrvinium pamoate is administered orally in a single dose of 5 mg of pyrvinium pamoate per kilogram of body weight. How many 50-mg tablets should be prescribed for a child weighing 88 lb?

187. The usual single adult dose of propranolol hydrochloride is 40 mg. Based on body surface area, what would be the dose for a child weighing 48 lb?

188. If two patients, each weighing 110 lb, were given the drug amikacin sulfate, one at a regimen of 7.5 mg/kg every 12 hours and the other 5 mg/kg every 8 hours, what is the difference in the total quantity of drug administered over a 24-hour period?

189. A study of vancomycin dosing in neonates showed that average peak serum vancomycin concentrations of 30 μg/mL are achieved following doses of 10 mg/kg of body weight. On this basis, what would be the expected serum concentration of the drug if a 2500-g child received 20 mg of vancomycin?

190. If the dose of a drug is 17.5 mg/m^2/day, how many milligrams of the drug should be administered daily to a patient weighing 65 lb and measuring 3 ft, 6 in. in height?

191. If the intravenous pediatric dose of dactinomycin is 2.5 mg/m^2/week, how many micrograms of the drug will a child having a BSA of 0.50 m^2 average per day of therapy?

192. The drug cyclophosphamide is administered for breast cancer at a daily dose of 100 mg/m^2 for up to 14 consecutive days. What would be the total quantity administered over the 2-week period for a patient measuring 5 ft, 2 in. in height and weighing 102 lb?

193. An adult accidentally swallowed 36 sodium fluoride tablets containing 2 mg of sodium fluoride (NaF, m.w.$-$42) per tablet.
(a) How many milligrams of fluoride were ingested?
(b) How many milliequivalents of sodium were ingested?

194. How many (a) millimoles, (b) milliequivalents, and (c) milliosmoles of magnesium sulfate (MgSO$_4$·7H$_2$O, m.w.$-$246) are present in 246 mL of a 10% (w/v) magnesium sulfate solution?

195. A certain hyperalimentation solution measures 1 liter. If the solution is to be administered over 6 hours and if the administration set is calibrated at 25 drops/mL, at what rate should the set be adjusted to administer the solution during the designated time interval?

196. An ampul contains 1.12 g of monobasic potassium phosphate (KH$_2$PO$_4$, m.w.$-$136) and 1.18 g of dibasic potassium phosphate (K$_2$HPO$_4$, m.w.$-$174). How many millimoles of total phosphate are present in the solution?

197. Calculate the net amount of a bill of goods for $5250, with a trade discount of 35% plus a 5% off invoice allowance and a cash discount of 2% for payment of the invoice within 10 days.

198. A certain nasal preparation is listed at $30.00 per dozen, less 40% and 10%. At what price per unit must the preparation be sold to yield a gross profit of 66⅔% on the cost?

199. A pharmacist buys a bottle of vitamin capsules at $15.75 less a discount of 40%. At what price must the capsules be sold to yield a gross profit of 40% on the selling price?

200. A pharmacist buys 10,000 capsules for $540.00, with a trade discount of $33\frac{1}{3}\%$ plus a 5% discount for quantity buying. At what price per hundred must the capsules be sold to realize a gross profit of 50% on the selling price?

201. A prescription specialty is purchased at $21.75 per 500 mL, less a trade discount of 34.5%. At what price must 60 mL of the specialty be sold to yield a gross profit of 50% on the selling price?

202. A prescription item costs a pharmacist $26.00. Using a markup of 25% on the cost plus a professional fee of $4.50, calculate the price of the prescription.

203. What would be the price of a prescription if a product costs $12.50 and the pharmacist applies a 30% markup on the cost plus a professional fee of $4.50?

204. If minoxidil topical solution is prescribed for a 30-year-old patient to treat male pattern baldness at a patient cost for the product of $60 per month, what would be the total cost over the patient's lifetime, assuming (1) a 78-year life span and (b) a 6% inflation rate on the cost of the drug product? (Clue: at a 6% annual inflation rate, the cost of the drug would double every 12 years.)

205. The drug paclitaxel (Taxol®) is available in 30-mg vials costing $147 each. What would be the drug cost in administering paclitaxel at 135 mg/m² once every 3 weeks during a 9-week period to a 1.9 m² patient?

206. Sodium cloxacillin for oral solution should be constituted at the time of dispensing and stored in a refrigerator for maximum stability. If stored at room temperature, however, the half-life of the sodium cloxacillin solution is only 10 days. If the original concentration of the constituted solution was 250 mg/5 mL, how much sodium cloxacillin will remain per 5 mL after storage at room temperature for 25 days?

207. If 3 mL of diluent are added to a vial containing 1 g of a drug for injection, resulting in a final volume of 3.4 mL, what is the concentration, in milligrams per milliliter, of the drug in the injectable solution?

208. A nitroglycerin concentrate solution contains 5 mg of nitroglycerin in each milliliter. A 10-mL ampul of the concentrate is added to 500 mL of D5W and infused into a patient at a flow rate of 3 microdrops per minute. If the infusion pump system delivers 60 microdrops/mL, how many micrograms of nitroglycerin would the patient receive in the first hour of therapy?

209. If, in the previous problem, the patient was to receive nitroglycerin at the rate of 5 μg per minute, at how many milliliters per hour should the infusion pump be set to deliver this dose?

210. A hospital medication order calls for the addition of 20 mEq of sodium chloride to a liter of mannitol injection. How many milliliters of a 14.5% (w/v) sodium chloride additive solution should be used?

211. If an infusion pump system is calibrated to deliver 15 microdrops per minute, equivalent to a delivery rate of 15 mL per hour, how many microdrops would be delivered per milliliter by the system?

212. The loading dose of Dilantin® in children is 20 mg/kg administered at an infusion rate of 0.5 mg/kg/min.

(*a*) What would be the dose for a child weighing 32 lb?

(*b*) Over what period of time should the dose be administered?

213. Calculate the creatinine clearance for a 30-year-old male patient weighing 80 kg with a serum creatinine of 2 mg/dL.

214. Sodium phosphate P 32 solution is used intravenously in tumor localization in a dose range of 250 μCi to 1 mCi. Express this dose range of radioactivity in megabecquerel units.

215. A commercial product of thallous chloride Tl 291 contains 244.2 MBq of radioactivity. Express this radioactivity in terms of millicuries.

216. If 150 mg of a drug are administered intravenously and the resultant drug plasma concentration is determined to be 30 μg/mL, calculate the apparent volume of distribution.

217. The loading dose of theophylline for a child is 5 mg/kg of body weight. For each milligram per kilogram of theophylline administered, the serum theophylline concentration increases by approximately 2 μg/mL. Calculate (*a*) the loading dose for a child weighing 44 lb, and (*b*) determine the approximate serum theophylline concentration.

218. Each 1 mg/kg of phenobarbital will, on average, increase the serum concentration of the drug by 1 μg/mL.

(*a*) What will be the expected serum concentration after a loading dose of 2 mg/kg?

(*b*) What should be the loading dose for a 165-lb patient?

219. Express a patient's cholesterol level of 175 mg/dL in terms of millimoles per liter.

220. The drug alprostadil is administered to infants by intravenous infusion following dilution in dextrose injection. If one ampul, containing 500 μg of alprostadil, is added to the indicated volume of dextrose injection, complete the table by calculating (*a*) the approximate concentration of the resulting solutions and (*b*) the infusion rates needed to provide 0.1 μg/kg/min of alprostadil.

500 μg Added to mL of Dextrose Injection	Approximate Concentration of Resulting Solution (μg/mL)	Infusion Rate (mL/kg/min)
250	———	———
100	———	———
50	———	———
25	———	———

Answers to Practice and Review Problems

Note: Answers are given to all problems in Chapter 1 (Some Fundamentals of Measurement and Calculation) and Appendix J (Exponential and Logarithmic Notation); elsewhere, only the answers to odd-numbered problems are given.

CHAPTER I
Roman Numerals (Page 3)

1. (a) xviii
   (b) lxiv
   (c) lxxii
   (d) cxxvi
   (e) xcix
   (f) xxxvii
   (g) lxxxiv
   (h) xlviii
   (i) MCMLXXXIX
2. (a) Part 4
   (b) Chapter 19

   (c) 1959
   (d) 1814
3. (a) 45
   (b) 2
   (c) 48
   (d) 64
   (e) 16
   (f) 84
4. (a) 5, 15, 80, 4
   (b) $1\frac{1}{2}$, 40, 6, $\frac{1}{2}$

Common and Decimal Fractions (Page 8)

1. (a) $\frac{37}{32}$ or $1\frac{5}{32}$
   (b) $\frac{13}{600}$
   (c) $\frac{77}{480}$
2. (a) $\frac{209}{64}$ or $3\frac{17}{64}$
   (b) $\frac{1}{120}$
   (c) $\frac{5}{6}$
3. (a) $\frac{225}{48}$ or $4\frac{11}{16}$
   (b) $\frac{105}{4}$ or $26\frac{1}{4}$
   (c) $\frac{9}{2500}$
4. (a) $\frac{10}{1}$ or 10
   (b) $\frac{3}{10}$
   (c) $\frac{1}{12}$
   (d) $\frac{2}{3}$
   (e) $\frac{8}{15}$
   (f) $\frac{64}{1}$ or 64
5. (a) $\frac{48}{3}$ or 16
   (b) $\frac{1}{60000}$
   (c) $\frac{25}{2}$ or $12\frac{1}{2}$

6. (a) $62\frac{1}{2}$
   (b) 15
   (c) 64
   (d) 12,500
7. (a) $\frac{1}{32}$
   (b) $\frac{4}{5}$
   (c) $\frac{64}{1}$
8. (a) 0.125
   (b) 0.0002
   (c) 0.0625
9. 2.048
10. 1.565
11. 2000 doses
12. $\frac{1}{240}$ gr
13. $1\frac{1}{8}$ oz
14. 4.416 g

Ratio, Proportion, Variation (Page 14)

1.
(a) $\dfrac{3 \text{ (gallons)}}{\frac{1}{2} \text{ (gallon)}}$ or $\dfrac{12 \text{ (quarts)}}{2 \text{ (quarts)}}$

(b) $\dfrac{1 \text{ (yard)}}{\frac{2}{3} \text{ (yard)}}$ or $\dfrac{3 \text{ (feet)}}{2 \text{ (feet)}}$

(c) $\dfrac{\frac{1}{2} \text{ (mile)}}{\frac{1}{3} \text{ (mile)}}$ or $\dfrac{2640 \text{ (feet)}}{1760 \text{ (feet)}}$

(d) $\dfrac{4 \text{ (hours)}}{2 \text{ (hours)}}$ or $\dfrac{240 \text{ (minutes)}}{120 \text{ (minutes)}}$

(e) $\dfrac{2 \text{ (feet)}}{\frac{1}{2} \text{ (foot)}}$ or $\dfrac{24 \text{ (inches)}}{6 \text{ (inches)}}$

2. $259.20
3. 2 patients
4. 0.91 g
5. $\frac{9}{50}$ gr
6. $22.77
7. 48 mg
8. 40 lb
9. $9.67
10. 25.6 g

11. 41.25 g
12. 0.6 mL
13. 0.75 mg
14. 14 gr
15. 300 minims
16. 0.3 mg
17. 150 units
18. 32,000 mg
19. 44 mg
20. 1333 mL
21. 0.15 mL
22. 25 tablets
23. (a) 300 sprays
    (b) 450 mg
24. 16,000,000 units
25. 0.15 mL
26. 125,000 units
27. (a) 1.5 g
    (b) 1 mEq
28. 0.25 mg
29. 18.75 mL
30. 2.4 μg
31. 2 mg
32. 1.1 g
33. 2,500 units

Significant Figures (Page 20)

1. (a) Six
   (b) Four
   (c) Three
   (d) Three
   (e) Seven
   (f) One
2. (a) Two
   (b) Three
   (c) Two
   (d) Four
   (e) Five
   (f) Two
   (g) Four
   (h) Three
   (i) Two
   (j) Two
3. (a) 32.8
   (b) 200
   (c) 0.0363
   (d) 21.6
   (e) 0.00944

(f) 1.08
(g) 27.1
(h) 0.862
(i) 3.14
(j) 1.01
4. (a) 0.001
   (b) 34.795
   (c) 0.005
   (d) 6.130
   (e) 14.900
   (f) 1.006
5. 330.8 g
6. 38 gr
7. 40 gr
8. (a) 6.38
   (b) 1.0
   (c) 90.2
   (d) 240 gr
   (e) 6.0 g
   (f) 211 g
   (g) 0.072 gr

(b) 0.054 g
(i) 628
(j) 225
(k) 2.6
(l) 0.0266
(m) 140
(n) 24

9.   473 mL means ± 0.5 mL

473.0 mL means ± 0.05 mL
10. 0.65 g means ± 0.005 g
    0.6500 g means ± 0.00005 g
11. (a) 4.0 gr
    (b) 0.43 gr
    (c) 14.819 g
    (d) 12 minims
    (e) 350 gr

Estimation (Page 24)

Note: Estimated answers will vary with methods used. Some calculated answers are given in parentheses for comparison.

1.   Six zeros
2.   Four zeros
3.   Three zeros
4.   Two zeros
5.   20,500 *(19,881)*
6.   22,000 *(21,405)*
7.   14,500 *(14,320)*
8.   36,000 *(35,314)*
9. $240.00 *($253.19)*
10. $160.00 *($169.99)*
11. $20 \times 20 = 400$ *(374)*
12. $30 \times 30 = 900$ *(868)*
13. $8 \times 50 = 400$ *(384)*
14. $20 \times 38 = 760$ *(722)*
15. $30 \times 60 = 1800$ *(1736)*
16. $40 \times 77 = 3080$ *(3003)*
17. $40 \times 40 = 1600$ *(1638)*
18. $120 \times 90 = 10,800$ or $11,000$ *(11,500)*
19. $360 \times 100 = 36,000$ *(35,700)*
20. $473 \times 100 = 47,300$ *(48,246)*
21. $600 \times 200 = 120,000$ *(121,584)*
22. $600 \times 120 = 72,000$ *(73,688)*
23. $650 \times 20 = 13,000$ *(12,825)*
24. $1000 \times 13 = 13,000$ *(12,974)*
25. $7000 \times 800 = 5,600,000$ *(5,435,670)*
26. $1000 \times 1000 = 1,000,000$ *(1,042,956)*
27. $8000 \times 10,000 = 80,000,000$ *(82,286,560)*
28. $7000 \times 20 = 140,000$ *(136,477)*
29. $5000 \times 1000 = 5,000,000$ *(4,917,078)*
30. $2300 \times 6000 = 13,800,000$ *(13,875,543)*

31. $2\frac{1}{2} \times 14 = 35$ *($36\frac{1}{4}$)*
32. $800 \div 3 = 266$ *($266\frac{2}{3}$)*
33. $21 \times 7 = 147$ *($142\frac{2}{9}$)*
34. $\frac{3}{4} \times 800 = 600$ *(612)*
35. $840 \div 3 = 280$ *(283.76)*
36. $6 \times 7000 = 42,000$ *(41,557)*
37. $2 \times 700 = 1400$ *(1438.812)*
38. $0.02 \times 500 = 10$ *(9.4304)*
39. $(7 \times 7000) \div 100 = 490$ *(504.6426)*
40. $100 \times 0.0031 = 0.31$ *(0.3038)*
41. $6 \times 70 = 420$ *(411.079)*
42. $7500 \div 10 = 750$ *(728.8947)*
43. $170 \div 20 = 8.5$ *(9.0)*
44. $(\frac{2}{3} \times 165)$ or $110 \div 10 = 11$ *(11)*
45. $180 \div 100 \div 20 = 0.09$ *(0.08)*
46. $300 \div 15 = 20$ *(21.39)*
47. $16 \div 320 = \frac{1}{20}$ or 0.05 *(0.05)*
48. $3600 \div 4 = 900$ *(900)*
49. $8400 \div 7 = 1200$ *(1200.7)*
50. $1100 \div 100 = 11$ *(11)*
51. $9800 \div 5 = 1960$ *(2000)*
52. $1700 \div 6 = 283$ *(298.5)*
53. $0.01 \div 5 = 0.002$ *(0.002149)*
54. $200 \div 4 = 50$ *(48.6)*
55. $19 \div 0.25 = 19 \times 4 = 76$ *(73.9)*
56. $19 \div 50 = 38 \div 100 = 0.38$ *(0.409)*
57. $460 \div 8 = 57.5$ *(57.3)*
58. $4500 \div 0.50 = 4500 \times 2 = 9000$ *(9340)*
59. 90,000
60. 300
61. 3
62. 0.01 or $\frac{1}{100}$
63. 3.5

64. 100
65. 100
66. 20
67. 160
68. $3,750
69. $400

70. $450
71. $800
72. 0.9 g
73. 750 doses
74. $35
75. $55

Percentage of Error (Page 27)

1. 5%
2. 8%
3. 5%
4. 2.4%
5. 6.3%
6. 1.4%
7. 0.1%
8. 8.8%
9. 6.7%
10. 0.24%
11. $3\frac{1}{8}$ gr
12. 0.2 g

13. 8.33%
14. 160 mg
15. 10%
16. (*a*) No; (*b*) Yes; (*c*) Yes; (*d*) No; (*e*) No; (*f*) Yes
17. 4.6%
18. 6%
19. 1.1%
20. 0.1%
21. 0.02 g
22. 0.1 mg

Aliquot Method of Measuring (Page 35)

1. (*a*) 100 mL
   (*b*) 3 mg
2. Weigh ... 120 mg
   Dilute with ... 1380 mg
   to make ... 1500 mg
   Weigh ... 150 mg
3. Weigh ... 80 mg
   Dilute with ... 1520 mg
   to make ... 1600 mg
   Weigh ... 100 mg
4. Weigh ... 2 gr
   Dilute with ... 38 gr
   to make ... 40 gr
   Weigh ... 2 gr
5. Weigh ... 400 mg
   Dilute with ... 7600 mg
   to make ... 8000 mg
   Weigh ... 400 mg
6. Weigh ... 4 gr
   Dilute with ... 16 gr
   to make ... 20 gr
   Weigh ... 5 gr
7. Weigh ... 160 mg
   Dilute with ... 3840 mg
   to make ... 4000 mg
   Weigh ... 200 mg

8. Weigh ... 3 gr
   Dilute with ... 13 gr
   to make ... 16 gr
   Weigh ... 4 gr
9. Measure ... 3 mL
   Dilute to ... 10 mL
   Measure ... 2 mL
10. Measure ... 2 mL
    Dilute to ... 10 mL
    Measure ... 2 mL
11. Measure ... 5 mL
    Dilute to ... 8 mL
    Measure ... 2 mL
12. Measure ... 3 mL
    Dilute to ... 8 mL
    Measure ... 2 mL
13. Weigh ... 150 mg
    Dilute with ... 450 mg
    to make ... 600 mg
    Weigh ... 200 mg

CHAPTER 2

Interpretation of the Prescription or Medication Order (Page 43)

1. (a) Dispense twelve rectal supposi-
      tories.
   (c) Mix and divide into 40 pow-
      ders.
   (e) Mix and make ointment. Dis-
      pense 10 grams.
   (g) Mix and make solution con-
      taining 1 gram per tablespoon.
   (i) Mix and make powder. Divide
      into 100 doses.
   (k) Hydrocortisone, 20 mg
2. (a) Instill two (2) drops in each
      eye every four (4) hours as
      needed for pain.
   (c) Apply morning and night for
      pain as directed.
   (e) Take one (1) teaspoonful in
      water every 4 or 5 hours as
      needed for pain.
   (g) Take one (1) capsule with
      water at night. Do not repeat.
   (i) Place one (1) tablet under the
      tongue, repeat if needed.
   (k) Dilute with an equal volume
      of water and use as gargle
      every 5 hours.
   (m) Take one (1) tablet as needed
      for shortness of breath.
   (o) Take two (2) tablets every 6
      hours around the clock for uri-
      nary tract infection.
3. (a) 1½ grains of Secobarbital So-
      dium by mouth every day at
      bedtime. Repeat if there is
      need.
   (b) 1000 milliliters of 5% dex-
      trose in water every 8 hours in-
      travenously with 20 milliequiv-
      alents of potassium chloride
      added to every third bottle.

   (c) 10 milligrams of Prochlorpera-
      zine intramuscularly every 3
      hours, if there is need, for nau-
      sea and vomiting.
   (d) One teaspoonful of Minocy-
      cline Hydrochloride Suspen-
      sion by mouth four times a
      day. Discontinue after 5 days.
   (e) 10 milligrams of Propranolol
      Hydrochloride by mouth three
      times a day before meals and
      at bedtime.
   (f) 40 units of NPH 100-Unit In-
      sulin subcutaneously every day
      in the morning.
   (g) 250 milligrams of Cefaman-
      dole Nafate intramuscularly
      every 12 hours.
   (h) 15 milliequivalents of Potas-
      sium Chloride by mouth twice
      a day after meals.
   (i) 1 milligram of Vincristine Sul-
      fate per square meter of body
      surface area.
   (j) Administer 30 mg of flur-
      azepam at bedtime as needed
      for sleep.
   (k) Administer 20 milliequiva-
      lents of potassium chloride per
      liter in D5W (5% dextrose in
      water) at the rate of 84 milli-
      liters per hour.
   (l) Administer 2.5 grams per kilo-
      gram of body weight per day
      of amino acids in total paren-
      teral nutrition.
4. (a) 50 days
   (b) yes, compliance rate = 102%
5. 40 tablets

CHAPTER 3

The Metric System (Page 52)

1. 502.550 g or 503 g
3. 7.325 g
5. 114 g
7. 20,410 g per 25.4 mm
9. 750 μg
11. 50,000 tablets
13. 15,384 tablets
15. 5 g of norgestrel
    0.5 g of ethinyl estradiol
17. 6.25 g
19. 5 mL
21. (a) 8.33 mg or 8 mg
    (b) 433.33 mg or 433 mg
    (c) 75 mg

23. 66 times
25. 2.1 mL
27. 24 mL
29. 400 μg
31. 7.2 kg
33. 5000 μg
35. 125 mL
37. (a) 2.27 g
    (b) 15,384 tablets
39. 4980 megabytes
41. 0.125 g
43. 222 doses
45. 25
47. 0.4 mL

CHAPTER 4 (Page 72)

Note: In calculating the number of doses contained in a specified quantity of medicine, disregard any fractional remainder.

1. 800 doses
3. 10 mg
5. 15 mg
7. 200 mL
9. 20 mL
11. 2.4, thus 3 inhalers required
13. 12 days
15. Thirty-five 25-mg tablets
    Seventy 5-mg tablets
17. 45 mg
19. 180 mg
21. 0.25 mL
23. 0.6 mL
25. 2.2 mg
27. 9.55 mL
29. 30 mg
31. 12.5 mg
33. ½ teaspoonful (2.5 mL)
    10 days
35. 2 teaspoonfuls
37. 185 mL
    7 teaspoonfuls
    4½ teaspoonfuls

39. 3.825 or 3.8 mL
41. 10 tablets
43. 7.5 mL
45. 18.3 lb
47. 626 mg/kg
49. 44 lb
51. 1364 μg
53. 2.5 mL
55. 2 mg
57. 4.2 g
59. (a) 56.8 mg
    (b) 1.7 mL
61. 202.5 or 203 mg
63. 8.7 mg
65. 35.4 mg
67. 600 μg
69. (a) 125 mg
    (b) 100 mg

CHAPTER 5
Reducing and Enlarging Formulas (Page 83)

1. 45 mL
    0.9 g
    3.6 g
    ad 180 mL
3. 0.57 g
    0.34 g
    22.7 g
    272 g
    568 g
    568 g
    ad 2270 g or 5 lb
5. 2400 g
    400 g
    5000 g
7. 576.923 g
    115.385 g
    461.539 g
    346.154 g
9. 800 mL
    200 mL
    3000 mL
    4000 mL or 4 L

11. 5 g
    500 g
13. 4.73 g
    23.65 g
    3311 g
    ad 4730 mL or 10 pt
15. 2000 g
    150 L
17. 0.710 g
    0.851 g
    9.460 g
    ad 473 mL or 1 pt
19. 540 g
    140 g
    ad 10,000 mL or 10 L
21. 2000 kg
    500 kg

CHAPTER 6
Density, Specific Gravity, and Specific Volume (Page 91)

1. 0.812 g/mL
3. 1.133
5. 1.300
7. 1.253
9. 0.863

11. 3.237
13. 0.891
15. 1.110
17. 1.227
19. 1.212

Specific Gravity in Calculations of Weight and Volume (Page 94)

1. 116 g
3. 190.4 or 190 g
5. 9.2 kg
7. 99.83 g
9. 4.86 kg
11. 1646.5 g
13. 405.4 or 405 mL
15. 73.5 mL

17. 500 mL
19. 2231.5 or 2232 mL
21. 139.8 or 140 mL
23. 270 mg
25. $36.47
27. $40.73
29. 41.3 g

CHAPTER 7

Percentage and Ratio Strength Calculations (Page 109)

1.	3.0 g	(d)	0.25%
3.	7.5 g	(e)	0.03%
5.	(a) 1.5 g	(f)	0.025%
	(b) 0.45 g	57. (a)	1:1000
7.	1.67%	(b)	1:18,182
9.	25 g	(c)	1:125
11.	5%	(d)	1:500
13.	(a) 5.4%	59. (a)	1:1250
	(b) 1.4%	(b)	1:5000
15.	50,444 or 50,440 mL	(c)	1:1000
17.	500 mL	61.	1:200
19.	681.8 or 682 mL		0.0005%
21.	1% (w/v)	63.	1:588
23.	0.39%	65.	1:4730
25.	0.005%	67.	409 μg
27.	70.95 or 71 mL	69.	1:200 (w/v)
29.	378.5 or 379 mL	71.	1:31,250,000 (w/v)
31.	20 L	73.	0.05 μg
33.	25%	75.	0.03 %
35.	3153 mL		0.06 %
37.	882.1 or 882 g		0.125%
39.	200 g		0.25 %
41.	45.45 or 45.5%	77.	0.26%
43.	24.24%	79.	0.0077 mg%
45.	2%	81.	282 mg to 318 mg
47.	(a) 3%	83.	6.99 mmol/L
	(b) ½%	85.	170 mg/dL
49.	270 mg	87.	1.25 mg/mL
51.	2.5%	89.	40 mg/dL
53.	9.5%	91.	0.4%
55.	(a) 0.067%	93.	115 g
	(b) 0.01%	95.	10 μg
	(c) 0.4 %		

CHAPTER 8

Dilution and Concentration (Page 136)

1.	1:3200	17.	248 mL
3.	4%	19.	1 mL
5.	0.0159 or 0.016%	21.	5.5 mL
7.	32%	23.	4 mL
9.	1:315		4 mL
11.	6694.4 or 6694 mL	25.	28.2 mL
13.	4.7 mL	27.	100 mL
15.	5047 mL	29.	1667 mL

31. qs to make 4150 mL
33. 600 mL
35. 115.7 or 116 mL
37. 770.4 or 770 mL
39. 0.002%
41. 14.5%
43. 3632 g
45. (a) 4.89 g
    (b) 44 g
47. 200 g
49. 1.667 g
51. 0.01%
53. 8.05 mL
55. 59.04 or 59 g
57. 2 g
59. 31.9%

61. 54.3%
63. 9.09 mg/mL
65. 8:5
67. 3:17
69. 6:5:5
71.   800 g
      1200 g
      2400 g
       400 g
73. 100 mL
75. 170 mL
77. 75 mL
79. 5000 g
81. 71.2 mL
83. 0.947
85. 4500 mL

CHAPTER 9

Isotonic Solutions (Page 151)

1. 1.73%
3. −0.52°C
5. −0.036°C
7. 201 mg
9. 0.502 g
11. 4.5 g
13. 0.111 g

15. 0.470 g
17. 0.690 g
19. 4.6 mL
21. 0.186 g
23. 0.294 g
25. 43.6 g
27. 13 mL

CHAPTER 10

Electrolyte Solutions: Milliequivalents, Millimoles and Milliosmoles (Page 164)

1. 372.5 mg
3. 4 mEq
5. 0.298%
7. 200 mEq
9. 180.18 g
11. 20 mL
13. 2.5 mEq/mL
15. 10 mEq/L
17. 14 mOsmol
19. 20 mEq
21. 4.36 mEq/L
23. 25 mEq
25. 2.7 mEq
27. 4.5 mEq
    2.25 mOsmol
29. 154 mOsmol
31. 555.5 or 556 mOsmol

33. 4.7 mEq
35. 32 mEq
37. (a) 28.08 g
    (b) 60 mL
39. 296 mg
41. 24.16 or 24 mEq
43. 16 tablets
45. 713 mL
47. 200.6 or 201 mL
49. (a) 0.595 mEq/mL
    (b) 297.6 mEq
    (c) 1190 mOsmol/L
51. (a) 27.8 mL per hour
    (b) 549 mOsmol
53. (a) 100 mmol
    (b) 200 mEq
    (c) 300 mOsmol

CHAPTER 11

Constituted Solutions, Intravenous Admixtures, and Rate of Flow Calculations (Page 183)

1. 200 mL
3. (*a*) 228 mL
   (*b*) 228 mL
5. 0.64 mL
7. 0.6 mL
9. 13.3 mL
11. 0.57 mL
13. 1.8 mL
15. 71.4 mL
17. 2647.9 kcal
19. 3.92 mg/mL
21. 7.8 mL
    7.5 mL
    0.1 mL
    0.08 mL
23. 30.3 mEq
25. (*a*) 15 mL
    (*b*) 31.5 mmol

27. 1.1 mL
    52.8 or 53 mg
29. 69.4 or 69 drops per minute
31. 32.6 or 33 drops per minute
33. (*a*) 40.27 or 40 mEq
    (*b*) 83.2 or 83 drops per minute
35. 7.5 mL
37. (*a*) 31.25 or 31 drops per minute
    (*b*) 0.3 unit
39. Approximately 50 drops per minute
41. 8 mL per hour
43. (*a*) 24 mL per hour
    (*b*) 6 drops per minute
45. 40 minutes
47. 15.8 or 16 drops per minute
49. 2.92 or 3 mL per minute

CHAPTER 12

Some Calculations Involving Units, μg/mg, and other Measures of Potency (Page 192)

1. 0.45 mL
3. 0.6 mL
5. 400,000 units
7. 4 capsules
9. Dissolve 1 tablet in enough iso-tonic sodium chloride solution to make 8 mL, and take 3 mL of the dilution.
11. 0.3 mL

13. 17 units
15. 46.9 units
17. 1.36 mL to 2.72 mL
19. 64.1 mg
21. 80 mg/mL
23. 137.5 mg
25. 60 Protective Units
27. 0.5 mL

CHAPTER 13

Some Calculations Involving the Use of Prefabricated Dosage Forms in Compounding Procedures (Page 197)

1. Dissolve 1 tablet in enough dis-tilled water to make 60 mL, and take 10 mL of the dilution.
3. 2500 mL
5. 15 tablets
7. 19.2 tablets
9. 1.5 tablets

11. (*a*) 7 capsules
    (*b*) 1250 mg
13. 20 capsules
15. 40 tablets
17. 12 capsules
19. 6 capsules
21. 16 tablets

CHAPTER 14

Some Calculations Associated with Drug Availability and Pharmacokinetics (Page 212)

1. 1.75 mL
3. 0.33
5. 25 L
7. 0.408 hr^{-1}
9. 12.5%
11. 52.3 mg
    15.8 mg

13. 40 liters
15. 0.6
17. 14.7 μg/dL
19. (a) 4.9 L
    (b) 2.45 mg

CHAPTER 15

Some Calculations Involving Radioactive Pharmaceuticals (Page 220)

1. 18500 to 37000 Bq
3. 9.9 mCi
5. 370 MBq
7. 152 days
9. 0.0541 hour^{-1}
11. $\lambda = 0.04794$ day^{-1}
    $T_{1/2} = 14.5$ days

13. $\lambda = 0.01084$ day^{-1}
    $T_{1/2} = 64$ days
15. 77.3 μCi (2.86 MBq)
17. 0.17 mL
19. (a) 4.7 mCi (174.8 MBq)
    (b) 3.2 mL

APPENDIX A

The Common Systems (Page 229)

1. (a) 150 gr
    (b) 1050 gr
    (c) 530 gr
    (d) 90 gr
3. (a) 23 ⅓ʒ 8 gr, or 23 1Ə ½Ə 8 gr
    (b) 23 2Ə ½Ə 5 gr, or 23 ⅓ʒ 1Ə
        5 gr
    (c) 23 1ʒ 1Ə ½Ə, or 3ʒ 1½Ə
    (d) 1ʒ ½Ə 5 gr
    (e) 1ʒ ⅓ʒ 6 gr, or 1ʒ 1Ə ½Ə
        6 gr
5. 84 fʒ
7. 5600 tablets
9. $4.42
11. 1750 tablets
13. (a) ʒi, ʒii, Əii of phenylpropano-
        lamine
        ʒi, ʒss, gr ii of dextromethor-
        phan HBr
    (b) ⅛ gr
15. 43,750 tablets

Intersystem Conversion (Page 236)

1. 6.35 cm
3. 8.46 L
5. 2.92 or 3 minims
7. 6.6 lb per 1.0 inch
9. 0.000098 or ¹⁄₁₀,₀₀₀ inch
11. 12 tablets
13. 11.07 or 11 gr of codeine sulfate
    120 gr of acetaminophen
15. 2.6 mg (¹⁄₂₅ gr)
    6.5 mg (¹⁄₁₀ gr)
    1.3 mg (¹⁄₅₀ gr)
17. 8.07 or 8 gr of ferrous sulfate
    1.62 or 1.6 gr of elemental iron
19. 0.325 mg
21. 108 mg
23. 1.25 mg
25. 14.6 gr
27. 22,727 μg/lb/day
29. 24.2 mg/kg

APPENDIX B

Some Pharmacoeconomic Calculations (Page 245)

1. IV therapy, $32.00 per day, average

   Oral therapy, $0.74 per day, average
3. $427.64
5. Cefazolin —$ 9.00

   Cefaxitin —$24.96

   Ceftriaxone—$31.39
7. (a) 44.1%

   (b) 43.6%

   (c) 34.8%
9. $2.42
11. $1,117.20

13. $2.11
15. $99.00
17. $2.27
19. $4.69
21. $1.46
23. 41.3%
25. $2.75
27. $2.34
29. 2.18%
31. $3.90
33. $7.96
35. $12.60
37. $4.60

APPENDIX C

Graphical Methods (Page 257)

1. 5

   -1.67
3. (b) $y = -3.7x + 250$

   (c) 194.5 mg/5 mL

   (d) -3.7 mg/5 mL/day

   or -0.74 mg/mL/day

5. (d) $\log y = -0.028x + 1.78$

   (e) 11 days

   39 days

   (f) 0.944 day^{-1}

APPENDIX D

Basic Statistical Concepts (Page 267)

1. Mean: 127.8

   Median: 126

   Mode: 125
3. Mean: 100.7

   A.D.:   2.62

   S.D.:   3.22
5. Mean: 5.02%

   Median: 5.02%

   Mode: 5.05%
7. Yes. Because every button has an equal chance of being drawn,

every subject has an equal chance of being selected for the experiment.

9. $1:3$ in favor of the later check.
11. (a) 247.75 or 248 mg

    (b) Tablets weighing ± 19 mg of the average weight fall within the designated limit. Others do not.

APPENDIX E
Thermometry (Page 274)

1. 50°F
3. 39.2°F
5. 25°C
7. 37°C
9. 23°F to 572°F
11. 40°C
13. −40°C
15. 86°F to 95°F

17. 68°F
19. −4° and 14°F
21. 176°F
    179.6°F
23. 198°C
    −111.1°C
25. 4.4°C
27. 0.56°C

APPENDIX F
Proof Strength (Page 279)

1. 102.6 proof gallons
3. 490 proof gallons
5. 8,550 proof gallons
7. 125 wine gallons

9. $128.12
11. $427.50
13. $45.00
15. 36.1 proof gallons

APPENDIX G
Solubility Ratios (Page 281)

1. 1:5.25, or 1 g in 5.25 mL of water
3. 1:2.67, or 1 g in 2.67 mL of water
5. 5.88% (w/w)

7. 59.5 g
    178.57 or 178.6 mL
9. 1 g in 0.7 mL
11. 1 g in 0.55 mL

APPENDIX H
Emulsion Nucleus (Page 284)

1. (a) 125 g
    (b) 250 mL

3. (a) 625 g
    (b) 1250 mL

APPENDIX I
HLB System: Problems Involving HLB Values (Page 287)

1. 14.7
3. 10.7
5. 12.2
7. 73% of Tween 40
    27% of Span 40

9. 5.6 g of Span 60
    19.4 g of Tween 20

APPENDIX J

Exponential And Logarithmic Notation (Page 290)

Exponential Notation

1. (a) 1.265×10^4
   (b) 5.5×10^{-9}
   (c) 4.51×10^2
   (d) 6.5×10^{-2}
   (e) 6.25×10^{-8}
2. (a) 4,100,000
   (b) 0.0365
   (c) 0.00000513
   (d) 250,000
   (e) 8695.6
3. (a) $17.5 \times 10^7 = 1.75 \times 10^8$
   (b) $16.4 \times 10^{-4} = 1.64 \times 10^{-3}$
   (c) 6.0×10^0
   (d) $12 \times 10^7 = 1.2 \times 10^8$
   (e) $36 \times 10^2 = 3.6 \times 10^3$
4. (a) 3.0×10^3
   (b) 3.0×10^{-10}
   (c) 3.0×10^9
5. (a) 8.52×10^4, or 8.5×10^4
   (b) 3.58×10^{-5}, or 3.6×10^{-5}
   (c) 2.99×10^3, or 3.0×10^3
6. (a) 6.441×10^6, or 6.4×10^6
   (b) 6.6×10^{-3}
   (c) 6.94×10^3, or 6.9×10^3

Logarithmic Notation Page 296)

1. (a) 3.3512
   (b) 0.7214
   (c) 3.8451
   (d) 2.2739
   (e) $\overline{3}.4675$
   (f) $\overline{1}.8600$
   (g) 5.3324
   (h) $\overline{4}.1373$
   (i) 1.8047
   (j) 6.7924
2. (a) $2.827 \times 10^4 = 28,270$
   (b) $1.42 \times 10^1 = 14.2$
   (c) $2.139 \times 10^0 = 2.139$
   (d) $1.29 \times 10^{-1} = 0.129$
   (e) $6.154 \times 10^2 = 615.4$
   (f) $1.468 \times 10^2 = 146.8$
   (g) $1.062 \times 10^0 = 1.062$
   (h) $7.766 \times 10^{-3} = 0.007766$
   (i) $8.383 \times 10^1 = 83.83$
   (j) $1.329 \times 10^{-2} = 0.01329$
3. (a) 22,790
   (b) 7315
   (c) 14.76
   (d) 822.6
   (e) 17,090
4. (a) 7517
   (b) 197.6
   (c) 0.00517
   (d) 35.37
   (e) 13.75 or 13.8
5. (a) 79.36 or 79.4
   (b) 108.5 or 109
   (c) 292.8 or 293

APPENDIX K

Some Calculations Involving Buffer Solutions (Page 303)

1. 3.86
3. 4.56
5. 5.5
7. 6.91

9. 2.82:1
11. 0.03 unit
13. 8.2 g
    6.0 g

APPENDIX L

Chemical Problems (Page 307)

1. C: 64.81%
   H: 13.60%
   O: 21.59%
3. Na: 16.66%
   H: 2.92%
   P: 22.45%
   O: 57.97%
5. 1024 g
7. 178.5 or 179 mg
9. 30 mL
11. 2.1 g
13. 80.5 mg
15. 3.78 g

Review Problems (Page 316)

1.   13.3%
3.   0.06 g
     0.024 g
     3.0   g
     0.12 g
5.   6000 μg
7.   (a) 90 μg
     (b) 0.1 mg
9. $2.18
11. 2.54 g
13. $0.79
15. 329.5 or 330 mg
17. 0.25 g
19. 17.5 mg
21. 7.3 mg
23. 30.68 or 31 mL
25. 275 mg
27. 105 mL
29. (a)   3.3 mg
     (b) 160   mg
     (c)   16   mL
31. 720 mg
33. 60 tablets
35.   30 mg
     200 mg
37. 2 tablets
39. 0.525 g
41. 50 μg
43. 200 mL

45. 8 hours
47. 82.7 or 83 mg
49. 17.6 mg/kg
51.   113.5 g
      181.6 g
      681   mL
      181.6 g
     1112.3 g
53.   546 g
        54 g
     ad 600 g
55.   7.57 g
           3.785 g
         378.5   mL
        1324   mL
     ad 3785   mL
57. 80 g
59. (a) 1.313
     (b) 0.762
61. 3704 mL
63. 181.6 or 182 mL
65. 160 mL
67. $7.56
69. (a) 0.2%
     (b) 1:500
71. 16 tablets
73. (a) 86.1%
     (b) 64.9%
     (c) 1.327
75. 2.9 g
77. 4 capsules
     1%
79. (a) 0.6 g
     (b) 12   g
81. 0.03%
83. 6.08% w/v
     25%
85. 30 mg
87. 2%
89. 1:500,000
91. 2.27 g
93. 10 tablets
95. 4.633 g
97. 12 tablets
99. 1230.8 or 1231 mL
     2769.2 or 2769 mL

101. 2752.7 or 2753 mL
103. 4455 ml
105. 5 mg%
107. 0.015% (w/v)
109. 62.5 or 63 tablets
111. 144 mg
113. 1.156 g
115. (a) 1.269 g
     (b) 25.4 or 25 mL
     (c) 221°F
117. 96.72 or 96.7 g
119.   361 g
       1580 g
121. 12.4 mL
123. 5 mL
125. 372.5 g
127. 1 mEq per 100 mL
129. 2.5 mEq
131. 16.8 mEq
133. 67.2 g
135. 1410 g
137. 183.75 g
139. 4.2
141. 1.7:1
143. 0.4:1
145. 0.83 mL
147. Mean 325.2   mg
     A.D.   5.18 mg
     S.D.   7.14 mg
149. No
151. 35.7
153. $769.50
155. 0.075 g
157. 2523.3 or 2523 g
     2523.3 or 2523 mL
159. 1 g in 18.75 mL
161. 236.5 g
     473 mL

163. 27.2 g
     86.3 g
165. 15 tablets
167. 28.8 or 29 granules
169. ⅜ tablet
     Dissolve 1 tablet in enough iso-
     tonic sodium chloride solution to
     make 8 mL and use 3 mL of the
     solution.
171. Use all of a 2-mL (80 mg) sy-
     ringe and 0.75 mL (30 mg) of a
     1.5-mL syringe.
173. 5000 mOsmol
175. 83.3 or 83 drops per minute
177. 30.45 or 30 drops per minute
179. 63.6 or 64 drops per minute
181. 54.2 or 54 drops per minute
183. 125 μg
185. 25 drops per minute
187. 20.1 or 20 mg
189. 24 μg/mL
191. 178.6 or 179 μg
193. (a) 32.6   mg
     (b)   1.71 mEq
195. 70 drops per minute
197. $3,177.04
199. $15.75
201. $3.42
203. $20.75
205. $3,770.55
207. 294 mg/mL
209. 3.06 mL per hour
211. 60 microdrops/mL
213. 61 mL per minute
215. 6.6 mCi
217. (a) 100 mg
     (b)   10 μg/mL
219. 4.52 mmol

Index

TABLE OF ATOMIC WEIGHTS[1]

Name	Symbol	Atomic number	Weight (accurate to 4 figures[2])	Approximate weight
Actinium	Ac	89	*	227
Aluminum	Al	13	26.98	27
Americium	Am	95	*	243
Antimony	Sb	51	121.8	122
Argon	Ar	18	39.95	40
Arsenic	As	33	74.92	75
Astatine	At	85	*	210
Barium	Ba	56	137.3	137
Berkelium	Bk	97	*	247
Beryllium	Be	4	9.012	9
Bismuth	Bi	83	209.0	209
Boron	B	5	10.81	11
Bromine	Br	35	79.90	80
Cadmium	Cd	48	112.4	112
Calcium	Ca	20	40.03	40
Californium	Cf	98	*	251
Carbon	C	6	12.01	12
Cerium	Ce	58	140.1	140
Cesium	Cs	55	132.9	133
Chlorine	Cl	17	35.45	35
Chromium	Cr	24	52.00	52
Cobalt	Co	27	58.93	59
Copper	Cu	29	63.55	64
Curium	Cm	96	*	247
Dysprosium	Dy	66	162.5	163
Einsteinium	Es	99	*	252
Erbium	Er	68	167.3	167
Europium	Eu	63	152.0	152
Fermium	Fm	100	*	257
Fluorine	F	9	19.00	19
Francium	Fr	87	*	223
Gadolinium	Gd	64	157.3	157
Gallium	Ga	31	69.72	70
Germanium	Ge	32	72.59	73
Gold	Au	79	197.0	197
Hafnium	Hf	72	178.5	179
Helium	He	2	4.003	4
Holmium	Ho	67	164.9	165
Hydrogen	H	1	1.008	1
Indium	In	49	114.8	115
Iodine	I	53	126.9	127
Iridium	Ir	77	192.2	192
Iron	Fe	26	55.85	56
Krypton	Kr	36	83.80	84
Lanthanum	La	57	138.9	139
Lawrencium	Lr	103	*	260
Lead	Pb	82	207.2	207
Lithium	Li	3	6.941	7
Lutetium	Lu	71	175.0	175
Magnesium	Mg	12	24.31	24
Manganese	Mn	25	54.94	55
Mendelevium	Md	101	*	258
Mercury	Hg	80	200.6	201
Molybdenum	Mo	42	95.94	96

[1] Derived from the table recommended in 1981 by the Commission on Atomic Weights of the International Union of Pure and Applied Chemistry. All atomic weight values are based on the atomic mass of $^{12}C = 12$.

[2] When rounded off to 4-figure accuracy,, these weights are practically identical to the similarly rounded-off weights in the older table based on oxygen = 16.0000.

(continued)